Substance Abuse Treatment and the Stages of Change

Also from the Authors

Addiction and Change:
How Addictions Develop and Addicted People Recover
Carlo C. DiClemente

Assessment of Addictive Behaviors, Second Edition
Edited by Dennis M. Donovan and G. Alan Marlatt

Changing Addictive Behavior: Bridging Clinical and Public Health Strategies
Edited by Jalie A. Tucker, Dennis M. Donovan, and G. Alan Marlatt

Group Treatment for Substance Abuse: A Stages-of-Change Therapy Manual
Mary Marden Velasquez, Gaylyn Gaddy Maurer,
Cathy Crouch, and Carlo C. DiClemente

Relapse Prevention: Maintenance Strategies in the Treatment
of Addictive Behaviors, Second Edition
Edited by G. Alan Marlatt and Dennis M. Donovan

Substance Abuse Treatment and the Stages of Change

Selecting and Planning Interventions

SECOND EDITION

GERARD J. CONNORS
CARLO C. DiCLEMENTE
MARY MARDEN VELASQUEZ
DENNIS M. DONOVAN

THE GUILFORD PRESS
New York   London

© 2013 The Guilford Press
A Division of Guilford Publications, Inc.
370 Seventh Avenue, Suite 1200, New York, NY 10001
www.guilford.com

Paperback edition 2016

Printed in the United States of America

This book is printed on acid-free paper.

Last digit is print number: 9   8   7   6   5

The authors have checked with sources believed to be reliable in their efforts to
provide information that is complete and generally in accord with the standards
of practice that are accepted at the time of publication. However, in view of the
possibility of human error or changes in behavioral, mental health, or medical sciences, neither the authors, nor the editor and publisher, nor any other party who
has been involved in the preparation or publication of this work warrants that the
information contained herein is in every respect accurate or complete, and they are
not responsible for any errors or omissions or the results obtained from the use of
such information. Readers are encouraged to confirm the information contained
in this book with other sources.

Library of Congress Cataloging-in-Publication Data

Connors, Gerard J. (Gerard Joseph), 1952-
  Substance abuse treatment and the stages of change : selecting and
  planning interventions / Gerald J. Connors, Carlo C. DiClemente,
  Mary Marden Velasquez, Dennis M. Donovan. — Second edition.
    pages cm.
  Includes bibliographical references and index.
  ISBN 978-1-4625-0804-4 (hardcover : alk. paper)
  ISBN 978-1-4625-2498-3 (paperback : alk. paper)
  1. Teenagers—Drug use. 2. Substance abuse—Treatment. I. Title.
RJ506.D78C66 2013
616.8600835—dc23
                                                        2012040524

To
Marissa
Lyn, Cara, and Anna
Jerry, Keith, Daniel, Heather, and Cali
Ann, Collin, and Angie

About the Authors

Gerard J. Connors, PhD, is Senior Research Scientist and former Director of the University at Buffalo Research Institute on Addictions. His clinical research interests include treatment of substance use disorders, patient–treatment matching, early interventions with heavy drinkers, the role of the therapeutic alliance in addictions treatment, and treatment outcome evaluation. Dr. Connors has authored or coauthored over 100 articles, book chapters, and books in the area of alcoholism and addictive behaviors.

Carlo C. DiClemente, PhD, is Professor in the Department of Psychology at the University of Maryland, Baltimore County (UMBC). He also directs the MDQuit Tobacco Resource Center and the Center for Community Collaboration at UMBC. Dr. DiClemente is the codeveloper of the stages-of-change model and the author of numerous scientific publications on motivation and behavior change with a variety of health and addictive behaviors. He is a recipient of the Innovators Combating Substance Abuse Award from the Robert Wood Johnson Foundation and the McGovern Award from the American Society of Addiction Medicine.

Mary Marden Velasquez, PhD, is Centennial Professor in Leadership for Community, Professional and Corporate Excellence and Director of the Health Behavior Research and Training Institute at the School of Social Work, University of Texas at Austin. Her work includes development of interventions in the areas of fetal alcohol spectrum disorder, alcohol and other drug abuse, group treatment for substance abuse,

HIV prevention, and smoking cessation. Dr. Velasquez is the author of numerous articles and book chapters on using brief interventions to facilitate treatment adherence and promote behavior change. She is a member of the Motivational Interviewing Network of Trainers.

Dennis M. Donovan, PhD, is Director of the Alcohol and Drug Abuse Institute and Professor in the Department of Psychiatry and Behavioral Sciences at the University of Washington School of Medicine. He has over 200 publications, including five books, in the area of alcohol and drug dependence. He served as President of the Society of Psychologists in Addictive Behaviors and is a Fellow of Division 28 (Psychopharmacology and Substance Abuse) and Division 50 (Society of Addiction Psychology) of the American Psychological Association.

Preface

It has been more than a decade since the first edition of this book was published. During this period of time, there has been a significant increase in the extent and importance of treatment for alcohol and drug use disorders as a major and integral part of health care and mental health services. In this context, professionals with a range of experiences and training, including alcohol and drug counselors, psychologists, social workers, and psychiatrists, are at the forefront of treating people with substance use disorders and their families. In addition to this diverse group of treatment providers, a variety of treatment techniques and interventions are used. While there certainly are advantages in this diversity in providers and treatments, integrating information about treatment and communicating it to all of the service providers who want it can be challenging. This book was originally conceived and written to reach the wide range of clinicians who treat substance use disorders, and that perspective remains central to this second edition. Throughout this book two issues remain fundamental. The first concerns the client's receptiveness or readiness to engage in the change process and use different methods of change, and the second concerns what constitutes those methods.

These issues are addressed in this volume through application of the stages-of-change model. The model offers an integrative framework for conceptualizing and implementing behavior change among substance abusers. Indeed, the stages-of-change model continues to be one of the most visible, popular, and influential models in the addictions field, and the concepts introduced by the stages-of-change model have become part of the lexicon of substance abuse treatment providers.

In this second edition, we further our efforts to integrate the present themes with treatment interventions and to provide a vehicle for the application of the stages-of-change model to the treatment of substance use disorders.

There are several noteworthy features of the second edition. Predominant among them is a markedly expanded coverage of the processes of change. We describe in detail how the client's engagement in stage-relevant processes of change is central to successful movement through the stages of change. In addition, the chapters have been updated to reflect the literature published on the stages of change over the past decade and current thinking on the stages, theoretical as well as clinical. Finally, the group treatment chapter has been markedly revamped and we have added a new chapter that describes representative applications of the stages-of-change model in "real-world" settings.

It is our hope that these efforts taken together will benefit clinicians in their continuing efforts with clients suffering from substance use disorders.

Acknowledgments

This second edition could not have been conceived and developed without the support and assistance of a number of people. We thank Howard T. Blane for his support and guidance. At The Guilford Press, we are very much indebted to Jim Nageotte, Senior Editor, for all of his support and editorial expertise; to Jane Keislar, Senior Assistant Editor; and to Jeannie Tang, Senior Production Editor. In addition, Mark Duerr, Michael Maher, and Tom Umberger provided patient and expert assistance in the development and preparation of the manuscript. Finally, we would like to thank our families for the support and encouragement they provided throughout this endeavor.

Contents

1

Background and Overview

Alcohol and drug use[1] is a common occurrence in today's society, with such use often associated with a variety of medical, psychological, and social problems (Galanter & Kleber, 2008). As we discuss later in this chapter, the financial costs to society are extremely high, and the human suffering is considerable. For these reasons society has looked to treatment as one way to modify an individual's substance use and its concomitant problems.

This book is a practical guide to treatment of alcohol and drug use disorders in adults that is based on the most current theory and research. We devote this chapter, as a foundation, to highlighting the prevalence of drug use and the consequences of harmful drug use. We then discuss efforts to formally define patterns of alcohol and drug use that are identified with people who participate in professional treatment programs. Following that, we note that treatment has been given a lot of attention in the alcohol and drug fields because of the urgency felt to change alcohol and drug use patterns that are harmful to individuals, society, or both. Accordingly, we then introduce the stages-of-change model, a conceptual approach to behavior change that has had a substantial impact on the treatment of substance abusers and is used as a focal point for crystallizing the diverse information presented in this volume.

---

[1]In this volume we use the terms "alcohol and drugs" or "drugs" as mutually *inclusive* terms. In fact, to say "alcohol and drugs" is redundant, since alcohol *is* a drug. However, because of the ways in which reports of basic and clinical research and other literature in the field have been written or organized, we will at times distinguish between alcohol and other drugs. We also should note that alcohol and other drugs typically are talked about by the population in general as though they are distinctly different.

1

ALCOHOL AND DRUG USE

The emphasis of this book is on alcohol and drug use that is excessive and results in problems in functioning. A step toward understanding such drug use patterns is to view an individual's use in the context of drug use in society in general. Along these lines, the national surveys of alcohol and other drug use that have been taken periodically over the past several decades are instructive.[2]

In the 2010 National Survey on Drug Use and Health (Substance Abuse and Mental Health Services Administration, 2011), data about drug use in the United States were collected from participants from the civilian, noninstitutionalized population aged 12 years or older. The data include overall prevalence of use during the past year and past month for different drugs, including alcohol and tobacco cigarettes. In this case, "use" means the respondent used that specific drug in question at least once during a particular time period (usually the last 30 days or past year). Several findings stand out. First, alcohol (used by 66% in the past year) leads the use list, followed by cigarettes (used by 27%) in a distant second place. Marijuana and hashish (at 12%) head the list of illicit drug use. These relationships hold up both for use in the past year and for use in the past month.

In terms of illicit drug use (a category including marijuana/hashish, cocaine [including crack], heroin, hallucinogens, inhalants, or prescription medications used in a manner not prescribed), current (i.e., past month) use was reported by 8.9% of the sample. The most commonly used illicit drug in the past month was marijuana, currently used by 6.9% of the sample. Current use of other illicit substances was considerably lower: 2.7% for nonmedical use of prescription-type psychotherapeutic drugs and less than 1% for cocaine (0.6%), hallucinogens (0.5%), and methamphetamine (0.2%). The presentation of percentages, however, sometimes underappreciates the numbers of individuals involved. For example, the 2.7% current use rate for prescription-type psychotherapeutics used in a manner not prescribed represents seven million individuals across the United States.

---

[2]For this discussion we use data from the 2010 National Survey on Drug Use and Health (Substance Abuse and Mental Health Services Administration, 2011). In this survey, interviews were completed with over 68,000 persons age 12 years or older in the civilian, noninstitutionalized population of the United States. Although the sample did include persons living in places like shelters, rooming houses, and college dorms, it did not include those who were in jail or military personnel on active duty. Overall, the national household surveys provide the best single description of frequency and quantity of different drug use in U.S. society.

For alcohol use, the survey revealed than just over half (52%) of the sample aged 12 or older reported being past-month drinkers of alcohol, translating into an estimated 131.3 million people. Almost one-quarter of the population (23.1%) reported having participated in binge drinking (with binge drinking defined as having five or more drinks on at least one occasion during the previous month).

The survey also gathered useful information on substance abuse, substance dependence, and treatment. In 2010, an estimated 8.7% of the population were classified with substance abuse or dependence in the past year, based on criteria specified in the fourth edition of the *Diagnostic and Statistical Manual of Mental Disorders* (American Psychiatric Association, 1994). Over two-thirds of these individuals (67.8%) were dependent on or abused alcohol but not illicit drugs; the remainder were either classified with dependence on or abuse of both alcohol and illicit drugs (13.1%) or with dependence on or abuse of illicit drugs but not alcohol (19.0%). The illicit drug with the highest level of past year dependence or abuse was marijuana, followed by pain relievers and cocaine.

Finally, in terms of treatment, it was estimated that 9.3% of those surveyed (representing 23.5 million individuals) needed treatment for an illicit drug use or alcohol use problem. Only 2.6 million of these 23.1 million individuals needing treatment actually received treatment (representing 1.0% of the sample overall and 11.2% of those identified as needing treatment). Thus, the vast majority of individuals identified as needing treatment for an illicit drug or alcohol use problem did not receive treatment during the previous year. Noteworthy is that among those classified as needing treatment but not receiving treatment, only 5.0% reported that they actually felt they needed treatment for their illicit drug or alcohol use problem.

The national survey data provide clinicians with the best single frame of reference to evaluate and interpret substance use by their clients.[3] Quality of the interpretation tends to improve with attention to subgroup differences. That is, any given client's pattern of substance use

---

[3]In the treatment of substance use disorders there is inconsistency among professionals in their use of the words "patient" or "client" to refer to individuals presenting for treatment. Often the term chosen depends on the treatment setting—that is, individuals in hospital inpatient settings are more likely to be referred to as "patients" while persons receiving treatment in outpatient community clinics are more likely to be referred to as "clients." In this volume we use the terms "patient" and "client" as synonymous to refer to an individual who is in formal treatment for his or her substance use problems.

can best be viewed in the context of what is typical for his or her subgroup as defined by characteristics such as age or gender. Of course, this principle might be applied to a range of sociodemographic (e.g., years of education) and other characteristics of the person. Substance use problems occur across all classes and groups in individuals and there is no typical substance abuser. However, knowledge of the norms of substance use for a client's subgroup can help the clinician and client to plan treatment goals and to anticipate the likely obstacles and supports in achieving and maintaining them.

THE PRICE OF DRUG USE

The consequences of alcohol and drug abuse are costly. "Cost-of-illness" studies provide a detailed estimate of the cost, in dollars, of a given illness or disease. In 2011, an economic study of the impact of illicit drug use on U.S. society was released by the U.S. Department of Justice (2011). Using data for 2007, the cost of illicit drug use totaled over $193 billion. This cost estimate was attributable to illicit drug use as gauged in three principal areas. The first, representing a cost estimated at $61.4 billion, was crime, predominantly capturing criminal justice system costs. The second principal area of cost, at $11.4 billion, was health. Major contributors in this area were hospital and emergency department costs for both nonhomicide and homicide cases and specialty treatment costs. However, the largest cost associated with illicit drug use, at $120.3 billion, was in the domain of productivity. This principal area included labor participation costs, incarceration costs, premature mortality costs, and specialty treatment costs for services provided at either the state or federal level.

The Department of Justice study only considered illicit drug use (including nonprescription use of prescription medications) and did not include alcohol use in its calculations. The additional costs associated with alcohol use in the United States are estimated to total $185 billion annually (Harwood, 2000). The majority of these costs are associated with reduced, lost, and forgone earnings, with the remainder attributed to costs associated with medical consequences and alcohol treatment and with lost workforce productivity, accidents, violence, and premature death.

The combined annual costs associated with alcohol and illicit drug use in the United States thus are in excess of $375 billion, a monumental figure using any standard. And the United States is not alone in experiencing enormous costs associated with alcohol and illicit drug use. Indeed, significant economic impacts of alcohol use and of illicit drug use have been reported globally (e.g., Baumberg, 2006; Rehm, Taylor, & Room, 2006; Thavorncharoensap et al., 2009). Looking only at alcohol consequences, the World Health Organization (2011) has estimated that approximately 2.3 million people die each year from the harmful use of alcohol, representing about 3.8% of all deaths in the world. Over half of these deaths occurred as a consequences of noncommunicable diseases, such as cancers, cardiovascular disease, and liver cirrhosis. Indeed, the World Health Organization estimates that 4.5% of the global burden of disease, as measured in disability-adjusted life years, is a consequence of harmful alcohol consumption.

It is noteworthy that although the economic impact of substance use extends well beyond the substance user, there are consequences closer to home for the families and significant others around the user. In the case of alcohol, for example, Casswell, You, and Huckle (2011) found that greater degrees of exposure to a heavy drinker are associated with lower health status and personal well-being on the part of the family member/significant other, even after controlling for demographic variables and the family member/significant other's own drinking. Comparable findings have been reported by Livingston, Wilkinson, and Laslett (2010).

Taken together, the estimated costs of alcohol and other drug abuse are staggering. While cost-of-illness studies are recognized as imprecise, such research nevertheless brings home the striking level of significant and far-reaching consequences that providers are addressing in alcohol and drug treatment. Moreover, financial cost-of-illness studies barely tap into the cost in human suffering related to substance abuse.

A BRIEF INTRODUCTION TO TREATMENT

As with many of the other concepts in this field, treatment has been variously defined. We use the definition arrived at by consensus in the Rinaldi and colleagues (Rinaldi, Steindler, Wilford, & Goodwin, 1988) Delphi Survey study. According to that study, the definition of treatment was agreed to be an "application of planned procedures to identify and change patterns of behavior that are maladaptive, destructive, or health injuring; or to restore appropriate levels of physical, psychological, or social functioning" (Rinaldi et al., 1988, p. 557).

With this definition, it is easy to imagine many different procedures that could be called "treatment." The majority of procedures that are used in the treatment of the substance use disorders can be broadly classified into individual treatment, marital/couple/family treatment, and group treatment. We discuss each of these modalities in detail in subsequent chapters. Note that the major modes of treatment are practiced in different settings, including inpatient/residential, partial hospital, and outpatient. In addition, we discuss the use of brief interventions in a variety of opportunistic settings.

THE STAGES-OF-CHANGE MODEL

A person's resistance to a given treatment effort has been a long-standing and sometimes frustrating problem for clinicians. In particular, individuals who present for treatment of substance use disorders have the reputation among clinicians of being unduly resistant or unwilling to change. Therefore, it would be useful to have a model or theory that would help to address the problem of how to match an individual's treatment to his or her commitment to change and personal journey through the process of change. One way to achieve this end would be to have a roadmap of the course of change in general and then to coordinate the treatment procedure that best fits where the person is in the course of change. Such a chart would be descriptive of a model of change.

In fact, several stages-of-change models have appeared in the psychotherapy literature over the years (e.g., Horn, 1976; Kanfer, 1986; Rosen & Shipley, 1983). We have chosen to use the Prochaska and DiClemente (1982, 1984, 1992) "stages-of-change" model as our preferred way of addressing a person's readiness for change. This model was developed from research on the treatment procedures or techniques that were identified in theories of change and that people use in modifying a particular problem behavior. We have selected this model from among the other possibilities for three reasons. First, the model describes dimensions of the change process in terms of stages and also describes how coping activities or processes of change interact with these stages. Second, it has generated more research than other models, and much of that research has pertained to people trying to change their patterns of substance use. Finally, this research has provided evidence for the validity of the stages-of-change construct and for its clinical utility (e.g., DiClemente, 2003, 2005b, 2006).

During the past 30 years the stages-of-change model itself has undergone changes to some degree, mainly as a result of the now fairly extensive research findings on the model that have been published. However, the changes in the model relate more to content than to underlying concept so that the ideas that originally generated the model remain largely intact. The most detailed versions of the model are presented by Prochaska and DiClemente (1992), DiClemente and Prochaska (1998), and DiClemente (2003).

The current model posits five stages of change, called, from earliest to latest, precontemplation, contemplation, preparation, action, and maintenance.[4] People who are in the precontemplation stage show no evidence of intent to change a problem behavior. They may be unaware that their behavior is a problem, or aware that it might be but unwilling to do anything about it, or may be discouraged about changing the behavior as a result of past failed attempts to do so. Individuals in precontemplation tend to see the behavior as having more positives than negatives for them and therefore judge that the behavior is under control or at least manageable. More importantly, they lack the interest and concern that would lead to a serious consideration of change.

During the contemplation stage, individuals are considering changing a particular behavior. Thoughts about change might include specific personal cost and benefits related to the behavior and what the consequences of change might entail. Individuals in contemplation are more visibly concerned and distressed about their problem behaviors than are those in precontemplation and have begun to weigh the positives and negatives of the current behavior and the change. They also are more likely to search for information relevant to the problem behavior and possible solutions.

The preparation stage represents people who have made a decision and are ready to change. These individuals intend to change soon and have begun to make small changes or to incorporate their experiences of previous tries at change in their planning for the current attempt to change. As noted in DiClemente et al. (1991), people in the preparation stage may have begun to increase self-regulation and to change the problem behavior. The key task for these individuals is committing to

---

[4]This discussion draws heavily on a chapter by Prochaska and DiClemente (1992). The stages presented are but one component of a broader transtheoretical model of behavior change (Prochaska, 1984; Prochaska & DiClemente, 1982) that also addresses levels of change and the process of change, components of which are discussed as appropriate in other sections of this volume.

and prioritizing the change efforts and creating an effective, acceptable, and accessible plan (DiClemente, 2003).

When people are in the action stage, behavior change clearly has begun and the plan implemented. Accordingly, individuals in the action stage need skills to implement specific behavior change methods they included in their plan and revise the plan as needed. They also need to be aware of various psychological (cognitive, behavioral, emotional) events that may work against their efforts at behavior change. Furthermore, there is a need to learn ways to prevent major reversals, such as an abstinent alcoholic taking a drink and returning to prechange patterns and levels of alcohol use. Such skills are essential to maintaining the desired change in a problem behavior and are especially important in changing alcohol and drug use disorders. According to Prochaska and DiClemente (1992), the action stage lasts an average of about 6 months in people working to change their substance use.

The last major stage of change is maintenance. In this stage individuals sustain and strengthen any changes they have made in the problem behavior. The change behavior becomes the new normative behavior and is integrated into the lifestyle and lifespace of the individual. In this regard, such changes, even after 6 months, may not be well established and may take a few years to be "secure."

We should pause here to highlight several fundamental points about the stages of change. First, as may have been clear in our presentation of the stages, the stages describe attitudes, intentions, and behaviors about change (Prochaska & DiClemente, 1992) as well as a series of tasks that the individual is confronted with during the change process (DiClemente, 2003). Second, the "change" sought after represents a specific targeted behavior and goal, such as abstinence from alcohol use or cocaine use. That is, commitment to change one behavior, such as alcohol use, may say nothing about commitment to change another, such as cigarette smoking. Commitment to reduce use of a particular substance, like alcohol, differs from commitment to abstain. Third, the model is used to describe voluntary change processes rather than mandatory or coerced change, in which the individual has or believes he or she has no option regarding engagement in his or her problem behavior. Moreover, the model is assumed to apply to efforts to change with or without the help of formal treatment and that the client's change process occurs before and after as well as during treatment. And last, each stage refers to a period of time and to specific tasks one must complete before moving to the next stage. People may differ in the amount of time they spend in a stage, but the activities and processes involved to progress from one stage to the next one are similar for everyone.

Table 1.1 summarizes each of the stages of change and the features associated with it. The first column describes the stages, the second describes what is needed to move forward, and the third highlights some considerations, strategies, and processes of change relevant for matching. Interventions that are most effective in each stage are a major topic of this book and of ongoing research projects by a number of investigators. For precontemplation, we have also highlighted "negative" interventions in that we suggest what *not* to do. Clearly the field needs to do more research on increasing the commitment to change in individuals who do not see they have a problem that is causing themselves or others distress. In the alcohol and drug treatment field such lack of awareness is commonly referred to as "denial" (a topic addressed in greater detail in Chapter 2). Imposing action-oriented behavioral change methods is not as likely to be as effective with individuals in precontemplation or contemplation as with those at other stages. Moreover, in response to the concept of the stages of change, a variety of verbal persuasion approaches and techniques, such as motivational interviewing (Miller & Rollnick, 1991, 2002), have been developed that have demonstrated considerable potential for eliciting interest and concern and dealing with ambivalence so clients can advance through the precontemplation and contemplation stages.

The second column heading of Table 1.1 summarizes what has to happen for a person to progress to the next stage of change. As we noted, the model assumes that these tasks must be accomplished or events must occur for progress to be made toward sustained change. It is also important to realize that these tasks can be accomplished more or less well so that moving forward has both qualitative as well as quantitative dimensions. Decisions, for example, can be based on well-formed and strong considerations or impulsive and extrinsically driven ones. The quality of the decision making as well as the strength of the decision will affect successful movement through the stages. Central to this movement through the stages of change is the client's engagement in stage-relevant processes of change. As described by DiClemente (2003), processes "represent the internal and external experiences and activities that enable individuals to move from stage to stage" (p. 32). Although there may be others, there are 10 identified processes. Five

TABLE 1.1. Stages of Change and Associated Features

Stage of change	Main characteristics of individuals in this stage	To move to next stage	Intervention match
Precontemplation	• No intent to change • Problem behavior seen as having more pros than cons	• Acknowledge problem • Increase awareness of negatives of problem • Evaluate self-regulatory activities • Create interest and concern	• Do *not* focus on behavioral change • Use motivational strategies
Contemplation	• Thinking about changing • Seeking information about problem • Evaluating pros and cons of change • Not prepared to change yet	• Make decision to act • Engage in preliminary action	• Consciousness raising • Self-reevaluation • Environmental reevaluation
Preparation	• Ready to change in attitude and behavior • May have begun to increase self-regulation and to change	• Set goals and priorities to achieve change • Develop acceptable and effective change plan	• Same as contemplation • Increase commitment or self-liberation
Action	• Modifying the problem behavior • Learning skills to prevent reversal to full return to problem behavior	• Apply behavior change methods for average of 6 months • Increase self-efficacy to perform the behavior change	• Methods of overt behavior change • Behavioral change processes
Maintenance	• Sustaining changes that have been accomplished	• Integrate change into lifestyle	• Methods of overt behavior change continued

Note. Data from Prochaska and DiClemente (1983, 1992) and DiClemente (2003).

have been categorized as experiential processes because they reflect internal thought processes and perceptions. The other five processes of change have been categorized as behavioral; they focus on actions and behaviors that operate in service of behavior change. The experiential processes are particularly relevant to accomplishing the tasks of the early stages of change, while the behavioral processes are particularly relevant to the later stages of change. The 10 processes of change are presented in Table 1.2. We will be referring back to these processes frequently throughout this volume.

Intervention matching involves focusing both on what the provider does and what activities or experiences the client needs to engage in to complete the tasks of the stage and move forward. The interaction of the stages and client processes of change are central to this model and will be described more fully in later chapters. In the third column of Table 1.1 some of the processes of change as well as provider strategies are highlighted for specific stages of change. For example, although developing awareness and knowledge about the problem and the solution is critical in all preaction stages, consciousness raising is critical in the contemplation stage to process decisional considerations. Similarly, self-reevaluation involves looking at oneself and changing the way one sees the problems or the solution. For example, the person asks the question "How does cigarette smoking or getting drunk make me feel about myself?" (Prochaska & DiClemente, 1983). Environmental reevaluation, on the other hand, entails reviewing how the problem in question affects the people and situations in the person's life space.

Note that at the earlier stages of change, overt behavior change methods are not the best match for the person. Better timing for such methods would be when the individual is in the action and maintenance stages, although there may be some initial use of behavior change methods in the preparation stage. Examples of these initial methods are varied and include use of behavioral processes of change including a helping relationship, counterconditioning, reinforcement management, and stimulus control (Prochaska & DiClemente, 1983).

Although we describe a person's progress through the stages of change as linear (one stage leads to the next), in practice people commonly regress and/or cycle back from an advanced stage to an earlier one. The stages-of-change model represents a cyclic progression for most changers—that is, individuals may go back to earlier stages of change after reaching a later one. This may occur a number of times before the

TABLE 1.2. Processes of Change

Experiential processes

- *Consciousness raising.* The client gains information and knowledge that increases his or her awareness about him or her, the current behavior pattern, and/or the potential new behavior.

- *Emotional arousal/dramatic relief.* The client experiences a significant, often emotional, reaction about the status quo and/or the new behavior. Clients often become motivated to initiate change efforts when their emotions are aroused by either external or internal stimuli.

- *Self-reevaluation.* The client studies and evaluates how the status quo and/or the new behavior relate to his or her personal values. As such, the client performs a thoughtful and emotional reappraisal of the behavior and begins to visualize the kind of person he or she might be after making a positive change.

- *Environmental reevaluation.* The client assesses the positive and negative effects that the status quo and/or new behavior will have upon others and the environment. The client is often motivated by the realization that his or her substance use has not only negatively affected him or her but also other, external areas (such as people in his or her life and the environments in which he or she function).

- *Social liberation.* The client notices and increases social alternatives that are in support of behavior change. Through this process, the client can be seen as utilizing resources in the environment to alter and maintain changes in behavior.

Behavioral processes

- *Stimulus control.* The client alters or avoids stimuli and cues that could trigger or encourage substance use. For example, the client who has maintained an association between a specific environment (such as a bar or a particular social situation) and substance use will be less likely to engage in substance use if he or she avoids such situations.

- *Counterconditioning.* The client begins making new connections between internal and environmental cues and substance use and/or substituting new, competing behaviors and activities in response to cues previously associated with substance use.

- *Reinforcement management.* The client starts rewarding his or her positive behavior changes (and as warranted eliminating reinforcements for substance use). The rewards themselves might be as concrete as going to a movie or buying a desired book, or it may be simply experiencing the positive consequences associated with not using substances.

- *Self-liberation.* The client develops a belief in his or her ability to make choices and change behavior, and acts on that belief by making and maintaining a commitment to that course of action.

- *Helping relationships.* The client seeks and nurtures relationships that provide support, care, and acceptance with respect to the behavior change endeavor. These relationships can be with family, friends, or peers.

Note. Based on Velasquez, Maurer, Crouch, and DiClemente (2001) and DiClemente (2003).

person makes it into the maintenance stage for good. In the addictions, cycling or recycling is normative—individuals often "successfully" attempt to change a problem numerous times before the change is stable (Brownell, Marlatt, Lichtenstein, & Wilson, 1986). Mark Twain's comment that "Quitting smoking is easy—I've done it many times" is an apt description of recycling hopefully on the road to successfully sustained change. In Chapter 9 we expand the stage of maintenance to include the critical topic of relapse. Although an individual can relapse while still in the action stage, the problem of relapse traditionally has been thought of and discussed most in the context of maintenance of change.

An excellent illustration of the typical course people take in changing addictive behavior was presented by DiClemente (2003) and is reproduced here in Figure 1.1. The cyclical model reflects the time-tested observation that the course of change is not linear.

The cyclical model reflects another critical facet of change that gives hope to changers and clinicians alike. Even though clients may

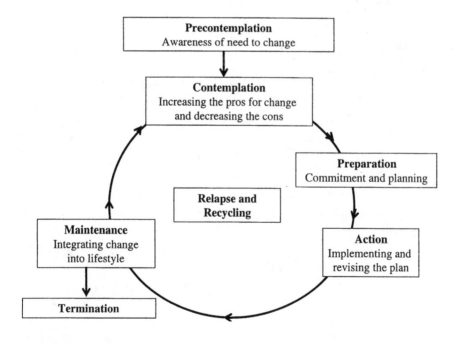

FIGURE 1.1. A cyclical representation of movement through the stages of change. From DiClemente (2003, p. 30). Copyright 2003 by The Guilford Press. Reprinted by permission.

work and make progress to a later stage of change, they often experience problems that send them back to an earlier one. However, in most cases, the person does not go all the way back to the precontemplation stage. Instead, he or she typically reverts to the contemplation or preparation stage for varying periods of time before advancing again. Most often, this represents a learning process and something is learned from a relapse so that the person does not fall all the way back to the cycle's entrance and learns something important about what is missing or what is needed to adequately complete the tasks of the stages. Of course, the challenge is to get people out of the cycle of advance–revert–advance and into the exit of the cycle. Terminating this change process is labeled "termination" in Figure 1.1—the point at which the person feels secure in his or her maintenance of change.

The stages model presents an excellent way to organize the vast amount of information that is available on treatment of substance use disorders. The model is based on clinical research and has important implications for clinical practice. We elaborate on these implications throughout this volume.

SUMMARY

• Alcohol and drug use are common among the general population. Use varies with several social and demographic variables, such as age, gender, and race.

• The effects of alcohol and other drug use cost society staggering sums of money and impose enormous human suffering on millions of individuals.

• Treatment has been defined in many ways. In this volume, we use the definition set forth by Rinaldi et al. (1988), namely, the "application of planned procedures to identify and change patterns of behavior that are maladaptive, destructive, or health injuring; or to restore appropriate levels of physical, psychological, or social functioning."

• The content of treatment and a person's receptiveness to change and treatment are fundamental to successful behavioral change. This volume utilizes the stages-of-change model to conceptualize the process of change and as a basis for deriving treatment content and implementing treatment strategies. The stages of change include five stages, called precontemplation, contemplation, preparation, action, and maintenance, each with a unique set of tasks, attitudes, and behaviors. The termination of this process occurs when the person is secure in his or her maintenance of change.

• Movement through the stages of change is facilitated by the client's engagement in stage-relevant experiential and behavioral processes of change.

2

The Stages of Change

Chapter 1 provided an overview of the stages-of-change model. In this chapter we discuss each of the stages of change in greater detail. As we noted in Chapter 1, the stages represent what DiClemente (2003) has described as "the motivational and dynamic fluctuations of the process of change over time" (p. 25). As part of our description of these stages, we present and analyze clinical scenarios. These case scenarios are intended to illustrate, from a stages-of-change perspective, what clinicians may expect from individuals who present for evaluation or treatment with a substance use disorder.

Following this, we shift our attention to some general clinical issues relevant to the respective stages of change. In terms of the precontemplation, contemplation, and preparation stages of change, we focus in particular on the critical tasks of each stage and the general concepts of denial and resistance. These concepts are pertinent to the precontemplation, contemplation, and sometimes the preparation stages because they are commonly viewed in the field as crucial obstacles to engaging in the processes of change needed to take the initial steps to address a problem. Traditional perspectives on denial and resistance are reviewed and their presumed relationship to treatment outcome discussed. This is followed by a presentation on some recent reformulations of denial and resistance. Particular emphasis is placed on motivational techniques and their relevance to the treatment of clients with substance use disorders in the earlier stages of change. Finally, we address the tasks and some of the clinical issues that arise in working with clients in the action and maintenance stages.

THE PRECONTEMPLATION STAGE

As implied by the term, individuals in the precontemplation stage are either ignoring or unaware of their alcohol or drug use problem, or if aware of them are not thinking seriously about making changes in their substance use. Prochaska and DiClemente (1984) have offered suggestions about several factors that can contribute to a person's being in precontemplation. One is that such individuals tend to be uninformed about the effects of their substance use on themselves or on others. An example would be the alcohol or marijuana abuser who in a solitary manner engages in heavy use but is ignoring or unaware of the potential long-term negative effects of such use, such as respiratory disorders.

Although some substance abusers are unaware of the dangers associated with their drug use, others, according to Prochaska and DiClemente (1984), simply are not receptive to indications that their alcohol or drug use is a problem. Such an attitude frequently has been conceptualized as "denial" or "resistance," which is discussed in greater detail later in this chapter. However, DiClemente and Velasquez (2002) and DiClemente (2003) have identified activities and experiences that help individuals stay in precontemplation in terms of the five R's: reveling ("I am enjoying this too much"), reluctance ("I really do not want to change"), rebellion ("No one can make me change"), resignation ("I cannot change"), and rationalization (the client's personal rationale why this is not a problem or "I do not need to change"). The precontemplation stage can also describe individuals who seek clinical services but who do so solely to placate others and not really to make changes in their alcohol or drug use (DiClemente, 2003; McConnaughy, DiClemente, Prochaska, & Velicer, 1989; Prochaska & DiClemente, 1984). Some general characteristics of persons in the precontemplation stage are listed in Table 2.1.

Much of the early research on the stages-of-change model was conducted with smokers, many of whom would meet the criteria for nicotine dependence (American Psychiatric Association, 1994). In one study DiClemente et al. (1991) reported on the characteristics of smokers volunteering for a smoking cessation program involving brief interventions. As part of the study, persons classified in precontemplation were compared to those in contemplation and to persons prepared for action taking. For the purposes of this study, those in precontemplation were defined as smokers who were not giving serious consideration to

TABLE 2.1. Common Characteristics of Individuals in the Precontemplation Stage

- Not interested or concerned about problem or need to change
- Defensive
- Resistant to suggestion of problems associated with their drug use
- Lacking awareness of a problem
- Uncommitted to or passive in treatment
- Engaging in little if any activity that could shift their view or perspective
- Consciously or unconsciously avoiding steps to change their behavior
- Often pressured by others to seek treatment
- Feeling coerced and "put upon" by significant others
- Not convinced that the negative aspects of their substance use outweigh the positive

Note. Adapted in part from DiClemente (2003) and Prochaska and DiClemente (1983, 1984).

stopping smoking during the upcoming 6-month period. DiClemente et al. (1991) found that the smokers in precontemplation, relative to those in contemplation and to those ready to change, reported fewer previous attempts at quitting, fewer concerns about quitting, more temptations to smoke, less confidence about quitting, and more advantages and fewer disadvantages of smoking. The smokers in precontemplation also used fewer coping activities or processes of change related to smoking cessation (e.g., consciousness raising, self-evaluation, counterconditioning). Not surprisingly, and supportive of the stages-of-change model, the persons in precontemplation made fewer attempts at quitting than did the other participants. These differences continue to be reflected in large-scale population studies of smokers (DiClemente, Delahanty, & Fiedler, 2010)

The precontemplation stage also has been studied among alcohol abusers. DiClemente and Hughes (1990) assessed stages of change with a large group of adults initiating outpatient alcoholism treatment. The clients were assessed not to be in need of detoxification or of an extended inpatient treatment regimen. They all completed a questionnaire, the University of Rhode Island Change Assessment Scale (URICA), that measures stages of change (see Chapter 3). Based on their responses to the questionnaire items, these clients fell into one of five "profiles" based on patterns of scores reflecting precontemplation, contemplation, action, and maintenance attitudes, experiences, and activities. The profiles were labeled "precontemplation," "ambivalent," "participation," "uninvolved," and "contemplation." Two of these groups have relevance to our understanding of persons in precontemplation. The first included clients labeled simply as being in precontemplation. These clients scored above average on the precontemplation scale and below average on the contemplation, action, and maintenance scales. As such, these are individuals who do not view themselves as having a problem with alcohol, are not contemplating change, and are not taking steps to effect changes in their drinking. According to DiClemente and Hughes (1990), the clients in this precontemplation group reported lower levels of concern about their alcohol use and lower scores on two alcoholism scales (general alcoholism and alcoholic deterioration) of the Alcohol Use Inventory (Horn, Wanberg, & Foster, 1987), relative to clients falling into groups characterized by more contemplation and action regarding their alcohol use. Nevertheless, level of drinking among the clients in precontemplation was comparable to that of clients thinking about changing or already initiating change, and their reported levels of withdrawal symptoms were also comparable.

The precontemplation cluster has been replicated by Carney and Kivlahan (1995) in their study of over 400 male polydrug users entering addictions treatment at a Veterans Administration hospital. Using a similar clustering procedure to study these clients' responses on the URICA measure, Carney and Kivlahan (1995) identified a group of polydrug users who were high on the precontemplation scale and low on the contemplation, action, and maintenance scales. Thus, a population of individuals in precontemplation is readily identifiable across alcohol and other drug abusers.

We noted earlier that being in precontemplation does not preclude entry to treatment for a substance use disorder, although generally the person does not acknowledge a problem and is arriving mainly to placate others. This would appear to be the case for the persons identified as being in precontemplation by DiClemente and Hughes (1990) and by Carney and Kivlahan (1995), all of whom were nevertheless seeking admission to addictions treatment programs.

Another cluster of individuals identified by DiClemente and Hughes (1990) was labeled "ambivalent." The ambivalent clients scored particularly high on the precontemplation scale (higher than the clients in the precontemplation cluster described earlier) but also above average on the contemplation, action, and maintenance stages. As such, this is a seemingly paradoxical group. On the one hand, they are predominantly characterized by precontemplative attributes. On the other hand, they also are above average on contemplation and action attributes. Given this pattern of apparent conflict, DiClemente and Hughes (1990) have characterized this cluster of clients as "somewhat reluctant or ambivalent about changing their alcohol-problemed behavior" (p. 223). Although high in precontemplation, they appear to be closer to contemplating change than the clients in the precontemplation group. This pattern of scores on the URICA scales was also found in a subgroup of the poly-drug users studied by Carney and Kivlahan (1995).

Taken together, individuals in precontemplation appear to be unaware or actively using strategies to resist becoming aware of their substance use problem. In fact, one study of smokers in precontemplation actually demonstrated that individuals who had higher harm mini-mization (rationalizing) scores used fewer cognitive processes of change compared to those with lower scores (Daniels, 1998). Ironically, they do appear frequently at treatment settings—but usually in response to external pressures such as family, job, or legal ultimatums. The pro-cesses of change most associated with movement from precontempla-tion to contemplation (see Table 2.2) include consciousness raising, emotional arousal/dramatic relief, self-reevaluation, and environmental reevaluation. In many ways, the focus on these processes is intended to envision the severity of the problem and the possibility of change (DiClemente, 2003).

Case Example of a Client in the Precontemplation Stage

Sam W is a 28-year-old married man who was seen at an outpatient drug treatment program for an intake evaluation. This initial appoint-ment was scheduled by his wife, Joan, who had indicated to the tele-phone receptionist that Sam's use of crack cocaine was out of control and that he needed treatment.

Sam appeared 15 minutes late for his intake evaluation. He was wearing slacks and a sports shirt and was well groomed. His wife accompanied him, but she preferred to wait for him in the waiting room and did not participate in the session. Sam began the session by stating "for the record" that he was not experiencing any problems associated with his drug use and that his wife was simply being narrow-minded and attempting to control him. He admitted that he was using mari-juana and crack cocaine, but he asserted that both were being used recreationally and not problematically.

TABLE 2.2. Processes of Change Predominantly Associated with Stage Movement

From precontemplation to contemplation	From contemplation to preparation	From preparation to action	From action to maintenance	Staying in maintenance
Consciousness raising	Self-reevaluation	Self-liberation	Self-liberation	Self-liberation
Emotional arousal/dramatic relief	Environmental reevaluation	Stimulus control	Stimulus control	Stimulus control
Self-reevaluation	Social liberation	Counterconditioning	Counterconditioning	Counterconditioning
Environmental reevaluation		Helping relationships	Reinforcement management	Reinforcement management
			Helping relationships	Helping relationships
				Social liberation

Note. From Velasquez, Maurer, Crouch, and DiClemente (2001, p. 10). Copyright 2001 by The Guilford Press. Reprinted by permission.

He described his marijuana use first. He had started smoking in high school, had continued in college, and had maintained his use over the years since. Sam reported that currently he smokes two joints several evenings during the week (usually after using cocaine with friends earlier in the evening) and three to four joints on either Friday or Saturday evening (but not both). He stated that marijuana relaxed him and took the edge off after a long day at work. He also indicated that marijuana helped him to fall asleep at night and that not smoking contributed to a restless night and irritable feelings the following day. When asked to indicate differences in himself on days he did not smoke versus days he did smoke, he replied that on smoking days he was more comfortable with himself and his world.

As implied above, Sam's current marijuana use was related in part to his cocaine use. Sam had first used crack cocaine in college, around a dozen times per year during his sophomore and junior years. He experienced a "scary high" when he used the cocaine ("scary" in the sense that he did not feel in control), but he asserted that this distress was more than offset by a euphoric feeling. He stopped using cocaine after his junior year because he had begun dating Joan, his wife-to-be, who did not use cocaine and was not comfortable with him using it.

Sam and Joan married 4 years ago, several years after they had met. They married 1 year after Sam's graduation with a degree in business accounting and immediately following Joan's graduation with a degree in nursing. They moved to a medium-sized city near their college town, where Sam accepted a position with an insurance company and Joan began working the evening shift at a public hospital. They were feeling good about their new jobs, but, according to Sam, they responded to their success differently. Joan devoted a considerable amount of energy to advancing her career and took courses toward a master's degree in nursing. Sam, on the other hand, felt he had delayed gratification long enough. He wanted to live more in the here-and-now. He began meeting with coworkers after work (while Joan was working her evening shift) to use crack cocaine. His use, and corresponding expenditures, increased gradually. Now, a year later, he was spending more time away from home, was getting less sleep, and was feeling occasional nervousness. He admitted to occasional use of speedball, a mixture of cocaine and heroin, to reduce jittery nerves associated with coming down from cocaine highs. He also reported experiencing more and more anxiety and nervousness when using the cocaine. Joan over this period became progressively more conscious of Sam's erratic behavior, his missed time from work, and his increased spending habits. They both became aware that their marital relationship had deteriorated, although not to the point where either had voiced a desire for a separation or divorce. Their relationship had become characterized by a sense of detachment rather than closeness.

In summarizing his impressions of his current situation, Sam reiterated that he did not believe his drug use was a problem for him. Instead, he viewed it as his wife's problem, an outgrowth of her rigidity and overcontrolling style. He had agreed to come to the clinic simply to appease Joan and to get her to "lighten up." He cited evidence indicating he was not a drug abuser: no arrests, no problems at work (although he had been passed up for promotion on two occasions during the past 18 months), and no apparent health problems. He discounted as inconsequential his poor work attendance, spending time away from home using cocaine with his coworkers, difficulties maintaining cash flow, and a pervasive tired-out feeling. He left the session saying that he had met his obligation to his wife by coming and that he saw no need to continue contacts with the clinic.

The background material presented by Sam and his behavior throughout the intake session provided a number of signs of a drug abuser in the precontemplation stage. First of all, he was defensive and resisted any suggestions that his drug use was causing problems for him. Indeed, he felt that the problem was not his drug use, but rather the conservative and narrow viewpoints of his wife. He also was able to describe his use and some negative consequences without showing much concern. He was, however, feeling pressure from his wife to seek treatment, and that was really the only reason he had attended the intake session. He was not invested in pursuing counseling, or even further evaluation, and clearly not interested in change.

THE CONTEMPLATION STAGE

An individual in the contemplation stage has begun thinking about changing his or her behavior but has not made a firm decision to change and is not yet engaged in actual behavior change strategies. Among substance abusers, contemplators are seriously pondering quitting or reducing their substance use. However, ambivalence about the problem and the change abounds. Frequently their thoughts about change emanate from an awareness (internally or externally generated) of the disadvantages of continued alcohol or drug use. Such thoughts sometimes dovetail with positive thoughts about a drug-free lifestyle and alternate with thoughts about the good things about using and the barriers to change. This evaluative balancing of the risks and benefits, the advantages and disadvantages of both the substance use and the behavior change, is the most central aspect of the contemplation stage (DiClemente, 2003).

The person in contemplation has been described in more detail by Prochaska and DiClemente (1982) and DiClemente (2003). They characterized these individuals as recognizing the existence of a problem, working to understand or make sense of it, and feeling distress and discomfort over this problem recognition. The person in contemplation is seeking to achieve a sense of mastery or control over the situation through a cognitive reappraisal.

An alcohol or drug abuser can remain in the contemplation stage for an indefinite period of time. The fact that a substance abuser enters treatment does not necessarily mean that he or she has left the stage of contemplation and has moved into the action stage. For many clients, entering treatment does not reflect action but rather a continuation of contemplation. When in treatment such clients are not necessarily resistant and can be open to discussing their concerns even if not ready to initiate action. These and some other common characteristics of persons in the contemplation stage are summarized in Table 2.3.

The descriptions of persons in contemplation in Table 2.3 have been borne out in clinical research. We return to DiClemente et al.'s (1991) large-scale study on the process of smoking cessation. A large number of the individuals that DiClemente et al. (1991) studied were classified

TABLE 2.3. Common Characteristics of Individuals in the Contemplation Stage

- Seeking to evaluate choices and understand their behavior
- Distressed
- Desirous of exerting control or mastery
- Thinking about making change
- Ambivalent
- Have not begun taking action and are not yet prepared to do so
- Frequently have made attempts to change in the past
- Evaluating pros and cons of their behavior
- Evaluating risks and benefits of making changes in their behavior

Note. Adapted in part from DiClemente et al. (1991), DiClemente and Hughes (1990), and Prochaska and DiClemente (1984, 1992).

as being in the contemplation stage. These individuals were smokers who reported that they were considering quitting during the following 6 months. They had not quit for more than a day during the past year and did not foresee quitting during the upcoming 30 days. Relative to the smokers in precontemplation, the smokers in contemplation had a history of more attempts to quit smoking, reported more concerns about wanting to quit, said they had fewer smoking temptations, had more confidence in their ability to quit, and identified fewer advantages and more disadvantages to smoking. The smokers in contemplation also described having previously resorted to more activities associated with quitting smoking. At a 1-month and 6-month follow-up, DiClemente et al. (1991) found that the smokers in the contemplation stage, relative to those in the precontemplation stage, had initiated more quit attempts overall and that the percentage of contemplation-stage smokers who made a quit attempt in the past 30 days was greater than that for the sample of the smokers in precontemplation. DiClemente and Hughes (1990) identified a sample of contemplation-stage drinkers in their study on alcohol abusers entering treatment. Those in the contemplation stage scored highest on the contemplation items from the Stages of Change Scale and lowest on precontemplation and action. A similar profile was found for a subgroup of the polysubstance abusers in the Carney and Kivlahan (1995) study. Thus, in both studies, the clients in contemplation were thinking about behavior change, but despite the fact that they were seeking treatment they scored below average on the action scale.

Individuals in contemplation in general are devoting serious thought to making a behavior change but have not made a firm decision to take action. Contemplation is not always a brief interim stage preceding movement into preparation and action. While many shift from contemplation to preparation and action, there are those who remain in contemplation for extended periods of time and others who move back into precontemplation. One of the challenges facing the clinician is helping the contemplative client to move toward preparation and subsequently action. The change processes most centrally associated with the transition from contemplation to preparation are self-reevaluation, environmental reevaluation, and social liberation (see Table 2.2). These processes can help activate the decisional process and shift the balance toward change. However, if the individual's costs–benefits analysis remains in equilibrium or shifts against change, he or she can get stuck or regress.

Case Example of a Client in the Contemplation Stage

Maureen J is a 46-year-old divorced woman presenting at a community mental health center with concerns about her use of alcohol. She reports that she began drinking at around age 17, and says that she is drinking more than she would like and is thinking about quitting.

Regarding her background, Maureen is the oldest of three daughters. Her father was alcohol-dependent, and one of her sisters is a recovering alcoholic. There is no family history of psychiatric or drug problems. Maureen reports that she used some marijuana, LSD, and cocaine when she was in her 20s but not since. She married her high school sweetheart shortly after they graduated. They divorced when she was 32, and they had no children. For the past 12 years Maureen has been working in a factory that produces windshield wipers. She has no history of psychiatric problems and has no previous treatment for alcohol abuse.

Maureen's drinking shows little variation from week to week. Almost all of her drinking occurs in a local tavern that is close to where she works and lives. Maureen is friendly with a number of other patrons there, some of whom are from work and some from other settings. On Mondays she generally is abstinent. On Tuesdays, Wednesdays, and Thursdays she typically consumes three to five bottles of beer each day. On weekends she drinks more heavily, about 10 to 12 beers daily. She acknowledges that in her drinking career she has experienced drinking binges while on vacations, has made rules to curtail drinking, tried to quit several times in the past, has missed work because of hangovers, and has experienced withdrawal from alcohol, predominantly in the form of mild shakes. Maureen saw these as fairly normal, stating that her drinking really is not much different from that of her friends. However, she is worried about several consequences of her drinking, specifically several recent blackouts, concerns expressed by her mother about her drinking, and feedback from her employer that she seemed to be missing more time from work recently and was not as sharp and on top of things during the morning as she had been in the past. In addition, although she has never been arrested for an alcohol-related offense, she drives home while under the influence of alcohol several times a week. These recent events, taken together, have put her in a position of thinking more about her alcohol use and the possibility of quitting. This is countered, in her mind, by the fact that she really has not been "burned" by her drinking and by her belief that important relationships with her friends will be negatively affected if she is not drinking and thus is not "one of the gang." As such, she is unclear as to what she needs to do and about what she wants to do about her drinking. For that reason, she contacted the clinic to discuss these questions with a counselor.

Maureen's presentation reflects several characteristics commonly seen among persons contemplating a change in their drinking behavior. First and foremost, she is thinking about making a change, although she is ambivalent about the need to change and is concerned about how abstinence would influence her current lifestyle and relationships with her friends. She is experiencing some distress (e.g., family concerns, employer comments on her missed time from work, driving under the influence of alcohol), although the fact that she has not experienced any major (from her point of view) negative consequences of drinking has lessened the impact of these events. In essence, she is in the midst of con-templating the pros and cons of her behavior and of making changes in her decisional balance that will determine whether she moves forward toward action or remains in contemplation or moves back to precon-templation.

THE PREPARATION STAGE

Individuals in the preparation stage are planning to initiate change in the near future and in many cases have learned valuable lessons from their past attempts at change and from failures associated with those efforts (Prochaska & DiClemente, 1992). The client in this stage has resolved the decision-making challenges faced during contemplation and has committed to a change plan soon to be implemented (DiClemente, 2003). Some common characteristics of persons in the prepara-tion stage are shown in Table 2.4.

The inclusion of the preparation stage in the stages-of-change model has had an interesting history. Such a stage, called "decision making," was originally proposed between contemplation and action. However, the analytic procedures used early on to evaluate data collected on the stages-of-change model suggested a four-step model (precontemplation, contemplation, action, and maintenance) (McConnaughy, Prochaska, & Velicer, 1983; McConnaughy et al., 1989). Later analyses, using an alternative data analytic approach felt to be more applicable, provided stronger support for the importance of and necessity for the preparation stage (DiClemente et al., 1991; Prochaska, DiClemente, & Norcross,

TABLE 2.4. Common Characteristics of Individuals in the Preparation Stage

- Intending to change their behavior
- Ready to change in terms of both attitude and behavior
- On the verge of taking action
- Engaged in the change process (possibly making small changes like cutting down)
- Prepared to make firm commitments to follow through on the action option they choose
- Making or having made the decision to change
- Open to planning and creating a personal change plan

Note. Adapted in part from DiClemente and Prochaska (1998), DiClemente et al. (1991), Prochaska and DiClemente (1992), and Prochaska, DiClemente, and Norcross (1992).

1992). Consequently, the present structure of the basic model includes five stages: precontemplation, contemplation, preparation, action, and maintenance.

Insights on clients in the preparation stage are provided in the study described by DiClemente et al. (1991), the investigation of processes of smoking cessation introduced earlier. The participants in that study who were classified as being in the preparation stage met two criteria: planning to quit within the next 30 days and having made a 24-hour quit attempt in the past year. Relative to those in precontemplation and contemplation, those in the preparation stage had a history of more prior attempts at quitting and had more quit attempts in the past year. In addition, those in preparation had higher levels of confidence in their ability to stop or maintain nonsmoking and of efficacy to abstain from smoking, relative to those in precontemplation and contemplation. Evaluations of the pros and cons of smoking also differed as a function of the stage of change. In this regard, those in preparation rated the positives of smoking lower than those in precontemplation or contemplation. They also rated the negatives of smoking higher than did those in the precontemplation or contemplation stages.

When reevaluated 1 and 6 months later, individuals initially classified in the preparation stage were found to be engaged in a variety of activities associated with quitting smoking, and doing so to a greater degree than those previously classified as either in precontemplation or contemplation. For example, those in preparation at baseline had initiated more quit attempts overall during follow-up and had a greater percentage of individuals having made quit attempts and currently not smoking.

Consistent with the above behavioral indicators was the finding by DiClemente et al. (1991) that the individuals in preparation were engaging in a greater variety of experiential and behavioral change processes, relative to those in precontemplation or contemplation. In terms of experiential processes, those in preparation scored higher on the processes of consciousness raising (e.g., seeking information about the addictive behavior, increasing awareness about one's problem behavior), environmental reevaluation (assessing the impact of the behavior on one's surroundings), and self-reevaluation (a personal reappraisal, in both affective and cognitive terms, of the problem and its impact on the person). In the domain of behavioral processes, those in preparation scored higher on self-liberation (choosing and committing to change), counterconditioning (making changes in the conditioned stimuli that influence behavior), reinforcement management (altering the contingencies that influence behavior), stimulus control (restructuring the environment to reduce the likelihood of a particular conditioned stimulus occurring), and emotional arousal/dramatic relief.

Taken together, individuals in preparation are high on dimensions related to both contemplation and action. This pattern was reflected in the DiClemente and Hughes (1990) presentation of a "participation" profile among alcoholics. Clients in this group were low on precontemplation and high on contemplation and action. A nearly identical pattern was found by Carney and Kivlahan (1995) among polysubstance abusers. Accordingly, the processes of change viewed as particularly relevant to the movement from preparation to action include self-liberation, stimulus control, counterconditioning, and helping relationships (see Table 2.2).

Case Example of a Client in the Preparation Stage

Tim L is a 34-year-old single man who attended an intake session at an outpatient drug treatment program. He was self-referred and had called to set up the appointment several days earlier. As part of a telephone prescreen, Tim indicated that he had been abusing amphetamines for years.

Tim presented at the intake session appearing tired and drained. Nevertheless, he was responsive and fully engaged throughout the session. He began immediately with a description of his current drug use. Specifically, Tim outlined a daily pattern of amphetamine use designed to aid him in dealing with a variety of daily tasks and activities. He reported that 2 years earlier he decided to enroll at a local junior college. At the time, he had been working an evening shift (4:30 P.M.–1:00 A.M.) at an office supply warehouse, loading trucks that would depart the following morning to make deliveries to local businesses throughout the city. In addition, Tim was working several hours a day (up to six or eight on days he did not have classes) as a car mechanic at a friend's garage, being paid "off the books." During school sessions, he sought to enroll in classes scheduled for the morning hours.

Tim reported that his use of the amphetamines, purchased regularly from a "safe contact who didn't work the streets," was an effort to "keep him going" and "on top of things." He reported that he generally felt this strategy was working, but that increasingly he was feeling "on edge," "irritable," and "just plain zapped." Although not described in his telephone prescreen, Tim at the intake also described daily use of marijuana, generally one or two joints when he got home at night. Further, he reported that throughout the day he was "almost always" drinking coffee and, when permissible, smoking cigarettes.

Tim's decision to contact the clinic was a difficult one because, he reported, it suggested he wasn't in charge of the situation. He was fearful that "everything would come crumbling down" and that his hopes of using his coursework to obtain a business or managerial position would not be realized. Tim suspected that his work at the supply warehouse was viewed as average at best, citing some tardiness and also periodic errors on getting orders onto the correct delivery trucks. However, he did not feel his employment was in jeopardy. At school he felt he was not performing up to his potential. He noted his social life was not affected because he didn't have one.

The decision by Tim to seek help coincided with several other decisions. First, he had decided to work at the garage only on days when he did not have classes. Second, he determined that his use of amphetamines needed to be terminated. He previously felt that he could simply reduce such use and tailor it to particular situations. He had made several efforts at reduction in the past, with no real effect. Third, while clear on the need to stop his use of marijuana and cigarettes as well, he wondered about the timing. Tim was concerned that stopping use of all three at once might make the termination of his main drug of concern more difficult. Finally, Tim reported that he had set the initiation of treatment as the starting point for making change, however recommended and scheduled by his counselor.

Several aspects of Tim's presentation stood out. He was clearly ready to change, certainly in terms of attitude and seemingly on the verge in terms of initiating a change in behavior. He had begun to take action by virtue of coming to his clinic appointment and being committed to a treatment plan. While not yet modifying his substance use, he was evidencing a firm commitment to the change process. Creating a viable change plan for his behavior prepares him to initiate action. To all outward appearances, he had engaged himself in the process of change and was prepared to proceed accordingly.

THE ACTION STAGE

As described by Prochaska, DiClemente, and Norcross (1992), "action is the stage in which individuals modify their behavior, experiences, or environment in order to overcome their problems" (p. 1104). In this regard, there are two central features that characterize persons in the action stage. The first is a firm and clear decision to change and commitment to that change. The second is the appearance of active behavioral manifestations of the commitment to change and the initiation of the change plan. Most typically these change attempts are reflected in individuals' efforts to make modifications in their behavioral patterns or in their environments. A listing of some characteristics common among people in the action stage is provided in Table 2.5.

Several studies have been conducted in an effort to empirically identify characteristics of people in the action stage. An early study by Prochaska and DiClemente (1983) involved the evaluation of over 850 persons who responded to newspaper articles and advertisements for a study on making changes in smoking behavior. Recent quitters, representing persons in the action stage, were defined as those who had quit smoking within 6 months of participating in the study. All subjects were evaluated according to the extent to which they were using different processes or mechanisms related to change. These processes, discussed in detail by Prochaska and DiClemente (1984), include consciousness raising, self-liberation, stimulus control, and helping relationships (relationships, including the therapeutic relationship, that provide support and inputs to making change). Persons in different stages of change would be expected to score differentially on these change processes. As an example, persons in precontemplation would be expected to score low on most of the change processes, since they are not thinking about

TABLE 2.5. Common Characteristics of Individuals in the Action Stage

- Client has decided to make change and reached the date to implement the change.
- Client has verbalized or otherwise demonstrated a firm commitment to making change.
- Efforts to modify behavior and/or one's environment are being taken.
- Client presents motivation and effort to achieve behavioral change.
- Client has committed to making change and is involved in behavioral change processes.
- Client is willing to follow suggested strategies and activities to change.

Note. Adapted in part from Prochaska and DiClemente (1984, 1992) and DiClemente and Hughes (1990).

change. Persons in contemplation, on the other hand, might be expected to score particularly high on consciousness raising.

In studying the individuals classified as being in the action phase, Prochaska and DiClemente (1983) found that these subjects scored highest on the processes of change labeled self-liberation, counterconditioning, stimulus control, reinforcement management, and helping relationships, relative to subjects classified as being in precontemplation or contemplation. Similar findings have been reported by Ahijevych and Wewers (1992). Prochaska, Velicer, DiClemente, and Fava (1988) showed that these five processes reflect a more general cluster of processes that includes activities with the aim of behavior change and of using others as resources for support and encouragement in the behavior change efforts.

Monitoring the extent of use of the varied processes of change across the stages-of-change model can provide information on when and where a particular process will be predominant. In conducting research on this topic, Prochaska, Velicer, Guadagnoli, Rossi, and DiClemente (1991) noted that reinforcement management is the first process that predominates for clients in the action stage. Prochaska et al. (1991) also found that the processes of self-reevaluation and stimulus control peak in the middle phase of the action stage, providing further support for viewing these processes as particularly relevant to this stage.

DiClemente and Hughes (1990) and Carney and Kivlahan (1995) identified an action stage profile in samples of alcohol and other substance abusers. Their clinical assessments in each case included administration of the URICA (described in Chapter 3) to determine scores on precontemplation, contemplation, action, and maintenance scales. One of the profiles that emerged from DiClemente and Hughes's analyses of the URICA scale scores reflected persons high on the action stage score. DiClemente and Hughes called this profile the "participation cluster." Because these clients scored well above average on both the action and contemplation scales, it seems they are invested in behavior change and are actively engaged in that effort. The clients also scored above average on the maintenance scale which really represents striving or struggling to maintain items. As would be expected, their scores on the precontemplation scale were low.

A subgroup of the polydrug users in the Carney and Kivlahan (1995) sample also exhibited a distinct pattern of scores that was similar to the participation cluster described by DiClemente and Hughes (1990): URICA scores were highest on the contemplation and action scales, above average on the maintenance scale, and well below average on the precontemplation scale. These polydrug users, then, can be described as clients who are not only thinking seriously about change but who also are actively engaged in the change process.

Of special relevance to the above, it has been demonstrated that client end-of-treatment profiles related to action activities (including stages-of-change scores measured using the URICA, processes of change, and self-efficacy) are predictive of posttreatment abstinence. In this regard, Carbonari and DiClemente (2000) used data gathered at the end of a 12-week course of treatment for an alcohol use disorder from 673 outpatients and 510 aftercare clients and classified their 12-month drinking outcome into one of three outcome groups: completely abstinent, some drinking but no heavy drinking, or continuing or returning to heavy drinking. The profiles of these three outcome groups on end-of-treatment stage-related attitudes and self-evaluations clearly distinguished the three outcome groups. The most consistent indications were reflected in contrasts between the profile components for the abstinent outcome group and the heavy drinking outcome group. Those in the abstinent outcome group scored higher on the URICA action scale, higher in confidence to abstain, lower in temptations to drink, and higher on use of behavioral processes of change (e.g., self-liberation, stimulus control, counterconditioning, reinforcement management, helping relationships), relative to those in the heavy drinking outcome group. The scores for the lighter drinking outcome group fell in between those of the other two groups. Although very different samples, the patterns of process-of-change variables were similar for both the outpatient and aftercare samples. Taken together, these findings suggest that individuals in the action stage have decided to make changes in their behavior, have committed to making these changes, and have begun taking action to effect the changes they want to achieve. Action-stage clients are motivated and ready to initiate steps to produce change, and the changes that occur in the action stage typically are the most dramatic and overt of those that occur in any of the other stages. The action phase most commonly lasts 3 to 6 months, the time needed to establish a new pattern of behavior that produces less relapse (DiClemente, 2003). Processes most centrally associated with movement from the action stage to maintenance are self-liberation, stimulus control, counterconditioning, reinforcement management, and helping relationships.

Case Example of a Client in the Action Stage

Paul J is a 34-year-old single man who attended an intake evaluation session at an addictions treatment center. He reported that he had been using multiple substances in various combinations since junior high school (currently he was using alcohol, cocaine, and marijuana). Further, he had decided that he wanted to be abstinent from all substance use, including alcohol, and immediately wanted to start taking the steps necessary to achieve this goal.

Paul's demeanor during his evaluation was serious, compliant, accommodating, and eager. He reported that he had used a variety of drugs since his junior high school years. The listing he provided included alcohol, marijuana, cocaine, LSD, peyote, stimulants, inhalants, and depressants. Paul noted that during different periods of his life he had been using different combinations of these drugs. For example, during junior high school he was using mainly alcohol and marijuana. During high school he began using cocaine regularly (around once a week). Immediately after high school he began spending much of his time with friends who were using inhalants and depressants. During his 20s his drug use predominantly revolved around the hallucinogens (e.g., LSD, peyote) and stimulants. Finally, Paul described that during the past 6 years his drug use had been restricted for the most part to almost daily use of marijuana and alcohol, and use of cocaine approximately four times a week. He noted that he occasionally would also use stimulants other than cocaine, but that such use was infrequent (maybe once a month, he estimated).

Paul's family, especially a brother and a sister, were concerned that his drug use was causing him to be "stuck" in his relationships and employment. Paul acknowledged that his drug use over the past decade had precluded the development of significant or long-term relationships with women (and often with friends more generally) and that he had difficulties maintaining a job. In fact, according to Paul, he had spent most of the past 10 years either underemployed, on unemployment benefits, or on welfare support. The status that bothered him most was underemployment because he felt he was capable of more challenging positions that would provide stimulation as well as better salaries. He noted, with some pride, that his drug use had not led to problems in his physical health (at least, as far as he was aware), accidents, or arrests. It was the absence of problems in these areas that he had used in the past as evidence that he did not have a problem with drug use.

Paul's current alcohol and drug use occurred with various combinations of acquaintances from a core group of around 15 persons. Sometimes he would get together with two or three of these individuals and they would (generally) go to someone's apartment to drink or use drugs. He would meet these people at one or two local spots where members of the group tended to congregate. Paul did not spend much time with these individuals beyond these specific drug use contexts. He would visit the local congregating settings in the mid- to late afternoon when not working, and after work when he was employed.

Paul at his intake session could not identify the precipitating circumstances that led to his decision to quit his alcohol and drug use. He did note that on numerous occasions in the past he had made the decision to terminate use of one or more—but not all—of the substances he was using at the time. For example, on a handful of occasions he had decided to stop using cocaine but did not feel at those times the need to make changes in his use of marijuana or alcohol. These past decisions regarding behavior change were short-lived, and Paul said that he did not believe his heart was in making long-term changes at that time. More often, he reported, he was responding to some acute illness associated with recent drug use or greater than usual complaints from his family.

This time, however, he said it was different. As he put it, now he "really" had decided to change and indeed had already implemented several steps in this regard. As an indication of this heightened commitment, Paul had not used any alcohol or drugs during the preceding

5 days and he had attended his intake session. Paul had also begun to attend meetings of Alcoholics Anonymous, and had begun to seek out and spend time with acquaintances not using drugs. Also unique to his current decision was the commitment to stop *all* drug use. Paul felt now that it was necessary for him to be abstinent from alcohol as well as all other substances.

Some of the more common characteristics of clients in the action stage were evident in Paul's intake presentation. First and foremost, he was verbalizing a firm decision to initiate and achieve behavioral changes in his use of alcohol and other drugs. Second, he was ready to collaborate with his counselor to initiate and continue steps to become sober. In fact, Paul had already initiated some steps on his own before his session and had been abstinent for several days. By all appearances he was motivated, committed, and in the midst of making changes.

THE MAINTENANCE STAGE

The stage of maintenance is characterized predominantly by two endeavors. The first is sustaining and further incorporating changes achieved during the action stage into a lifestyle, and the second is avoiding relapse. Persons in the maintenance stage have accomplished at least some minimal amount of change as a function of successful efforts exerted during the action stage and are on their way to developing a new stable pattern of nonusing behavior. A listing of some characteristics often reported by individuals in maintenance is given in Table 2.6.

Since sustaining change often entails continued use of techniques for initiating change, it is not surprising that the processes of change used most by persons in maintenance overlap with processes frequently

---

TABLE 2.6 Common Characteristics of Individuals in the Maintenance Stage

- Client is working to sustain changes achieved to date.
- Considerable attention is focused on avoiding slips or relapses.
- Client may describe fear or anxiety regarding relapse when facing a high-risk situation.
- Less frequent but often intense temptations to use substances or return to substance use may be faced.
- Beginning to build an alternative lifestyle that does not include the old behavior.

Note. Adapted in part from Prochaska and DiClemente (1984, 1992) and DiClemente and Hughes (1990).

observed in the action stage. As shown in Table 2.2, most noteworthy among persons in maintenance are the processes of self-liberation, stimulus control, counterconditioning, reinforcement management, helping relationships, and social liberation (see also Ahijevych & Wewers, 1992; DiClemente & Prochaska, 1982; Prochaska & DiClemente, 1983, 1986). The overlap in these predominant processes across the action and maintenance stages highlights that maintenance is not static but instead an active and vital endeavor.

Given the overlap in primary change processes, one might wonder about how to tell if a person is in action versus maintenance. For research purposes, investigators have operationalized the onset of maintenance as 6 months following some successful action, such as the last drug use or drink (e.g., Prochaska et al., 1992). Clinically speaking, action might be viewed as a period during which efforts are taken to effect change and get such change established, with maintenance occurring after initial change-related efforts have stabilized and a new pattern of behavior developed. The selection of this 6-month point was also guided by indications in the relapse literature that the vast majority of relapses occur during the first 6 months of a change.

Since addictive behaviors are complex, multifaceted problems, therapists and clients often work to break a problem domain down into more manageable components. For example, consider the case of a polydrug abuser who mainly uses cocaine, marijuana, and alcohol. He or she may further report that cocaine use is creating the majority of problems in his or her life but that eventually he or she wants to terminate all substance use. It may be that the therapist and client agree to focus on the cocaine use first and utilize successes in that arena to subsequently terminate the use of marijuana and alcohol. In such a scenario, the client might achieve abstinence from cocaine using a set of change strategies and utilize them successfully for an extended period of time such that they become part of a maintenance stage. Meanwhile, the client might start action-related strategies for cessation of marijuana and alcohol use. In this manner, he or she may be in a stage of maintenance regarding cocaine use but in an action state regarding marijuana and alcohol use.

While there may not be an unequivocal definition for when one departs from action and embarks on maintenance, there is more certainty on what represents a failure in either action or maintenance, and that is relapse. When a person relapses and returns to using a particular substance again, it is clear that there was a breakdown in the strategies that had been employed previously to sustain abstinence. At such a point, and as discussed in Chapter 1, such persons might attempt to "recycle" themselves by reinitiating contemplation, preparation, or action. Alternatively, some individuals might be sufficiently discouraged that they revert back to a stage of precontemplation. There is some controversy as to what constitutes a lapse versus a relapse. A *lapse* is a single event or a brief encounter with the prior behavior. A lapse indicates that there is a problem in the current change plan, a lapse of commitment or judgment, or a particularly challenging situation. Rapid recovery from a lapse often will keep the person in action or maintenance. A more significant return to use would signify *relapse*, according to DiClemente (2003).

A final issue surrounding the stage of maintenance is the question of whether a person ever successfully leaves this stage. In the abstract, the answer is yes, and termination of the change process can occur when the individual's temptations to use are at a level of zero and when the person's confidence about not using drugs is 100% (Prochaska & DiClemente, 1986) and there is little or no effort needed to maintain change. Individuals who begin to use after having achieved termination may be more reinitiating than relapsing (DiClemente, 2003). More practically, however, it probably makes some sense to view individuals as continuing to maintain and thus remaining aware of risks or challenges to their maintenance of a particular change in behavior.

Case Example of a Client in the Maintenance Stage

Angela M is a 47-year-old woman who quit drinking around 11 months ago. Prior to then she had been drinking heavily and problematically for over 20 years, experiencing over that period a variety of negative alcohol-related consequences.

Angela began drinking in high school, and her drinking at that time was limited to weekend drinking with friends. However, even then she reported she was drinking too much and over time began to experience hangovers and some difficulties remembering events from the preceding evening while drinking. Following high school she attended a local community college and continued drinking in this pattern, with the exception that she might also drink on some weekday evening as well. Despite taking many risks, she reports, she managed to avoid any alcohol-related arrests during this time, such as driving under the influence. Angela does note, though, that she probably would have done better in school and performed better on her part-time jobs had she not been drinking so much.

Throughout high school and while attending community college, Angela lived at home with her parents and one younger brother. While her parents were upset with the frequency of her drinking, she never had the sense they were particularly concerned about it. After completing her coursework, Angela took a position as an engineering technician, which entailed serving as an assistant to company staff working on building renovation plans. Since the job was not within commuting distance from her home, she moved into an apartment with a girlfriend she had known in college.

Angela reports that in the following years there were several changes in her drinking. For example, she found that she could consume relatively large amounts of alcohol, considerably more than her friends and acquaintances. She also found that she was consuming a larger array of alcoholic beverages, including strong mixed drinks. Finally, Angela reported that she was not convinced she had much "direction" in life and worried that she might not find a partner to settle down with.

Angela characterizes the next 20 years as a "blur," despite several notable life events. For example, she initiated four job changes, two of which were promotions professionally. The other two were for "changes in scenery." In addition, she met a man, Peter, whom she lived with for several years and then married when she was 37. Angela describes this relationship then and currently as the most valued aspect of her life.

The reason those 20 years were described as a blur is that her drinking continued to the point where she was consuming in excess of six standard drink equivalents of alcohol most evenings, and more on weekends. Peter also drank frequently, but rarely as heavily, and he only occasionally confronted her about her drinking. Gradually, though, Angela reported an awareness of more and more signals that she needed to cut back, the most pronounced being a pair of arrests for driving under the influence of alcohol at ages 40 and 42. After the first arrest, she reports she cut back considerably but gradually returned to her prearrest level of drinking. The second arrest was followed in time with three attempts at outpatient alcoholism treatment, at ages 42, 43, and 44. The first two treatment endeavors were "helpful" and led to a fair amount of abstinence and many fewer heavy drinking days.

However, the changes never lasted as long as she wanted—perhaps, she reports, because she was not fully committed to abstaining completely. Her third treatment, at age 44, "took hold" in that she found her resolve stronger than ever and her working relationship with her counselor particularly helpful and positive. They focused extensively on a number of approaches to achieving stable abstinence, including a detailed functional analysis of her drinking (the determinants, immediate and longer term consequences, expected negative effects and benefits of drinking, etc.), development of alternatives to drinking (including stress management, avoiding situations associated with previous heavy drinking, coping with cravings and urges, and drink refusal skills), the inclusion of Peter in portions of treatment to incorporate his support and encouragement, and the development of plans to prevent relapse or at least to minimize drinking, should a slip occur.

Angela's treatment entailed mostly weekly individual and group sessions for almost 10 months, followed by mostly individual sessions on a less frequent basis. While she experienced some setbacks, she generally rebounded quickly, and, perhaps more importantly, she felt she learned valuable "sobriety lessons" from such events. Eventually, she and her counselor determined that they comfortably could move to scheduling monthly appointments. They further agreed that Angela could call and touch base prior to the scheduled appointment time, and if all was going well they could cancel the appointment and reschedule for a month later.

It was at this point that Angela was phasing herself more fully into the maintenance stage. During recent years she had taken considerable action to cease her drinking, especially during her third outpatient treatment. Angela had incorporated a variety of change strategies that she had been using successfully, following an early period of trial-and-error in the application of these strategies. Now her attention was focused on what she called "cruise control," whereby she could step back from the vigilance associated with skill acquisition and application and instead let much of that behavior occur more naturally. She emphasized that "cruise control" still entailed paying close attention to her environment, including attention to her own thoughts and feelings. Further, Angela still spent time anticipating drinking situations and reviewing in advance her plans to deal with such situations. Even with close to a year of abstinence, she experienced periodic thoughts and temptations regarding alcohol use, although she was pleased that she could not really classify them as cravings. Finally, it was Angela's sense that she would always need to be in a state of full awareness regarding potential challenges to her abstinence and that she would never be in a position to take her sobriety for granted.

CLINICAL ISSUES RELEVANT TO THE PRECONTEMPLATION, CONTEMPLATION, AND PREPARATION STAGES

As we noted earlier, persons in the precontemplation and contemplation stages are not taking action toward changing their substance use. Individuals in preparation have made the decision and are already planning on making changes in their behavior, although some resistance may remain. The lack of decisional action unfortunately has been thought to reflect "denial" and/or "resistance," and traditionally it has been argued that a primary task of the clinician is to confront denial or resistance in order to break through it. Successful confrontation is presumed to set the stage for the individual to take action regarding his or her substance use disorder.

In this section, we discuss denial and resistance in greater depth. We first define the terms and then describe how they are assumed to be manifested in the treatment process. Next, alternative ways of conceptualizing denial and resistance are discussed. We emphasize motivational interviewing, which involves the use of a variety of clinical techniques to help individuals mobilize their own motivations and resources to overcome their ambivalence and begin to create behavioral change (Miller & Rollnick, 1991, 2002).

Denial

Although Paolino and McCrady (1977), among others, have called denial the most misused term in the substance abuse literature, denial traditionally has been a cornerstone of many models of rehabilitation for persons with substance use disorders. Chafetz (1970) identified denial as one of the alcoholic's most characteristic defense mechanisms. He wrote that "denial constitutes the main method by which alcoholics deal with life" (Chafetz, 1970, p. 10), and similar impressions have been offered regarding persons who abuse drugs other than alcohol (e.g., Washton, 1987). Further, clinicians say denial is among the most difficult problems they face in working with clients (Metzger, 1988). In fact, one proposed definition of alcoholism, published in the *Journal of the American Medical Association* (Morse & Flavin, 1992), included a component called "distortions in thinking, most notably denial" (p. 1012). The committee developing the definition used denial in their formulation "not only in the psychoanalytic sense of a single psychologic defense mechanism disavowing the significance of events but more broadly to include a range of psychologic maneuvers that decrease awareness of the fact that alcohol use is the cause of a person's problems rather than a solution to those problems. Denial becomes an integral part of the disease and is nearly always a major obstacle to recovery" (p. 1013).

Denial is rooted in the psychoanalytic literature on defense mechanisms, which are viewed as unconscious processes used by an individual to alleviate emotional conflict and anxiety. Vaillant (1977) organized the variety of defense mechanisms (e.g., distortion, projection, repression, suppression) according to the level of maturity they reflect and their importance to the degree of psychopathology. Denial was placed in the category of least mature defense mechanisms. As described by Vaillant (1977), denial's primary component is a distorted perception of reality. As such, denial entails negating or refusing thoughts, external feedback, and other forms of awareness about a behavior that, if fully conscious and "rational," would be intolerable to the individual.

Anderson (1981) provided one of the more comprehensive discussions of denial. He used the term "denial" to designate "a wide repertoire of psychological defenses and maneuvers that alcoholic persons unwittingly set up to protect themselves from the realization that they do in fact have a drinking problem" (p. 11), or by extension, a problem with any psychoactive substance. As with defense mechanisms more generally, denial was seen as an unconscious (unwitting) process. Moreover, denial can also operate within the substance abuser's family or other support systems.

Anderson (1981) identified a variety of the defensive maneuvers that are most typically observed, including simple denial, minimizing, blaming, rationalizing, intellectualizing, diversion, and hostility. In discussing these manifestations of denial, Anderson provided two of its other features. The first is that denial is automatic and not simply lying or willfully deceptive. Instead, the denial is an outgrowth of a firmly entrenched state of self-delusion. The second feature of denial, according to Anderson, is that it is progressive. He observes that "by the time an individual's illness is sufficiently advanced that the problem appears serious to others, an elaborate system of defenses has usually been built up" (p. 13). Thus, as the severity of alcoholism increases, the complexity and intractability of the denial increases comparably.

Resistance

Another term frequently encountered in the treatment literature on substance abuse is resistance. A hallmark construct in the psychoanalytic literature for decades, *resistance* was defined by Fenichel (1945) as "everything that prevents the patient from producing material derived from the unconscious" (p. 27). The concept of resistance is "understood in psychoanalysis as the process through which any action, emotion, or thought comes to interfere with the patient's becoming conscious . . . of previously unconscious mental processes and contents" (Liotti, 1987, p. 88).

More recently, therapists use the term "resistance" more generally to refer to client behaviors that they view as antitherapeutic (Turkat & Meyer, 1982). As such, resistance is seen as occurring on both conscious and unconscious levels. While resistance may have the goal of avoiding uncomfortable feelings such as anxiety or guilt, resistance also can refer to the client who is unmotivated for change. Representative of this view are Lazarus and Fay (1982), who state that "resistant patients are neither people who 'do not want help' nor are 'deliberate saboteurs,' but instead people for whom exploration and change are difficult, painful, and even dangerous" (p. 200).

In an effort to better specify the construct of resistance, several investigators have identified subcategories of resistance and have applied the term to particular diagnostic domains or therapeutic approaches. Sandler, Holder, and Dare (1970), for example, identified 10 forms of resistance that may occur during psychotherapy (e.g., transference resistance, resistance due to secondary gain, resistance related to specific behavior change techniques). In addition, Cavaiola (1984) proposed a set of stages of resistance that characterizes drunk-driving recidivists, and Weissberg and Levay (1981) applied Sandler et al.'s (1970) forms of resistance to conjoint sex therapy. Examinations of resistance in the context of particular therapeutic approaches have been provided for family therapy (Anderson & Stewart, 1983; Larson & Talley, 1977; Will, 1983), marital therapy (Gurman, 1984; Spinks & Birchler, 1982), and group therapy (Balgopal & Hull, 1973; Muhleman, 1987). Similarly, in addition to discussions of resistance in psychoanalytic psychotherapy (Chessick, 1974; Greenson, 1967), the construct has been described in relation to behavior therapy (Jahn & Lichstein, 1980), cognitive-behavioral therapy (Golden, 1983), and rational-emotive therapy (Ellis, 1983a, 1983b, 1984, 1985).

In the context of the stages-of-change model, individuals in precontemplation are sometimes, perhaps often, resistant to consideration of making changes in their behavior. Resistance and denial are not characteristics of a disease but are common human strategies for managing problems and change in our lives. These characteristics can be seen whenever individuals are faced with the need to change diet, leave abusive relationships, take medications, or manage addictive behaviors. They represent avoidant coping mechanisms that enable an individual to keep a pattern of behavior that is known and comfortable even if it is dysfunctional. The challenge for the therapist, according to DiClemente and Velasquez (2002), is to identify how the client is managing to resist change and to diffuse that hesitancy in a positive way. Such resistance to change among persons in precontemplation, as noted earlier in this chapter, has been summarized by DiClemente and Velasquez (2002) and DiClemente (2003) by five R's: reveling, reluctance, rebellion, resignation, and rationalization. The presence and influence of these forms of resistance to change, which can operate singularly or more often in combination with each other, serve to decrease use of helpful processes of change, like self-reevaluation, and keep the person stuck in the early stages of change. Finding ways to defuse and defeat these resistance-enhancing strategies is a critical focus for the therapist when dealing with precontemplation and contemplation.

Reconceptualizing Denial and Resistance

As noted above, denial and resistance are concepts frequently used to explain why clients do not succeed in treatment. As such, it is the client traits of resistance and denial that lead to a treatment failure. However, there are significant difficulties in empirically documenting the validity of a trait model in accounting for treatment responsivity (see Miller, 1985). Among the components of the trait model that have *not* been substantiated, according to Miller (1985), are that denial is more frequently seen among alcoholics than among other clinical populations and that denial is directly related to treatment outcome.

Miller (1985) and Miller and Rollnick (1991) have argued that the use of constructs such as denial and resistance has not advanced our knowledge about addictive behavior or its treatment. Instead, they view resistance specifically as a reaction to a client–therapist relationship that lacks agreement and collaboration rather than a client characteristic. In their recent conceptualization, Miller and Rollnick (2013) use the term "sustain talk" to describe what was previously thought of as client resistance. Sustain talk is client language that does not move in the direction of change, but instead indicates a client's stated reasons not to make a change in a particular behavior, thus maintaining the status quo.

As an alternative, they have focused on enhancing motivation. Miller (1985) notes that the term "motivation" frequently is viewed as the flip side of denial and resistance. So, according to Miller (1985), an important endeavor in the treatment of addictive behaviors is to work toward maximizing the occurrence of behaviors related to resolution of the substance use problem. In this regard, a "motivational intervention" would refer to any "operation that increases the probability of entering, continuing, and complying with an active change strategy" (Miller, 1985, p. 88). Miller (1985) originally outlined a series of motivational interventions that potentially could be used to promote change, including giving advice, providing feedback, setting goals, role playing, continuing contacts, manipulating external contingencies, providing choices, and decreasing the attractiveness of problem behavior. More recently, Miller and Rollnick (1991, 2002) summarized these and other strategies as "building blocks" that can be applied as part of the clinician's effort to engender productive change in an individual's addictive behavior. Essential strategies, described in detail in Miller and Rollnick (2002), are summarized by the acronym OARS, representing open questions, affirming, reflecting, and summarizing (see Table 2.7).

It is useful to describe several of these strategies in the context of the stages-of-change model, particularly the stages of precontemplation and contemplation. Individuals in precontemplation, as noted earlier, are characterized by lack of awareness of a drug problem and evidence that drug use is contributing to dysfunction. As a result, one objective of motivational interventions with clients in the precontemplation stage often is to make more salient the effects of their drug use on their lives and create interest and concern for change. Among those in contemplation who are ambivalent about the level of the problem or making change, a major goal of motivational interventions is to promote decision

TABLE 2.7. Essential Motivational Methods for Promoting Change among Persons with Addictive Behaviors

- *Open questions:* Asking open-ended questions
- *Affirming:* Affirming, supporting, and reinforcing the client
- *Reflecting:* Reflecting back to the client
- *Summarizing:* Providing statements that link together and reinforce material that has been discussed

Note. Adapted from Miller and Rollnick (2002). Copyright 2002 by The Guilford Press. Adapted by permission.

making and change language that emphasize the pros of reduced or zero use and the cons of continued use at existing levels and to encourage the taking of steps that will lead to action.

Motivational-enhancing interventions that focus on discussing and describing typical use, reactions of significant others, and objective feedback using biochemical measures are designed to decrease substance attractiveness and increase personal concern and awareness. These are most applicable in working with clients in either the precontemplation or contemplation stages. Decreasing the utility and attractiveness of the drug potentially makes it easier for those in precontemplation to become aware of and acknowledge the negatives of drug use. Similarly, engaging those in contemplation in a risk–reward analysis of their current behavior and discussing important values and goals that are at risk can tip the balance in favor of the disadvantages of drug use and consequently move them toward action to change their drug use.

Providing choice is another intervention with potential therapeutic relevance for persons in the stages of precontemplation and contemplation. In the case of those in precontemplation, identifying options for the client may help diffuse the resentments that arise when an authority figure or significant other has applied pressure on the client to seek treatment. If the client believes he or she has a choice in directions that can be taken, then the accompanying sense that he or she can prescribe and guide the course of action may result in initiating critical steps toward change. Similarly, the person in contemplation wavering about change may use the availability of several options as a way of initiating steps toward action.

These and numerous other intervention strategies are discussed in greater detail throughout this volume. For now, they are introduced in the context of interventions relevant to the processes of changing behavior.

CLINICAL ISSUES RELEVANT TO THE ACTION AND MAINTENANCE STAGES

The clinical tasks associated with working with clients in the action and maintenance stages are appropriately different from those faced when clients are in the precontemplation or contemplation stages. The preparation stage represents the transitional tasks that need to bridge decision making and action. As noted earlier in this chapter, the client in the action stage has begun to take steps to change behavior, and the client in the maintenance stage has reached some initial success in achieving his or her behavior change goals and is seeking now to maintain those gains and goals. Below we identify some of the issues that arise in working with clients in these two stages and preview some of the strategies that can be used in addressing these issues. These issues and strategies are discussed in much greater detail throughout the remainder of this volume.

Clients in the action stages generally have developed a plan for change and have begun to implement it. As highlighted by DiClemente (1991), they often use treatment to make a public commitment to action, to obtain some external confirmation of their plan, to seek support, to gain greater self-efficacy, to enhance skills, and in many cases to create artificial external monitors of their behavior. Helping clients increase their sense of self-efficacy is a particularly important task of the action stage. Helping them to use behavioral strategies to overcome temptations to use and to achieve and sustain success offers the behavioral foundation of efficacy. Focusing on clients' successful activities, reaffirming their decisions, and helping them to make intrinsic attributions of success also can increase their self-efficacy evaluations. A sampling of clinical strategies potentially applicable for use with clients in the action stage is shown in Table 2.8.

Clients in the maintenance stage are seeking to firmly establish their new behavioral patterns and avoid a return to substance use. Sustaining behavior change can be very difficult, initial success can breed overconfidence, cues for use are ubiquitous, and relapses often occur. A sample of strategies available for use with clients in the maintenance stage is shown in Table 2.9. These and other matters are discussed thoroughly in upcoming chapters on clinical interventions. The issue of relapse, and clinical responses to such events, is addressed in detail in Chapter 9.

TABLE 2.8. Representative Clinical Strategies Applicable to Clients in the Action Stage

- Maintain client engagement in treatment.
- Support a realistic view of change through small, successive, and successful steps.
- Acknowledge the difficulties encountered in the early stages of change (withdrawal, distress, discomfort).
- Help client identify high-risk situations through a functional analysis and develop appropriate coping strategies to overcome these.
- Assist client in finding new sources of reinforcement to support positive change.
- Help client assess whether he or she has strong family and social support.
- Promote seeking support from mutual help groups.

Note. From Miller (1999).

TABLE 2.9. Representative Clinical Strategies Applicable to Clients in the Maintenance Stage

- Help client identify and sample drug-free sources of satisfaction (i.e., develop new reinforcers).
- Support lifestyle changes that support freedom from dependence on substances.
- Affirm client's resolve and self-efficacy.
- Help client practice, apply, and sustain new coping strategies to avoid a return to drug use.
- Maintain supportive contact.
- Help client resolve any additional mental health, physical health, and life context problems.

Note. From Miller (1999).

SUMMARY

- Persons in the precontemplation stage generally are underaware, ignorant, or actively minimizing concerns about their drug use problem. If aware, they are not thinking seriously about their drug use or about making changes in it. Processes of change most central to movement from precontemplation to contemplation include consciousness raising, emotional arousal/dramatic relief, self-reevaluation, and environmental reevaluation.

- Researchers have identified a group of individuals labeled "ambivalent." These are individuals who rate highest on precontemplation but also above average on contemplation, action, and maintenance stages of change.

- Persons in contemplation have started to think about making changes in their behavior, but as yet have not made the decision to change or initiated actual behavior change strategies. Processes of change most associated with movement from contemplation to preparation include self-reevaluation, environmental reevaluation, and social liberation.

- Individuals in the preparation stage have resolved the decision-making issues faced in contemplation and are planning to initiate change in the near future. The change processes most associated with movement from preparation to action include self-liberation, stimulus control, counterconditioning, and helping relationships.

- Clients in the action stage are characterized by a firm decision to make change and by evidence of active, overt behavioral manifestations of the commitment to change. Processes of change most central to the transition from action to maintenance include self-liberation, stimulus control, counterconditioning, reinforcement management, and helping relationships.

- Research has identified a cluster of individuals who appear to be in the action stage. Based on the URICA, they score high on the contemplation and action stages of change and low on precontemplation.

- Clients in the maintenance stage are predominantly focused on sustaining changes and on avoiding relapse. Processes used considerably by persons in maintenance are self-liberation, stimulus control, counterconditioning, reinforcement management, helping relationships, and social liberation.

- Denial and resistance have been described as characteristics of substance abusers or the disease of addiction. However, these strategies are common ways individuals deal with life challenges and to avoid changes that they are not ready to make. Resistance represents counter-therapeutic behaviors directed toward minimizing uncomfortable feelings and the need for change.

- Focusing on ambivalence and the construct of motivation may be an alternative to focusing on denial and resistance. A variety of motivational interventions (offering advice, giving feedback, providing choices, and decreasing the attractiveness of problem behavior) and strategies that employ open-ended questions, affirmations, reflective listening, and summarizing offered in a collaborative, empathic, and evocative spirit and style have been identified by Miller and his colleagues that can address challenges of early stage tasks.

• Motivation, in terms of acknowledging problems, making decisions to change, increasing commitment, initiating change, and maintaining changes, is an important component of each of the stages of change.

3

Assessment

Assessment is a critical concern in all substance abuse treatment settings. However, operationalizing assessment, though widely practiced, is difficult. In this book we define *assessment* as the collection and use of information to obtain an understanding of an individual (or couple or family), usually for purposes of treatment planning, modification, and evaluation. Therefore, assessment may occur before, during, or following any defined period of treatment (e.g., Donovan, 1999; Donovan & Marlatt, 2005; Sobell, Sobell, & Nirenberg, 1988; Sobell, Toneatto, & Sobell, 1994).

Reviews and copies of many of the most important assessment measures used in alcohol and drug treatment are readily available.[1] Rather than reviewing all these measures, in this chapter we first will show ways to systematically identify an individual's stage of change. No matter how interesting the idea of "stage of change," it can have practical value only if it can be measured. We also will discuss how to assess specific coping mechanisms described as the five experiential and five

---

[1]Many of the measures described in this chapter are readily available, at no charge for downloading, at one or more of the following resources: the HABITS lab at the University of Maryland, Baltimore County (*www.umbc.edu/psyc/habits*); the Center on Alcoholism, Substance Abuse, and Addictions at the University of New Mexico (*casaa.unm.edu*); the Substance Use Screening and Assessment Instruments Database at the Alcohol and Drug Abuse Institute at the University of Washington (*lib.adai.washington.edu/instruments*); the website for the NIAAA *Assessing Alcohol Problems* monograph (*pubs.niaaa.nih.gov/publications/Assesing%20Alcohol/index. htm#contents*); the Healthy Lifestyles Guided Self-Change Program at Nova Southeastern University's (NSU) Psychology Services Center (*www.nova.edu/gsc/online_files.html*); and the measures companion website for *Treating Addiction: A Guide for Professionals* (Miller, Forcehimes, & Zweben, 2011) (*www.guilford.com/cgi-bin/cartscript.cgi?page=etc/miller11.html&dir=pp/ addictions&cart_id=897890.1358*).

behavioral processes of change that interact with the stages. From there, we will identify and discuss a variety of measures that have particular relevance to the assessment of individuals in different stages of change. The ultimate goal of this chapter is to increase understanding of how such assessments can be used to improve treatment planning for individuals in different stages of change, which is discussed in Chapter 4.

MEASURING THE STAGES OF CHANGE

As we noted in Chapter 1, the stages of change were developed to reflect attitudes, intentions, and behaviors associated with the process of changing a given behavior. According to this model, the change process is best represented by a series of discrete tasks, periods, or stages that a person completes and passes through on a successful journey to sustained change. Key features of stage models are the assumptions that discrete segments of a process can be defined and that each segment has an important role to play in the change process that can be identified and isolated.

Several instruments to measure stage of change (summarized by Carey, Purnine, Maisto, & Carey, 1999; DiClemente, Schlundt, & Gemmell, 2004; and Donovan, in press) have been developed. All involve respondents reporting on their perceptions, attitudes, and intentions toward change and often on their behaviors in the recent past relevant to changing the problem behavior. Current cognitions and behaviors as well as intentions regarding engaging in the behavior in the near future seem to be critical elements of these measures.

One of the original ways to evaluate and assign a person to a stage of change is to classify clients based on how they answer five simple questions. This measure is called the "staging algorithm" and is presented first since it was used in the seminal smoking cessation studies used to create and validate the stages. Thereafter we will discuss measures that are used when simple yes–no responses may be misleading, including the University of Rhode Island Change Assessment Scale, the Stages of Change Readiness and Treatment Eagerness Scale, and the Readiness to Change Questionnaire. These three measures provide a quantitative summary score for each stage of change assessed, based on the individual's responses to questionnaire items reflecting attitudes, behaviors, and intentions related to each stage of change. The resulting scores enable one to define a person as being in one "dominant" stage of change or to construct a readiness-to-change "profile" based on the individual's score for each of the stages. Finally, we review some alternate ways that have been used to assess stages including self-staging, and several brief "ladder" and goal-rating scales for gauging one's degree of readiness to change and using interview data. While some of these measures are not as useful for identifying an individual's particular stage of change, these measures do provide a snapshot of one's current readiness to change that often reflects stage status or tasks.

Staging Algorithm

In the staging algorithm procedure, respondents are asked to answer five simple questions with dichotomous yes–no responses. The combination of their responses is scored according to predetermined rules (Prochaska & DiClemente, 1992) that allow one to classify subjects as in precontemplation, contemplation, preparation, action, or maintenance. The questions concern (1) whether the subject still engages in the problem behavior (in this case, smoking); (2) whether he or she is considering quitting in the next 6 months; (3) whether he or she is planning to quit in the next 30 days; (4) whether he or she has stopped smoking for at least 24 hours in the past year, and, if he or she has quit; (5) for how long. Subjects can be classified in one and only one stage of change. The first discrimination is between those currently engaging in the behavior (smokers) and those who have quit, allowing the distinction between preaction stages (precontemplation, contemplation, and preparation) and action stages (action and maintenance). The distinction between action and maintenance is based on whether the individual has continued the change for more than 6 months (maintenance). Preaction stages are distinguished as follows. Individuals in precontemplation are those who are *not* considering change in the next 6 months. Individuals in contemplation are considering but not planning change in the next 30 days. Individuals in preparation are considering and planning change in the next 30 days. For added specificity, especially in some smoking studies, the preparation stage also included only those planning to quit and who have made a quit attempt in the past year, since this is often seen as a behavioral indicator of commitment to change. The staging algorithm has been used in studies that have provided strong evidence for the ability of stage of change to predict treatment outcomes, which is essential to the argument that stage of change has clinical utility (Belding, Iguchi, & Lamb, 1997).

However, it is best used with problems where the individual feels comfortable disclosing his or her intentions and goals.

University of Rhode Island Change Assessment Scale

In clinical and other settings where socially desirable responding is likely, clients often respond to algorithm questions in ways that they believe they should, distorting where they are in the process of change. With this in mind, McConnaughy, DiClemente, Prochaska, and Velicer (McConnaughy, Prochaska, & Velicer, 1983; McConnaughy, DiClemente, Prochaska, & Velicer, 1989) developed the University of Rhode Island Change Assessment Scale (URICA) as a method of classifying subjects in stages of change when a straightforward algorithm does not work. The scale consists of 32 items that have been shown to reflect four factors related to the stages of precontemplation, contemplation, action, and maintenance. The items describe attitudes, intentions, and behaviors associated with the stage-specific tasks related to changing a target behavior. Furthermore, in the original version URICA items are written generically, so they can apply to change for a range of behaviors or goals (cutting down on drinking or abstinence). The stem or introduction to the items determines which specific behavior is the target of the assessment. In the original psychometric studies that evaluated multiple target behaviors, separate sets of eight items load on or are associated with each stage of change. Table 3.1 shows samples of items that are associated with each of the four stages of change included in the URICA. Later studies focusing on alcohol problems used a 28-item version with seven items representing each stage (DiClemente & Hughes, 1990; DiClemente, Doyle, & Donovan, 2009). Briefer, 12-item versions of the URICA have also been used (Soderstrom et al., 2006).

In the area of substance abuse, the URICA has been used by specifying specific drugs (e.g., cocaine, marijuana, heroin, alcohol) or the more generic "illegal drugs" as the target. Some have instead substituted the specific problem substance in the actual items. It is preferable to assess specific substances whenever possible because when a client is using multiple substances he or she may not be ready to change one substance and not another; therefore, using the generic term may not capture the true stage for each substance.

Each of the items is responded to according to degree of agreement: strongly disagree (score of 1), disagree (2), undecided (3), agree (4), and

TABLE 3.1. Two University of Rhode Island Change Assessment Scale (URICA) Items for Each of Four Stages of Change

Stage of change	Items
Precontemplation	• As far as I'm concerned, I don't have any problems that need changing. • I guess I have faults, but there's nothing I really need to change.
Contemplation	• I think I might be ready for some self-improvement. • I wish I had more ideas on how to solve my problem.
Action	• I am finally doing some work on my problem. • Anyone can talk about changing; I'm actually doing something about it.
Maintenance	• I'm not following through with what I had already changed as well as I had hoped, and I'm here to prevent a relapse of the problem. • I thought once I had resolved the problem I would be free of it, but sometimes I find myself struggling with it.

Note. When used in the assessment of substance use, the instructional set would indicate that the client should respond to the items in the context of their general drug use or in the context of a specific substance (e.g., cocaine, alcohol, heroin). Alternatively, the scale items themselves can be modified to reflect a particular substance (e.g., the action item "I am finally doing some work on my problem" could be revised to "I am finally doing some work on my cocaine problem").

strongly agree (5). The items are scored in the "positive" direction for each stage, so that the higher the score a person receives for a stage, the "more" he or she endorses attitudes and behaviors particular to that stage. With eight items for each stage, the highest score a person can receive for a stage is 40 and the lowest is eight .

This brief introduction to the URICA shows that a person actually can be assigned a score for each of the stages of change. Such a method of scoring contrasts with the categorical approach to measurement of stage of change that involves assignment of a person to a discrete category of change. By receiving a score for each stage, individuals can be "clustered," or grouped, according to the pattern of scores on the four stage subscales (as described in Chapter 2). The clusters may be labeled either according to a "dominant" (according to score) stage of change or according to the researcher's or clinician's interpretation of what the pattern of subscale scores says about the person's attitudes toward or perceptions of changing the problem behavior (DiClemente & Hughes, 1990). Research that has been completed with this clustering approach has revealed excellent consistency in subscale score patterns among, for example, inpatients and outpatients with alcohol dependence and individuals receiving treatment at a weight loss clinic (Prochaska & DiClemente, 1992). Research on a sample of individuals presenting for outpatient alcohol treatment (Carbonari, DiClemente, Addy, & Pollack, 1996) has yielded alternative short forms of the URICA (two 12-item versions and a 24-item version). In addition, clinical researchers have been evaluating the use of a continuous "readiness to change" score that is calculated by summing the subscale scores for the contemplation, action, and maintenance stages and subtracting the precontemplation subscale score and reflects the stage profiles found in previous research. This readiness score has been found to predict abstinence from drinking outcomes among outpatients receiving alcoholism treatment (DiClemente, Carbonari, Zweben, Morrel, & Lee, 2001; Project MATCH Research Group, 1997a).

In summary, the URICA in its various versions has become the most common way of measuring stages of change in clinical settings where more direct assessment may be misleading. It also has been evaluated in dual diagnosis samples (Nidecker, DiClemente, Bennett, & Bellack, 2008; Pantalon, Nich, Franckforter, & Carroll, 2002) and with adolescents (Greenstein, Franklin, & McGuffin, 1999). The scale allows for identification of individuals by the pattern of their subscale scores. These patterns or profiles have been named either according to a dominant stage of change score or by interpretation of a combination of scores. The profile approach so far has revealed excellent consistency in stage-of-change score patterns across diverse populations. With this as a basis, clusters may then be correlated with other variables that are of conceptual or clinical importance. A single readiness score has been found to be related to stage profiles at baseline but may be difficult to use over time (DiClemente, Schlundt, & Gemmell, 2004).

Stages of Change Readiness and Treatment Eagerness Scale

The Stages of Change Readiness and Treatment Eagerness Scale (SOCRATES) was developed by Miller and his colleagues (Miller & Tonigan, 1996) and is analogous to the URICA in concept, even using some of the same items. The SOCRATES consists of 40 items constructed and scored in a way similar to the URICA. Respondents indicate their degree of agreement with an item and accordingly can receive a score from 1 to 5. The scores for eight items then are summed to give a scale score for each of five stages of change, namely, precontemplation, contemplation, determination/preparation, action, and maintenance. In this sense the SOCRATES yields a profile of stage scores and, like the URICA, can be used to identify a person's "dominant" stage. Table 3.2 presents sample items that constitute each of the five SOCRATES-identified stages of change.

Miller and Tonigan (1996) reported the development of a 19-item short form of SOCRATES that has good psychometric properties and research and clinical utility. The 19 items that constitute the brief SOCRATES were selected from among the 40 items making up the longer form. Analyses of responses to the brief SOCRATES items by a sample of individuals presenting for alcohol treatment showed that the briefer measure taps into three dimensions, called Taking Steps (to change drinking behavior), Recognition (that the respondent has an alcohol problem), and Ambivalence (about whether the respondent has an alcohol problem). Miller and Tonigan (1996) have recommended use of the brief SOCRATES over the longer version of the instrument. A drug use version of the SOCRATES is also available.

TABLE 3.2. Two Stages of Change Readiness and Treatment Eagerness Scale (SOCRATES) Items for Each of Five Stages of Change

Stage of change	Items
Precontemplation	• The only reason I'm here is that somebody made me come. • I am a fairly normal drinker.
Contemplation	• Sometimes I wonder if my drinking is hurting other people. • I don't think I have "a problem" with drinking, but there are times when I wonder if I drink too much.
Preparation	• I am a problem drinker. • I drink too much at times.
Action	• I have already been trying to change my drinking, and I am here to get some more help with it. • I have started to carry out a plan to cut down or stop my drinking.
Maintenance	• I am worried that my previous problems with drinking might come back. • Now that I have changed my drinking, it is important for me to hold onto the change I've made.

Note. Items may be adjusted to measure stage of change for drug use other than alcohol by substituting the drug(s) in question for references to drinking and alcohol.

Readiness to Change Questionnaire

There are actually two versions of the Readiness to Change Question-naire (RCQ). The original measure (the RCQ), developed by Rollnick, Heather, Gold, and Hall (1992), was created for use with individuals with risky drinking who presented in a setting for the treatment of medical problems. This scale used only some items from the URICA that evaluated the three stages of precontemplation, contemplation, and action. However, its applicability to individuals in addictions treat-ment settings appeared to be limited (Gavin, Sobell, & Sobell, 1998). In response, the second version of the RCQ was specifically developed for use with patients participating in a specialized treatment for alcohol use disorders. The RCQ-Treatment Version, or RCQ(TV), was developed by Heather, Luce, Peck, Dunbar, and James (1999) and later revised by Heather and Hönekopp (2008).

Both versions of the RCQ were based on Prochaska and DiCle-mente's ideas about stages of change and the URICA questionnaire. However, the RCQ and the RCQ(TV), each comprised of 12 items, are briefer than the URICA or SOCRATES. Like the SOCRATES, the RCQ and RCQ(TV) focus on readiness to change drinking behavior.

The RCQ is composed of 12 items, clustered into three stages (each with four items) called precontemplation, contemplation, and action. Table 3.3 (upper panel) shows sample items from the scale. Responses to each of the RCQ items can range from strongly disagree (score of −2), through 0, to strongly agree (score of +2). Therefore, for each stage of change a person's score can range from −8 to +8. As does the URICA, this scale places respondents on a continuum within each stage of change. Initial studies of the RCQ (Rollnick et al., 1992) show that it has good psychometric properties as well as the ability to predict treat-ment outcomes (Heather, Rollnick, & Bell, 1993).

The RCQ(TV), recommended by Heather et al. (1999) for use in addictions treatment populations, contains 12 items, with four items pertaining to each of three change stages: precontemplation, contempla-tion, and action. Table 3.3 (lower panel) provides a pair of sample items from each of these stages.

Responses to the RCQ(TV) items are provided on a 5-point scale ranging from 1 = strongly disagree to 5 = strongly agree. The actual scoring of the responses to each item was from −2 (strongly disagree) to +2 (strongly agree), similar to the RCQ, and the total for each scale could range from −8 to +8. The measure has been shown to have good

TABLE 3.3. Sample Items from the Readiness for Change Questionnaires Representing Each of Three Stages of Change

Stage of change items	
	Readiness for Change Questionnaire
Precontemplation	• It's a waste of time thinking about my drinking.
Contemplation	• I am at the stage where I should think about drinking less alcohol.
Action	• I am trying to drink less than I used to.
	Readiness for Change Questionnaire—Treatment Version
Precontemplation	• I am a fairly normal drinker. • There is nothing I really need to change about my drinking.
Contemplation	• Sometimes I think I should quit or cut down on my drinking. • I enjoy my drinking but sometimes I drink too much.
Action	• Anyone can talk about wanting to do something about their drinking, but I am actually doing something about it. • I have started to carry out a plan to cut down or quit drinking.

Note. Items may be adjusted to measure stage of change for drug use other than alcohol by substituting the drug(s) in question for references to drinking and alcohol.

psychometric properties (Heather et al., 1999; Heather & Hönekopp, 2008).

In a more recent development involving the RCQ, Epler, Kivlahan, Bush, Dobie, and Bradley (2005) presented a drinking algorithm to assess readiness to change drinking. Calling their measure the Reasons to Change Algorithm (RTC Algorithm), Epler et al. used just three of the RCQ questions: Has the amount you drink changed in the past 3 months?, Are you interested in drinking less?, and Do you think you drink more than you should? Based on responses provided, Epler et al. were able to classify respondents to either the precontemplation, contemplation, or action stages (as would have been determined through use of the full RCQ). As with the RCQ, the RTC Algorithm was recommended for use in primary care or medical settings.

Overall, progress has been excellent in validating the premise that people can be identified with a stage of change. Continued research will likely confirm the idea that, rather than a strict stage model of change, a combination of stage and continuum of readiness-for-change models will best describe individuals' preparedness for change (see, e.g., DiClemente, 2005b; Miller & Tonigan, 1996). Stages are not best conceptualized as containers or labels but as being associated with important tasks that when completed sufficiently will lead to sustained change (DiClemente, Holmgren, & Rounsaville, 2010). Despite the important and interesting questions about how to conceptualize a person's "location" in the change process, for ease of discussion and organization we will keep the discrete stage-of-change idea intact except where this simplifying approach misrepresents an idea or some information.

Readiness "Ladders"/Rating Scales

The measures presented above are the most commonly used for purposes of assessing an individual's status within the stages of change, particularly in research studies. However, it is not possible in all settings to administer one of these measures. In such situations, or when multiple assessments are scheduled over time (e.g., before or after each treatment session), readiness "ladders" or "ruler" rating scales have been designed to rapidly assess an individual's readiness to change. While these ladders or rulers often do not uniquely categorize individuals into one of the discrete stages of change, they do provide a useful metric of the person's readiness to change and an approximation of the stage of change (Biener & Abrams, 1991; Hogue, Dauber, & Morgenstern, 2010). Some have labels at different points in the continuum identifying stage tasks, others simply ask on a scale from 1 to 10 how ready are you to stop drinking or to cut down on your drinking or drug use.

Generally following the lead of Biener and Abrams (1991), who developed a "contemplation ladder" to assess readiness to consider smoking cessation, these ladders typically entail individuals indicating where they fall on a continuous scale in terms of their readiness to change a given behavior, such as drinking or drug use. The contemplation ladder developed by Biener and Abrams (1991), for example, was an 11-point Likert-type scale with a rating range from 0 = "no thoughts of quitting" to 10 = "taking action to quit," with other points labeled "thinking about quitting" and "planning to quit."

Other types of continuous measures involve a forced-choice response to a series of options that represent different stages of change. Pregnant women, for example, were asked to pick a response from a series of options or statements that represented different options for staying quit postpartum, which were used to determine their postpartum smoking stage of change (Stotts, DiClemente, Carbonari, & Mullen, 2000). A descriptive type of ladder developed specifically for assessment of readiness to stop using alcohol and drugs (separately assessed) was developed by Hogue et al. (2010). Response choices on their ladders ranged from 1 to 7, using for alcohol [drugs] the following descriptors: 1 = I do not have a problem with drinking [drugs], and I do not intend to cut down; 2 = I might have a problem with drinking [drugs], but I do not intend to cut down or quit now; 3 = I am thinking about cutting down on my drinking [drug use], but I am not thinking about quitting drinking [drug use] altogether; 4 = I am thinking about quitting drinking [using drugs] altogether, but I still have not made any definite plans; 5 = I am close to making a decision to quit drinking alcohol [using drugs]; 6 = I have decided to quit drinking alcohol [using drugs], at least for now; and 7 = I have decided to quit drinking alcohol [using drugs] and plan never to drink [use drugs] again.

Another representative brief assessment of readiness to change, in this case a ruler as opposed to a ladder, was presented by Velasquez et al. (2001). It is shown in Figure 3.1. Depending on the context, the question posed could be changed to address readiness to change one's drug use.

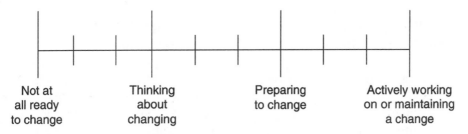

FIGURE 3.1. A sample readiness ruler. From Velasquez, Maurer, Crouch, and DiClemente (2001, p. 30). Copyright 2001 by The Guilford Press. Reprinted by permission.

ASSESSING PROCESSES OF CHANGE

As described in Chapters 1 and 2, the processes of change (both experiential and behavioral) are the mechanisms or coping activities that individuals engage in to complete stage tasks and transition from one stage to another in their efforts to modify problem behaviors. Accordingly, it will be important at every given point in the change process to attend not only to the particular stage task of a client but also to the extent to which clients are engaged in these processes. A convenient, reliable, and valid tool for the assessment of these processes is the Processes of Change Questionnaire (Prochaska et al., 1988), originally developed to assess and track processes related to smoking cessation. There have been a number of variations on this original measure for a variety of health and addictive behaviors.

Recommended for use in the present context are the alcohol and illegal drug versions of the Processes of Change Questionnaire; for each, there is a 40-item version and a briefer 20-item version with either two or four items for each of the 10 processes. Clients indicate, on a 5-point scale from 1 = never to 5 = repeatedly, the frequency of their use of a variety of thoughts, behaviors, and experiences that help them complete the tasks of the preaction stages as well as avoid the problem behavior (drinking or using illegal drugs) during the action and maintenance stages. Completion of the measure typically takes between 5 and 10 minutes. Table 3.4 shows a sampling of items from each of the five experiential and five behavioral processes of change. Usually experiential processes are more important in the early stages and behavioral in the later stages for modifying alcohol and substance abuse.

ASSESSMENTS WITH PARTICULAR RELEVANCE TO CLIENTS IN THE PRECONTEMPLATION, CONTEMPLATION, AND PREPARATION STAGES

Among the measures most relevant to the assessment of persons in the precontemplation, contemplation, and preparation stages are those used for substance abuse screening and for the identification and specification of quantity, frequency, and consequences of use as well as related problems (including measures designed for purposes of assessing actual alcohol and drug use and for making diagnostic determinations). Such basic assessments have as a goal the defining of the nature and extent of the pattern of substance use in a way that is descriptive, shows its

TABLE 3.4. Representative Processes of Change Questionnaire Items for the Five Experiential and Five Behavioral Processes of Change

Process of change	Items
	Experiential processes
Consciousness raising	• I read newspaper stories that may help me quit drinking. • I think about information that people have personally given me on the benefits of quitting drinking.
Emotional arousal/ dramatic relief	• I get upset when I think about illnesses caused by drinking. • Stories abut alcohol and its effects upset me.
Environmental reevaluation	• I stop to think about how my drinking is hurting people around me. • I am considering the idea that people around me would be better off without my problem drinking.
Self-reevaluation	• I consider that feeling good about myself includes changing my drinking behavior. • I become disappointed with myself when I depend on alcohol.
Social liberation	• I notice that people with alcohol problems are making known their desire not to be pressed to drink. • I see advertisements on television about how society is trying to help people not drink.
	Behavioral processes
Contingency management	• I do something nice for myself for making efforts to change. • I don't let myself have fun when I drink.
Counterconditioning	• I try to think about other things when I begin to think about drinking. • I do something else instead of drinking when I need to deal with tension.
Helping relationships	• I can talk with at least one special person about my drinking experiences. • I have someone whom I can count on to help me when I'm having problems with drinking.
Self-liberation	• I make myself aware that I can choose to overcome my drinking if I want to. • I make commitments to myself not to drink.
Stimulus control	• I remove things from my home or work that remind me of drinking. • I stay away from places generally associated with drinking.

Note. When used in the assessment of illegal drug use, the instructional set and items would reference drug use. The measures themselves, along with scoring information, are available through the website of the HABITS lab at the University of Maryland, Baltimore County.

full functional properties, and leads to diagnostic conclusions. The data from these assessments taken together can be used for two important intervention functions in addition to simply deriving a diagnosis. The first is to develop objective feedback for clients on their substance use and its consequences. This feedback is of clinical value generally. However, the motivational impact of these data when presented in an objective, motivationally enhancing manner is most important to clients in the precontemplation and contemplation stages of change, because in these stages individuals either underestimate or do not acknowledge a problem and are not firmly committed to changing it. The second important function of these types of assessments is to develop an understanding or hypotheses about what factors are maintaining the person's pattern of alcohol and drug use, which has direct relevance to treatment planning.

With the above as preface, we review in the following sections the major biological and self-report measures for identifying individuals who have alcohol or other drug problems. We concentrate on breath test, urinalysis, and blood test procedures for biological methods, and on the interview and questionnaire for self-report methods.

Biological Methods

Breath Testing

The most common assessment for the presence of alcohol in the system is the breath test. The breath test is popular because it is noninvasive, accurate when correctly used, portable, inexpensive, and quick and easy to administer. Because of all of these advantages, there have been concerted efforts to produce similarly convenient ways to measure the presence of other drugs using breath tests. Unfortunately, except for a carbon monoxide measure for tobacco smoking, a satisfactory method has yet to be developed for most drugs of abuse. Most breath tests provide a timeframe for detection that is limited to more recent use (past 4 to 12 hours) and depends on the amount of use.

The major rationale for the use of breath testing as a screening method is that it can serve as an indicator of possible alcohol problems that, if positive, would be followed up with additional assessment. For example, if an individual presented for an interview in some setting, or for some purpose other than substance abuse treatment, such as an appointment for medical care or for psychiatric care, the presence of alcohol in the person's system could be considered a sign of heavy drinking patterns and associated problems. A positive blood alcohol concentration indicated by the breathalyzer then would be evaluated further by other assessment techniques described below.

Breath testing also can serve as an important clinical tool in treating individuals for their already identified problems with substances. For example, routine breath testing of individuals before beginning each of their treatment sessions may encourage their sobriety and can be used as a point of intervention or a marker for offering incentives if the individual screens negative.

Urinalysis

Urinalysis probably is the most popular method of testing for the presence of drugs other than alcohol in the blood, although alcohol also can be detected by urinalysis. Urinalysis can, with cost differences, provide a qualitative (drug present or absent) or quantitative (how much drug, if it is present) measure of drug concentration. Urinalysis gives a measure of use over the past 2 to 3 days for most drugs of abuse, and over a week or longer in cases of heavy cannabis or phencyclidine use (Anton, Litton, & Allen, 1995; DuPont & Selavka, 2008).

Despite advancements in the use of urinalysis procedures over the past several decades (DuPont & Selavka, 2008; Maisto, McKay, & Connors, 1990), there remain several major considerations in the use of urinalysis. This is particularly true because of the now widespread use of urinalysis in different settings. The first point to consider is the interpretation of any single test outcome. One true, positive outcome, for example, is not evidence for current drug intoxication or impairment, or of frequency and duration of drug use. In this regard, individual user differences in the potency of drug used, in the administration of the drug, and in the rates of drug absorption, distribution, and metabolism, as well as actual use, may affect a true positive finding. As a result, drawing conclusions from just one test is not good practice.

Another concern is the problem of false positive and false negative findings. A false positive result can occur by "confusing" the analytical method. For example, an individual may use a legal substance (poppy seeds) that imitates some drug of abuse (narcotics), which would result in a positive finding for the drug of abuse. A false negative finding usually is the more common concern of people doing the testing. Such findings often occur through the user's deliberate efforts to invalidate a test, such as by using a nonuser's urine sample or by adulterating the urine sample to interfere with its analysis. A false negative finding also may result from the tester's failure to appreciate the span of time of previous drug use that urinalysis can detect. For example, a person may have used cocaine daily and heavily for up to 6 days before urinalysis. And, in response to the question "How much cocaine have you used in the past week?," the user may reply, "None." The urine test would corroborate the "none" response.

In summary, urinalysis can be an accurate tool for identifying and following up with individuals with alcohol or drug problems. However, its value depends on following well-specified procedures in its use. Although laboratory analysis is most accurate, there are a number of dipstick products marketed that can indicate positive findings for a variety of drugs of abuse. If there are any questions, positives obtained in this manner can be verified with urinalysis.

Blood Tests

The methods we have described so far all are ways to detect the presence of alcohol or other drugs in the blood and thus are measures of recent use. Of course, blood samples can be analyzed directly for this same purpose. However, blood samples also can be analyzed for evidence of longer term (recent weeks to years) heavy alcohol use. This can be done, first, by testing for elevation of liver enzymes, which is correlated with heavy alcohol consumption in the past month. The tests in this category that are used commonly include aspartate aminotransferase (AST), alanine aminotransferase (ALT), gamma-glutamyltransferase (GGT), and carbohydrate deficient transferrin (CDT) (e.g., Allen, Sillanaukee, Strid, & Litten, 2003; Anton et al., 1995).

All four of these tests may be significantly elevated (compared to the normal range values) with past heavy drinking. GGT and CDT appear to be the more sensitive tests for assessing changes (whether increases or decreases) in alcohol consumption (Anton et al., 1995). Although these blood tests have received the most attention as screening and identification methods, particularly in medical settings, they also often are used in the treatment and evaluation of individuals already identified as having alcohol problems.

A test for GGT, AST, ALT, or CDT should not be used alone as a screening method, for several reasons (Leigh & Skinner, 1988). First, the test may be affected by using drugs other than alcohol, so there is not excellent specificity (for alcohol) of these biochemical tests. This is a problem not only for what are typically called the drugs of "abuse"; for example, MCV may be elevated by cigarette smoking. Another problem is that when the person tested is in good physical health, the test is far less likely to be elevated even if recent heavy drinking did occur. Relatedly, the tests have good specificity in general population studies but do less well in discriminating between persons with alcohol dependence and medically ill patients without an alcohol use disorder (Anton et al., 1995). This is because test values may be elevated by disease processes that have little to do with high alcohol use. Third, the degree of elevation of the tests and quantity of alcohol consumed does not follow a simple linear pattern. So, for example, as quantity of alcohol increases, enzyme elevation does not increase proportionately throughout the range of values that are possible. Therefore, the relationship between alcohol consumption and blood test score is complex. Relatedly, there are large differences among individuals in the relationship between alcohol use and lab test scores. Finally, lab test scores alone may discriminate most productively between individuals who are light, nonproblem drinkers and those who already have suffered serious consequences from heavy alcohol use. However, it has been much more difficult to reliably identify individuals with mild to moderate impairment due to alcohol. A good screening method should be able to identify cases with less severe alcohol problems.

These problems should not be taken to imply that biochemical measures of recent heavy drinking should be discarded altogether. Rather, the weaknesses of the tests point up the necessity of using them in conjunction with other measures (Anton, Lieber, Tabakoff, & CDTect Study Group, 2002; Babor & Higgins-Biddle, 2000). In this regard, relevant recommendations have included using combinations of laboratory tests (Allen et al., 2003; Leigh & Skinner, 1988) and using laboratory tests with such measures as screening questionnaires and a client's clinical record (Allen et al., 2003; Anton et al., 1995; Niles & McCrady, 1991; Leigh & Skinner, 1988).

Self-Report Screening Methods

Screening methods that involve responding to questions from an interviewer or to items on a questionnaire about the use of alcohol and associated consequences are well established and researched for the detection of alcohol problems. However, there are far fewer measures available for the identification of individuals with other drug problems. Although several instruments have the stated purpose of identifying drug abuse in adults, many (exceptions include the Drug Abuse Screening Test, the ASSIST, and the AUDIT, reviewed below) are viewed as being too long to be of practical value as brief screeners in most clinical settings. In this section we review the most important and widely used self-report alcohol and drug use disorder screening measures.

Michigan Alcoholism Screening Test

The Michigan Alcoholism Screening Test (MAST) was developed by Selzer (1971) in order to provide a quick, systematic, quantifiable way to "diagnose" alcoholism that could be administered by professionals and paraprofessionals alike. In fact, the MAST more accurately is seen today as a method that helps to identify—not to diagnose—individuals with alcohol problems.

The original MAST consists of 25 items relating to primarily negative consequences (whether physical, psychological, family, or legal) of alcohol use. Each item is answered by checking "Yes" or "No." Items are weighted, which means that responses to some items suggesting the presence of an alcohol use disorder receive more points (in a range of 1 to 5) than do other responses. A total score of 0 to 53 is possible, with a score of 5 or higher suggestive of alcohol dependence. The MAST can be self-administered, taking about 5 to 10 minutes, or it can be administered by an interviewer, which takes about 15 to 20 minutes (Jacobson, 1989). Examples of MAST items are "Do you feel you are a normal drinker?," "Have you ever lost a job because of drinking?," and "Have you ever gotten into trouble at work because of your drinking?"

It is obvious from the foregoing sample items that the MAST "pulls" for problems with alcohol. Depending on whether the testing situation encourages or discourages accurate reporting of consequences related to alcohol use, this has led to an over- or underidentification of alcoholism. Jacobson's (1989) summary of the large volume of research on the MAST suggests, however, that maintaining a cutoff score of 5 overidentifies. He advises adjusting the cutoff score to as high as 12, depending on preference for a test more sensitive in identifying alcohol dependence or a test that is better at specifying a person who does not have problems with alcohol.

One feature of the MAST that contributes to overidentification of current alcohol problems is exemplified by the sample MAST items listed above. There is a lack of a consistent time referent for the items: Some items refer to current status ("Do you feel you are a normal drinker?"), while others refer to a lifetime ("Have you ever gotten into trouble at work because of your drinking?"). Therefore, if the interest is in identifying people with current alcohol problems only, this lack of a consistent time referent would tend to result in a higher number of false positives. One way around this problem, if the MAST is administered by an interviewer, is to ask the respondent "when?" if he or she answers positively to a "lifetime referent" test item (see Jacobson, 1989).

The great popularity of the MAST led to two briefer versions, the 13-item Short Michigan Alcoholism Screening Test (SMAST) and the 10-item Brief Michigan Alcoholism Screening Test (BMAST) (Selzer, Vinokur, & van Rooijen, 1975, and Pokorny, Miller, & Kaplan, 1972, respectively). The Self-Administered Michigan Alcoholism Screening Test (Swenson & Morse, 1975) is another MAST derivative. Jacobson (1989) argues that these MAST modifications have "reasonable" reliability and validity, but Gibbs's (1983) review suggests that the MAST is more reliable. These comments notwithstanding, the high face validity (or obviousness) of the MAST and its derivatives suggests that the degree of validity may closely reflect the degree of response bias potential in the context of test administration.

Drug Abuse Screening Test and the Alcohol, Smoking and Substance Involvement Screening Test

As the acronym suggests, the Drug Abuse Screening Test (DAST) is the MAST counterpart for problems with drugs other than alcohol. This test was developed by Skinner (1982), and the original version consisted of 28 items that are answered "Yes" or "No." The current version of the DAST includes the 20 items that discriminated criterion groups most productively in validation studies. Analogous to the MAST, the DAST primarily focuses on the consequences of drug use and can be self-administered or administered by an interviewer. The DAST is also analogous to the MAST in the inconsistent time references of the DAST's 20 items. Some examples include "Have you used drugs other than those required for medical reasons?," "Do you abuse more than one drug at a time?," and "Does your spouse (or parents) ever complain about your involvement with drugs?" A briefer, 10-item version of the DAST also is available (Skinner, 1982).

The DAST items are not assigned any weights, so that a person's score for the test is the simple sum of the number of items answered in the direction of increased drug problems. Therefore, scores can range from 0 to 20. Unlike the MAST, no formally developed cutoff scores (for identifying persons with drug problems) are available. However, the initial validation study of the DAST that Skinner (1982) completed suggests that scores of 6 or higher are indicative of drug problems. Furthermore, as DAST scores increase, the implication is that the individual's drug problems are more severe (see Babor, 1993).

The Alcohol, Smoking and Substance Involvement Screening Test (ASSIST) (World Health Organization ASSIST Working Group, 2002; World Health Organization, 2010) was developed to identify substance use and associated problems in primary health care settings. It is composed of eight items that can be administered by a health worker in around 5–10 minutes. The measure is designed to screen for use and consequences associated with use of tobacco products, alcohol, cannabis, amphetamine-type stimulants, sedatives and sleeping pills (benzodiazepines), hallucinogens, inhalants, opioids, and "other drugs." The score derived for each substance falls into a low-, moderate-, or high-risk category. The ASSIST captures information on lifetime use of each substance as well as use and associated problems over the last 3 months. The measure has strong psychometric characteristics (Humeniuk et al., 2008). One important consideration with all current drug abuse screens is that they often focus on illegal drugs of abuse instead of misuse or illegal use of prescription medications, which represents a very significant current problem. More recently, the National Institute on Drug Abuse has proposed use of a modified version of the ASSIST as part of its recommended protocol for screening for drug use in general medical settings.[2]

CAGE and Some Very Brief Screening Measures

The CAGE (Mayfield, McLeod, & Hall, 1974) is the briefest of the self-report screening methods that we have presented so far. The test name is an acronym of letters of words in the only four items that make up the test: (1) "Have you ever felt you should Cut down on your drinking?," (2) "Have people Annoyed you by criticizing your drinking?," (3) "Have you ever felt Guilty about your drinking?," and (4) "Have you ever had a drink first thing in the morning (Eye opener)?" These four questions

---

[2]Available at *www.drugabuse.gov/publications/resource-guide/step-1-nida-modified-assist.*

are asked by an interviewer, taking only a few minutes at most. A cutoff score of two to three items answered "Yes" seems to work most productively for sensitive and accurate identification (Jacobson, 1989).

There are a couple of points that are important to note in using the CAGE. The first is that the high face validity and the paucity of items suggest that if a positive identification is made it should be corroborated, if at all possible, by another data source, such as the respondent's spouse, biochemical measures, history, or other more extensive screen. In this regard, such a practice has become common in using the MAST and derivatives because of their obvious intent to detect misuse among populations that are not eager to admit problematic use. The second point is that the CAGE questions have no time referent, so that, for example, an item could be answered positively because of events of 20 years ago but not currently. This suggests that, in some cases, the CAGE would yield too many positives in relation to *current* alcohol problems. As we noted in our discussion of the MAST, Jacobson (1989) suggests one way to solve this problem is to ask "when" or for more information for any question that is answered yes.

A method that Cyr and Wartman (1988) reported beats the brevity of the CAGE by two items in identifying alcohol problems. This study involved case identification of men and women who were admitted to a primary care unit of a large teaching hospital in southern New England. While the clients were waiting for their first appointment with their new physicians, they were interviewed for about 45 minutes regarding medical history, family history (for alcohol problems), health habits, and alcohol use. Essentially, the idea was to cover screening for alcoholism, risk factors for alcoholism, and standard alcohol history. After the interview was completed, a research assistant administered the MAST.

Cyr and Wartman used all the information they collected to see what interview information they collected predicted a "diagnosis" of alcoholism, as determined by MAST score (cutoff score of 5). It was found that two interview questions, "Have you ever had a drinking problem?" and "When was your last drink?" (a response of within the last 24 hours should be considered a positive indicator), together were excellent predictors of a positive identification on the MAST. A total of 91.5% of the MAST-identified persons with alcohol dependence answered one or both of these questions positively, while 89.7% of the MAST-identified persons without alcohol dependence answered negatively to one or both questions. This test performance outdistanced by far the predictive value of other interview questions, such as "How much do you drink?" and "How often do you drink?"

Other brief screening strategies also have been developed. Williams and Vinson (2001), for example, described use of a single question. Brown, Leonard, Saunders, and Papasouliotis (2001), in an effort to assess both alcohol and other substance abuse, developed the Two-Item Conjoint Screen (called the TICS). Another single-item screening test, developed to assess drug use in primary care settings, has also been proposed (Smith, Schmidt, Allensworth-Davies, & Saitz, 2010). The items associated with these brief screening strategies are shown in Table 3.5 (along with the three items of the AUDIT-C, which will be described momentarily).

Taken together, the emergence of these very brief screening methods has attracted a lot of attention because of the idea that it is possible to identify alcohol problems in a primary medical care setting with such a quick, efficient method. Of course, there are caveats before getting swept away by the results to date. First, quick screens are meant to cast a broad net in identifying potential problems and are not designed to provide diagnoses or identify only people who need additional treatment. Also, whether the results can be replicated with other samples and settings is still open to research. Yet the implications of these studies should be most appealing to case finders and supported the impetus to create Screening, Brief Intervention, and Referral tor Treatment (SBIRT) protocols in many healthcare settings to facilitate early identification and capitalize on teachable moments to influence drug and alcohol use (Babor et al., 2007; Madras et al., 2009).

Alcohol Use Disorders Identification Test

The Alcohol Use Disorders Identification Test (AUDIT) is a 10-item screening measure that was designed specifically for use in the medical treatment setting. In particular, the AUDIT was developed for use in primary care clinics, although research shows that it is suited for use in other settings as well, such as psychiatric clinics, the legal system, and the military (Allen & Columbus, 1995; Saunders, Aasland, Babor, de la Fuente, & Grant, 1993).

The response to each of the 10 items of the AUDIT is given a score, and the total score is derived simply by adding the individual's score for

TABLE 3.5. Brief Screening Approaches

Cyr and Wartman (1988):
- Have you ever had a drinking problem?
- When was your last drink?

Williams and Vinson (2001):
- When was the last time you had more than "x" drinks in 1 day? (where "x" = four for women and five for men)

Brown et al. (2001):
- In the past year, have you ever drunk or used drugs more than you meant to?
- Have you felt you wanted or needed to cut down on your drinking or drug use in the last year?

Smith et al. (2010):
- How many times in the past year have you used an illegal drug or used a prescription medication for nonmedical reasons?

AUDIT-C (Bush et al., 1998):
- How often do you have a drink containing alcohol?
- How many drinks containing alcohol do you have on a typical day when you are drinking?
- How often do you have six or more drinks on one occasion?

Note. For the Cyr and Wartman items, a positive response to the first item or a response of within the past 24 hours to the second would be considered a positive indication. For the Williams and Vinson item, a response of within the last 3 months would be considered positive. For the Brown et al. items, a positive response to either would be considered positive. For the Smith et al. item, a response of at least one time would be considered positive for drug use. For the AUDIT-C, the first item is scored as follows: "never" is 0 points, "two to four times a month" is 2 points, "two to three times a week" is 3 points, and "four or more times a week" is 4 points. For the second AUDIT-C question, "1 or 2" is scored 0 points, "3 or 4" is 1 point, "5 or 6" is 2 points, "7 to 9" is 3 points, and "10 or more" is 4 points. For the third AUDIT-C item, "never" is scored 0 points, "less than monthly" is 1 point, "monthly" is 2 points, "weekly" is 3 points, and "daily or almost daily" is 4 points. The scores for the three AUDIT-C items are then scored, and a score of 4 or greater for men and 3 or greater for women provides a positive indication.

each of the respective items. The minimum (cutoff) score for possible indication of alcohol problems is 8. Administration of the test takes only a few minutes, and its scoring even takes less time than that. Furthermore, research strongly supports the AUDIT's reliability and validity (Connors, 1995). In brief, the AUDIT is a more recently developed screening measure that is becoming increasingly popular because of its ease of administration and scoring, applicability to several different case-finding settings, and research support for its reliability and validity.

A more recently developed variation of the basic AUDIT is the AUDIT-Consumption, or AUDIT-C (Bush, Kivlahan, McDonell, Fihn,

& Bradley, 1998). The AUDIT-C is comprised of the first three questions of the AUDIT. Scores range from 0 to 12, and a positive result is indicated by a score of 4 or greater among men and 3 or greater among women (Bradley et al., 2003, 2007; Bush et al., 1998). The AUDIT-C items are provided in Table 3.5.

MacAndrew Scale

So far we have reviewed self-report methods of identification that are obvious in what they are designed to measure. The MacAndrew Scale (MAC) stands in stark contrast to these in that it has low face validity, that is, is not so obvious (given the questions). This scale, which was developed by MacAndrew (1965), has no items pertaining to alcohol, its use, or consequences related to its use. Instead, the MAC consists of 49 items from the Minnesota Multiphasic Personality Inventory (MMPI) that have been shown to discriminate empirically between persons with alcohol dependence and those in other groups. The MAC is self-administered, and respondents answer "true" or "false" to each item. The test takes about 15 minutes to complete.

During the 1980s the MMPI was revised, and in 1989 the MMPI-2 was published (Graham, 1999). The MAC scale is retained in the MMPI-2, with the same number of items, and is called the MAC-R(evised). The only difference between the MAC-R and the MAC is that four MAC items were replaced with four other items that discriminate between individuals who have alcohol problems and those who do not. Therefore, scores on the MAC-R may be interpreted similarly to scores on the MAC (Graham, 1999).

Craig (2005) reports that the MAC/MAC-R is sensitive to identifying people who actually have alcohol (and also substance abuse) problems, although its ability to discriminate decreases when other comorbid psychiatric conditions are also present. This implies that if a positive MAC score is obtained it should be corroborated by another data source. Craig suggests these cutoff scores for the MAC/MAC-R: > 25, positive for men, and > 23, positive for women.

To summarize this section, research has produced several self-report alcohol screening questionnaires that are brief, inexpensive, and easy to administer in virtually any clinical setting. Unfortunately, practical screening instruments that focus on other drugs of abuse are not nearly so common. However, with the advent of SBIRT there are a number of very brief screens being developed for inclusion in medical settings that have not yet been extensively studied for sensitivity and specificity.

It is important to note that the goals and the context of the screening may affect which measure is selected. For example, Connors and Volk's (2003) review shows that in studies directly comparing the two instruments, the MAST tends to be more sensitive than the CAGE but that the CAGE may perform better than the MAST with elderly primary care clients.

Intake Interview and Structured Diagnostic Interview Schedules

Intake Interview

The mainstay measure of almost all substance abuse treatment programs is the personal intake interview. The common core across all intake interviews is questions regarding substance use history, patterns, and consequences, although the specific format and content of such interviews vary considerably from one treatment program to another. More recently, accreditation agencies are specifying what must be included in these interviews (e.g., history of sexual abuse and trauma) and determining the nature or extent of the intake.

Questions about substance use history generally emphasize onset of use, perceived years of problem use of alcohol or other drugs, context of substance use, reasons for substance use, family history of alcohol or other drug problems, patterns of substance use, and quantity and frequency of alcohol and other drug use. Questions on consequences of substance use usually emphasize the domains of physical and psychological health, social and marital/family relationships, job performance, and legal factors (especially arrests related to substance use, such as driving under the influence).

One important area of questioning in intake interviews is symptoms of physical dependence on alcohol or other drugs. For example, for alcohol, questions might be asked about current or lifetime occurrence .of hangovers, shakes (tremors), seizures or convulsions, "loss of control" drinking, hallucinations, delirium tremens, memory impairment and blackouts, tolerance, and drinking to quell withdrawal symptoms. Finally, intake interviews often include inquiries about past attempts to resolve substance use problems, such as efforts to reduce use without the help of formal treatment, attendance at self-help groups (e.g., Alcoholics Anonymous, Narcotics Anonymous), or the use of formal treatment.

The intake interview is the source of information that is used in the vast majority of substance abuse treatment settings as the main source of diagnosis. Because they tend to reflect the treatment philosophy of a program staff and any idiosyncratic needs of a program, clinical intake interviews generally are characterized by their lack of standardization in interview content, format, and administration. The result is that it is impossible to compare with any faith intake data for different treatment settings or even for different respondents in the same treatment settings.

One obvious way around this difficulty is to standardize. An example of such an intake interview is the Comprehensive Drinker Profile (CDP; Miller & Marlatt, 1984). The CDP was designed to enable systematic collection of data on the use of alcohol and on other areas of life functioning, including other drug use. Part of what makes the CDP standardized is that it is accompanied by a manual to guide interview administration and interpretation of responses. The CDP earns the "comprehensive" part of its name, as it includes questions on client demographics, family and living situation, employment, education, drinking history (including development of the alcohol problem, current drinking pattern, and alcohol-related problems), other substance use, medical and psychiatric history, and motivation for treatment. The CDP takes about 50 minutes to administer. If a shorter interview is desired, the Brief Drinker Profile also is available.

Structured Diagnostic Interview Schedules

These measures may be viewed as "specialized" intake interviews, as they are geared specifically to collecting data for the purpose of categorization in a system of psychiatric nomenclature. Formal diagnosis may be of considerable help in treatment planning, and it is generally required in any case in accredited substance abuse treatment settings. The advantage in the use of formal measures in arriving at diagnosis is the same as we described in discussing the CDP, namely, a better opportunity for reliability and validity in the information gathered. We include formal diagnosis in this section of the chapter (as opposed to the following section on action and maintenance) because diagnosis is potentially relevant to case identification, as selected diagnostic instruments have been designed for evaluating individuals who might appear outside the substance abuse treatment setting.

The four instruments that we have selected to present in this section pertain to diagnosis of substance use disorders as well as other adult psychopathology. The instruments originally were developed primarily for epidemiological and clinical research purposes but often are used clinically to the benefit of treatment planning. They take about 60 to 90 minutes to administer in their entirety. Naturally, just administering sections on substance use can take considerably less time. Times for administration vary with the respondent, as "skip options" are available if the respondent "screens out" of any disorder. Furthermore, interviews may be administered in person or by computer.

Table 3.6 provides some specific details about four diagnostic interviews commonly used by substance abuse clinicians and researchers: the Diagnostic Interview Schedule (DIS), the Structured Clinical Interview for DSM-IV (SCID), the Psychiatric Research Interview for Substance and Mental Disorders (PRISM) (formerly known as the SCID Alcohol/Drug Version), and the Alcohol Use Disorders and Associated Disabilities Interview Schedule (AUDADIS). Using the information in Table 3.6 to compare the instruments shows that choice of a diagnostic measure depends on the answers to questions about purpose of making diagnoses, characteristics of interviewers and respondents, resources for staff training, and requirements for reliability and validity. Much more detail is available on each of the instruments listed in Table 3.6 by writing to different sources on the measures (contact information is provided in Hasin, 1991, p. 299, and Allen & Wilson, 2003). It should be noted that the two major diagnostic nomenclature systems—the *Diagnostic and Statistical Manual of Mental Disorders* (DSM) and the *International Classification of Diseases* (ICD)—are periodically revised, and the diagnostic tools described above updated accordingly.

Multivariate Measures

Many excellent measures of single variables or factors that are relevant to assessment in substance abuse treatment settings have been developed. For example, single-variable measures concern only one construct, such as expectations about alcohol and drug effects, self-esteem, or social support. Because of the large number and variety of single-variable measures in the substance abuse treatment area, we will not attempt to review them here; several reviews are available for the interested reader (e.g., Allen & Wilson, 2003; Donovan, in press; Donovan & Marlatt, 2005). For our purposes, the listing in Table 3.7 of recommended areas of measurement of individuals presenting for drug or alcohol treatment

TABLE 3.6. Major Standardized Diagnostic Instruments

Instrument	Main features	Training required for administration
Diagnostic Interview Schedule (DIS)	• Fully structured, designed for administration by nonclinicians • Newer version linked to DSM-IV criteria	• Read manual, complete homework assignments, attend 1-week training session.
Structured Clinical Interview for DSM-IV (SCID)	• Semistructured, designed for use by experienced clinical interviewers • Linked to DSM-IV criteria	• Read brief user's guide, watch 6-hour videotape. Option of SCID trainer visit to training site (interviewers assumed to be already experienced and knowledgeable in clinical interviewing).
Psychiatric Research Interview for Substance and Mental Disorders (PRISM)	• Semistructured, based on standard SCID but more structured • Designed to improve the reliability of psychiatric diagnoses among persons with alcohol and other drug problems • Focuses on comorbidity of substance and mental disorders • Emphasis on reliable assessment of community residents (thus milder symptoms) as well as patients • Interviewers should have clinical skills and knowledge of diagnostic criteria	• Study of PRISM training manual, rating of videotaped interviews, 2 days of role playing and lectures on the PRISM, watching and rating additional videotaped interviews, further role playing with trainers, audiotaping own interview for review by trainers.
Alcohol Use Disorders and Associated Disabilities Interview Schedule (AUDADIS)	• Fully structured, designed for use by nonclinicians • Also may be used in clinical settings • Linked to criteria of DSM-III-R; for alcohol and other drug diagnoses, uses criteria of DSM-III, ICD-10, and DSM-IV • Allows assessment of symptoms over a broad range of severities • Especially good for evaluating relationship between substance use and other psychiatric disorders • Must be administered in person	• Use of self-study materials, 5 days of classroom training, and completion of trainer-observed interviews.

Note. Data from Hasin (1991) and Maisto, McKay, and Tiffany (2003).

gives a good idea of the number of single-factor measures that are available, given that most areas of assessment have many such measures associated with them.

In keeping with our emphasis on multivariate models of substance abuse, we will discuss two self-report measures that are designed to capture multiple dimensions of substance use and related problems. These are the Alcohol Use Inventory and the Addiction Severity Index.

Alcohol Use Inventory

The Alcohol Use Inventory (AUI; Horn et al., 1987; Wanberg, Horn, & Foster, 1977) is a 228-item test that was developed to measure multiple features of alcohol use and consequences in individuals presenting for treatment of alcohol problems. The items, which are presented in a multiple-choice format, reflect 24 scales, or factors. The test takes about 35 minutes to complete and can be computer- or hand-scored.

TABLE 3.7. Recommended Areas to Assess in Individuals Presenting for Treatment of Alcohol or Other Drug Problems

- Specific quantities of alcohol or other drugs used, and the frequency of their use
- Predominant mood states and situations antecedent and consequent to substance use
- Usual and unusual substance use circumstances and patterns
- History of alcohol and other drug withdrawal symptoms
- Medical problems associated with or exacerbated by substance use
- Identification of possible difficulties the patient may have in initially refraining from substance use
- Extent and severity of previous substance use problems
- Multiple drug use
- Reports of frequent thoughts or urges to drink or take drugs
- History of previous responses to alcohol or drug treatment and self-initiated periods of abstinence
- Review of the positive consequences of substance use
- Other life problems
- Indicants of tolerance to alcohol or other drugs
- Past or present indicants of liver disorder
- Motivational readiness to change
- Barriers to treatment involvement
- (For alcohol use) Risks associated with considering a nonabstinent treatment goal

Note. Adapted from Sobell, Sobell, and Nirenberg (1988); Sobell, Toneatto, and Sobell (1994); Maisto, O'Farrell, Worthen, and Walitzer (1993); and Donovan (in press).

The 24 AUI scales were derived through extensive research. The scales reflect the respondent's style of alcohol use, the benefits he or she perceives to receive from drinking, negative consequences of drinking, and awareness that the respondent has about his or her alcohol problem and concerns about it. Note that this last area of evaluation, which actually is one scale of the AUI, fits nicely as a precontemplation/contemplation stage measure, as it is directly relevant to the central questions of those stages of change.

One of the outstanding features of the AUI that warrants mention is that it can be used to match individuals to specific treatment settings (e.g., inpatient or outpatient) or to treatment modalities (e.g., individual or family). Therefore, the AUI is one of the few assessments available in the substance abuse area that take direct steps toward being treatment-prescriptive. In the user's guide for the AUI (Horn et al., 1987), the authors discuss how the test results can be used for specific, individualized treatment planning. An excellent example of how AUI data can be used to identify "profiles" of alcohol abusing clients was recently provided by Rychtarik, Koutsky, and Miller (1998, 1999).

In summary, the AUI is a well-developed, well-evaluated, and clinically valuable multivariate measure of alcohol use and related consequences. Full appreciation of the AUI's development, content, and use can be obtained by study of the test guide (Horn et al., 1987). Currently it is one of the most useful multivariate measures available for individuals who present for alcohol treatment.

Addiction Severity Index

In contrast to the AUI, the Addiction Severity Index (ASI) was designed for use with individuals who present for alcohol or other drug treatment. The ASI is a structured personal interview that was designed to measure the severity of problems in five different areas that are typically affected as part of individuals' alcohol or other drug abuse: medical, employment, legal, family relations, and psychiatric. Severity of both alcohol and other drug use also is measured. The ASI was developed for use in treatment planning upon clients' admission to treatment and as a measure of change during and following treatment (McLellan et al., 1992; McLellan, Luborsky, Woody, & O'Brien, 1980).

In each of the areas of functioning that is measured with the ASI, questions are asked on the number, frequency, and duration of the problem symptoms, both in a client's lifetime and in the past 30 days. From these basic data, two different scores are derived. First, the individual receives a composite score in each area based on answers given to each of the items that constitutes an area of functioning. These scores reflect problem area severity and are arithmetically derived from key interview items comprising each area. Clients' perceptions of problem severity also are obtained for each area by asking them to rate both the severity of the problem and their need of further treatment for it. Lastly, after the interview is completed, the interviewer is asked to judge the severity of each problem area by rating the need for further treatment, based on responses to individual items and on the client's perception of need for treatment and how troubled he or she is by the problem in question.

Since the ASI was published in 1980, it has become a popular instrument in alcohol and drug treatment settings in the United States, Canada, and Europe. In general, reliability and validity data are good, and they hold up across different client populations defined by age, sex, race, and primary drug problem. In addition, the psychometric properties of the ASI have been shown to be sound when evaluated in several European nations.

The ASI takes about 50 to 60 minutes to complete by a competent interviewer. (There is also a briefer version, called the ASI-Lite, which typically takes less than 30 minutes to administer.) Requirements for learning to give the ASI are minimal, with the ability to communicate effectively with people who present for substance abuse treatment the basic necessity. Training is possible through use of an on-site training package that is available from the test developers. Also available are self-report and computerized versions.

To summarize, the ASI is a multivariate measure of severity of substance use and related areas of functioning. It is an excellent measure to use for assessment of individuals who present for alcohol or other drug treatment and can be an important part of feedback development and treatment planning.

Measures of Alcohol and Other Drug Use

Alcohol Consumption

The desired features of a measure of alcohol use are that it provide reliable, valid, and precise information on quantity of use, frequency of use, and patterns of use over specified time periods. Such time periods typically range from 30 days to 1 year before treatment admission. This collection of desirable measure features, along with a specified time period of at least 30 days, would allow for measurement of alcohol use that would be most helpful in treatment planning and that would enable sensitive measurement of changes in drinking during treatment and following its termination.

In the area of alcohol research and treatment many and varied measures of alcohol use have been developed. For clinical use, one measure that has emerged that has our set of desirable features is the Timeline Followback (TLFB) interview (Sobell, Maisto, Sobell, & Cooper, 1979; Sobell & Sobell, 1992, 1996, 2008). In the TLFB interview, respondents are given a calendar and asked to provide estimates of their daily alcohol consumption over a given period of time. Research on the TLFB has included study of intervals of up to 360 days before the interview day. Respondents are helped in their recall of daily drinking by the use of memory aids, including the use of a visual calendar, the listing of key dates (holidays, birthdays, etc.) on the calendar, the use of a standard drink conversion card (i.e., the quantities consumed of different alcoholic beverages are converted to "standard drinks"), and the identification of extended periods of drinking certain amounts, including no drinking.

Often the first reaction of interviewers and interviewees alike is that obtaining reasonable estimates of daily drinking for as far back as 1 year is pure fantasy. However, with only a minimum of training it becomes clear to new interviewers that such data can be reliably gathered and that it reflects estimates of critical patterns of drinking over time. This has been demonstrated by the TLFB's impressive track record of successful use in both clinical and research settings since its publication in 1979.

Essentially, the scores that are derived from the daily drinking TLFB protocol are summary (over some period of time) indices. These may include, for example, percentage of days engaging in a given level or quantity of drinking, such as abstinence or heavy drinking days, maximum number of drinks on a day, or average number of drinks a day. In addition, information about temporal patterns in drinking can be derived (e.g., weekend, daily, or binge drinker). In effect, the initial collection of daily drinking data makes possible the use of a wide variety of summary variables that are specifically suited to the clinician's or researcher's needs.

Since the TLFB's appearance, research on its reliability and validity has been published extensively by both its developers and others. The data are consistently good in this regard, across different treatment settings and populations. The TLFB has become even more accessible with the publication of a manual that describes the TLFB's development and instructions for its administration, a training video, and software for computer administration of the TLFB (Sobell & Sobell, 1996). It is important to emphasize, however, that TLFB data are psychometrically sound only for the summary variables that we referenced earlier. Therefore, single-day estimates of drinking do not have research evidence to support their reliability and validity; as we discuss later, given the limitations of memory, such precision in retrospective measures probably should not be expected.

Form 90 Family of Instruments

As part of the design of the multiple-site treatment-matching study called Project MATCH (Project MATCH Research Group, 1997a), the strengths of the TLFB and the alcohol consumption section of the Comprehensive Drinker Profile (described earlier in this chapter) were combined to create a new measure of alcohol consumption called the Form 90 (Miller & DelBoca, 1994). Like the TLFB, the Form 90 is a structured interview that has the goal of recording retrospective self-reports of daily alcohol use. As its name implies, Form 90 is designed to collect information about the past 90 days. It yields information that is highly similar to that of the TLFB, but adds the ability to estimate what blood alcohol concentrations the individual reached on his or her drinking days. (Of course, making such estimates requires that the interviewer also obtain information from the respondent about the time course of alcohol consumption events.) Other differences between the TLFB and Form 90 primarily involve methods of administration to allow more efficient data collection when repetitive patterns and episodes of drinking are apparent in the respondent's drinking behavior. Psychometric assessments of the Form 90 have been positive (Tonigan, Miller, & Brown, 1997). As with the TLFB, a manual for the Form 90 is available (Miller, 1996), as is supporting computer software.

Other Drug Use

In discussing measurement of different variables relevant to substance abuse treatment, we have presented actual measures. However, in this section of self-report measures of consumption of drugs other than alcohol, we make an exception to that. As we discuss later, although there are examples of comprehensive measures of drug use, none is widely accepted. For this and other reasons that will become apparent in our discussion, we will not present examples of measures. It would seem to be more useful to review briefly the nuances and problems in measuring drug use, as well as to make recommendations in doing so. Clinicians then may apply these recommendations to their own assessment needs.

The desired features of a self-report measure of drug use are the same as those we listed for alcohol, with the addition of the need to measure route of administration of the drug and the combined use of more than one drug. Unfortunately, there are complexities in getting accurate information on drug use from an individual and in interpreting the information that is obtained that are not problems in measuring alcohol consumption (Maisto et al., 1990; Martin & Wilkinson, 1989). These difficulties include, first, that sometimes it may be impossible to obtain data on quantities of street drugs sold, because often users do not know how much pharmacologically active ingredients are in the drugs they buy, and sometimes do not even know what drug they are buying. A second problem is in interpreting the data when multiple drugs are used: How should the data be combined to arrive at a single "drug use index"? It is no problem to combine the alcohol consumed in beer, wine, and hard liquor, because alcohol is common to the three types of beverages. But it is another matter to arrive at an analogous total-use index for other drug use. The question is important, because a total-use index would provide a quantitative statement about pretreatment drug use and would be a reference for measuring change from that level. Fortunately, there have been attempts to derive indices of total drug use, and we discuss these below. A last point also concerns interpretation of multiple drug use, including alcohol. In this regard, use of different drugs should not be seen as independent behaviors. Drugs may interact pharmacologically, resulting in an alteration of effects that are experienced by a given drug that may be different than what is experienced when that drug is taken alone. Also, behaviorally the use of one drug may be the antecedent or subsequent event of using another. For example, individuals may not use cocaine unless they already have drunk a certain amount of alcohol. Or alcohol may be consumed following cocaine use to attenuate cocaine's stimulant effects.

Because of these and other complexities, methods of measuring drug use are far behind those in measuring alcohol use. Nevertheless, research has provided three useful guidelines for measuring drug consumption (Addiction Research Foundation, 1993). These principles are, first, to avoid using broad categories for drugs that are used frequently in the population of interest. Because there is no single generally accepted way to classify drugs, categorizations of them may be arbitrary. It is important to keep in mind that when categories are broad there may be differences of importance among drugs within a category, both in pharmacology and psychological and physical effects, as well as the problems that may result from use. Therefore, if a class of drugs is of major interest to the clinician or researcher, it is necessary to measure each drug as specifically as possible. It always is possible to form larger classifications later but difficult to do the reverse.

Another guideline in measurement is first to obtain information on the frequency of drug use. As we noted, accurate information on quantity of drug use may be difficult or impossible to obtain. Some use times of administration, amount of money spent, and days of use to estimate quantity and frequency of use. Finally, besides frequency and, possibly, quantity information, it is important to obtain data on information such as route of administration, patterns of use, and the use of prescription medications.

It is fortunate that there have been a few good drug use measures developed for obtaining accurate data on lifetime and current street and prescription drug use. Illustrations of many of the most useful measures are provided in Addiction Research Foundation (1993). In addition, the TLFB and Form 90 may be used to collect information (primarily frequency data) on drug use other than alcohol (e.g., Ehrman & Robins, 1994; Miller, 1996; Sacks, Drake, Williams, Banks, & Herrell, 2003). These or other available drug use measures should be reviewed carefully before selecting one, with the idea of choosing the one that most productively addresses the clinical or research questions at hand for a given client population.

Once a measure of drug use is selected, there are somewhat different paths to follow for evaluation of single and multiple drug use. These paths are summarized in Figure 3.2. The problem is relatively simple when single drug use is the problem. In that case, with the use of structured and standardized interviews, there is little difficulty in collecting information on drug use frequency and route of administration. Once such data are obtained, they can be interpreted in a straightforward way. Furthermore, it then will be possible to measure change, say, in frequency of use over time. If it is possible to obtain accurate information on quantity of use, those data should be obtained as well, as a "bonus." The problem for multiple drug use differs because there is the need to obtain a drug use summary index so that a quantitative reference of change is available. As we explained, no generally accepted summary index has been developed, so the goal is to derive one that most productively suits the clinician's or researcher's specific needs.

To conclude our discussion of measuring drug use, no single standard self-report measure exists. It is unlikely that one will emerge any time soon, as patterns of drug use vary widely and are complex, drugs come and go and return again in popularity or availability, and different populations use different drugs differently (e.g., compare the use of prescription drugs by adolescents and the elderly). For now, clinicians will need to obtain the information that is needed for a specific setting and purpose as accurately as possible and then interpret the data in a way that makes the most sense for the population in question.

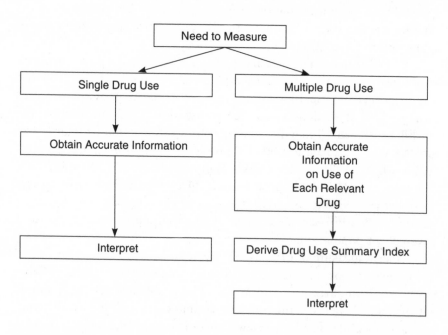

FIGURE 3.2. Flow chart of procedures to follow in measuring and interpreting single and multiple drug use.

Self-Monitoring: Self-Report of Current Behavior

Self-monitoring typically focuses on information for a behavioral assessment of current substance use, such as antecedents to use, frequency of use, patterns of use, and consequences of use. In self-monitoring, these data are not obtained by direct observation but by the person's monitoring and self-report of what is happening in his or her natural environment (e.g., Lemmens, Tan, & Knibbe, 1992; Sobell, Bogardis, Schuller, Leo, & Sobell, 1989).

When done properly, that is, the behavior is recorded when it occurs or at latest at the end of the day of occurrence, self-monitoring avoids the memory problems inherent in retrospective self-report methods of consumption such as the TLFB. And self-monitoring data are far more detailed than data collected when using retrospective measures. Self-monitoring can also become an excellent feedback mechanism providing information and increasing motivation. As such, self-monitoring provides an excellent assessment tool. It also is an excellent method to use in evaluating ongoing substance abuse treatment (e.g., Sobell et al., 1994). There are a few drawbacks to self-monitoring, however. The currency of the data is bought at the expense of obtaining information on longer term past use. Therefore, self-monitoring obviously is not the method of choice when the interest is in learning about a client's substance use in the past 6 months. Another problem with self-monitoring is getting clients, or research subjects for that matter, to comply consistently with the request that they provide information about current substance use.

Summary

The large majority of clinical measures that have been developed in the alcohol and drug fields, including those discussed above, have been designed to obtain a better description and understanding of individuals, whether done briefly and efficiently in the context of screening or in greater detail with clients seeking treatment. In either case, the information gathered will be available for application in providing feedback to individuals about their alcohol and/or substance use and in the development of treatment plans for those seeking clinical services.

As noted earlier in this chapter, the provision of feedback to individuals based on assessment instruments such as those identified above is perhaps best utilized in working with individuals in precontemplation and contemplation to increase interest and concern or to tip decision considerations regarding the pros and cons of their substance use and their commitment to change. As we discuss in greater detail in the chapter on individual treatment (Chapter 5), providing feedback is a powerful tool for intervening with individuals in these two stages of change. In a similar manner, information gathered using these approaches can be used as well with individuals in the preparation stage, where the person is engaged and committed to the change process and needs to develop a viable plan of action that takes into consideration the dimensions of the problem, the consequences, the environment, and the personal skills of the individual. Here assessment data can be used for consolidating and building upon that commitment to the change process and in the development of a particular plan of action for that individual. As is always the case, the purpose of the assessment and the key constructs that the clinician wants to evaluate as well as the assessment burden on the client must be considered in choosing assessments (Gastfriend, Donovan, Lefebvre, & Murray, 2005).

ASSESSMENTS WITH PARTICULAR RELEVANCE TO CLIENTS IN THE ACTION AND MAINTENANCE STAGES

The tasks of treatment differ as a function of the person's stage of change, as we describe more in upcoming chapters (such as Chapter 5 on individual treatment and Chapter 6 on group treatment). Similarly, the focus of assessment often will vary as a function of the stage of change and often accuracy of self-report improves as individuals become more convinced of the problem and invested in the solution. Information gathered using the previously presented measures can be used by the therapist and client to generate hypotheses or deductions about the client's substance use and factors associated with its development and maintenance. These assumed connections need to be constantly reevaluated and there are some specialized assessments analyzing important dimensions of use that become particularly relevant to individuals in the action and maintenance stages of change. The results of these specialized assessments are used to develop more refined treatment interventions for a given individual. Accordingly, this section has two major parts. First, we discuss how the assessment measures applied in the context of clients in the precontemplation, contemplation, and preparation stages of change can be used in the specialized assessment of clients who progress into the action and maintenance stages. Second, we discuss considerations in the assessment of relapse risk and self-efficacy.

Specialized Assessment

Several examples will help to clarify the use of more specialized levels of assessment for clients who progress into the stages of action and maintenance. The first would most likely occur while a person is in treatment and in the action stage of change. Suppose that the Comprehensive Drinker Profile (CDP) was administered to the person as part of the formal intake assessment. In addition to more normal assessments of readiness and processes of change, Section "C" of the CDP is called "Motivational Information" and concerns reasons for drinking and the effects a person experiences when he or she drinks alcohol. Two items in Section C consist of open-ended questions, respectively, about thoughts or feelings that tend to trigger a desire to drink and situations or a set of events that might result in the person's drinking. These two items and the remaining wide-ranging items of the CDP are typical of assessments conducted in the precontemplation, contemplation, and preparation stages; however, psychological and situational triggers to drink can be evaluated in considerably more detail in assessments associated with the action and maintenance stages. Measures of drinking situations, self-efficacy, and temptation to drink, as well as measures of craving (Donovan, in press) offer more detailed information in real time that can inform treatment and change strategies through the preparation, action, and maintenance stages.

One specialized assessment asks the individual to complete the Inventory of Drinking Situations (IDS; Annis, 1982a; Annis, Graham, & Davis, 1987). The IDS is a questionnaire that is designed to measure "high-risk" situations or triggers for heavy drinking. The original IDS consisted of 100 items, although a 42-item version is available (Isenhart, 1991, 1993). (A 50-item drug version, called the Inventory of Drug-Taking Situations [IDTS; Annis & Martin, 1993a; Annis, Turner, & Sklar, 1997] is also available.) The IDS and IDTS measures provide a risk profile of eight factors: unpleasant emotions, physical discomfort, pleasant emotions, testing personal control, urges and temptations to drink, conflict with others, social pressure to drink, and pleasant times with others. If there is consistency in the present example between the CDP trigger responses and the IDS, these data could be made the basis of a specialized coping skills training intervention.

We can readily offer a second example of specialized assessment that would be most useful with a person in the action stage of change. As part of a structured diagnostic interview, the mental status exam may suggest that a polysubstance abuser who has been adequately detoxified has short-term memory impairment but no deficits in longer term memory or in other areas of cognitive functioning. Further testing of this possibility would be critical, as the presence of short-term memory deficits could have considerable influence on how a treatment is administered or affect the content of treatment. A specialized assessment, therefore, would be indicated. In this case, it would make sense after detoxification to administer to a person interested in engaging in treatment and quitting substance use the Wechsler Memory Scale—Revised or some other cognitive assessment instrument, which would result in data on different types (short-term, long-term, verbal, and visual are examples) of memory function. In addition, administration of the Wechsler Intelligence Scale for Adults—Revised (WAIS-R) would enable an extensive evaluation of general intelligence or cognitive functioning important for planning and implementation of action plans.

An example of another specialized assessment applicable to the action and maintenance stages focuses on skills. Most drug and alcohol treatment programs involve participation in a social skills group. Systematic behavioral observation of the individual in that group can suggest difficulties in resisting friends' pressure to drink or use drugs. Therapists might well predict that potential relapse situations for that person would include those in which there might be considerable peer-group pressure to use substances, such as at parties. Therefore, these predispositions would be important to know at the beginning of the action or maintenance (of sobriety) stage of change and in developing an individual's aftercare or discharge plans.

More generally, the therapist might want to have the person complete the Situational Confidence Questionnaire (SCQ; Annis, 1982b, 1987; Annis & Graham, 1988). The SCQ is a counterpart to the IDS, asking the respondent to indicate how likely he or she will be able to cope with a variety of situations without drinking heavily. The original SCQ consisted of 100 items (now there also are 42- and 39-item versions of the test, along with an even briefer eight-item version called the Brief Situational Confidence Questionnaire [Breslin, Sobell, Sobell, & Agrawal, 2000]) that were created to measure an individual's self-efficacy in coping with different situations without drinking heavily. While the IDS attempts to determine the relative cue strength for drinking in each situation, the SCQ attempts to determine individuals' current level of confidence in their ability to encounter each of these situations without drinking heavily. A 50-item version for other drugs, called the Drug-Taking Confidence Questionnaire (DTCQ; Annis & Martin, 1993b), also has been developed. The items on the SCQ (and DTCQ) generally parallel those on the IDS (and IDTS), and the SCQ yields a profile on the same eight dimensions used in the IDS. Wherever the individual shows less confidence or "self-efficacy" (Bandura, 1977) to cope with different situations without using alcohol or drugs is where relapse theoretically is most probable.

A client's responses on the SCQ can be used to monitor the development of the client's self-efficacy in relation to coping with specific drinking situations (identified and prioritized by use of the IDS) over the course of treatment or with increasing sobriety. Self-efficacy would be expected to increase across treatment; this appears to be the case (e.g., Burling, Reilly, Molzen, & Ziff, 1989; Miller, Ross, Emmerson, & Todt, 1989; Rychtarik, Prue, Rapp, & King, 1992; Sitharthan & Kavanagh, 1991). Burling et al. (1989), for example, found that self-efficacy increased during the course of inpatient treatment and was higher for those individuals who were abstainers at a 6-month follow-up than for those who had relapsed. The assumption that higher levels of self-efficacy would be associated with lower levels of relapse or posttreatment drinking has been supported (e.g., Rychtarik et al., 1992; Sitharthan & Kavanagh, 1991; Solomon & Annis, 1990), although this has not been a universal result (e.g., Mayer & Koeningsmark, 1991). Nevertheless, profiles for the SCQ (and also for the IDS) may be valuable aids in treatment planning and evaluation (Cunningham, Sobell, Sobell, Gavin, & Annis, 1995).

A final measure with unique relevance to the present topic is the Alcohol Abstinence Self-Efficacy Scale (AASE), developed by DiClemente, Carbonari, Montgomery, and Hughes (1994) to assess vulnerability to drink and efficacy to abstain. They noted that efficacy needs to be assessed for the particular behavior goal of the individual and that efficacy to avoid heavy drinking or remain abstinent when facing drinking cues differs. Thus, the SCQ's focus on heavy drinking may not be an appropriate measure to assess self-efficacy in abstinence-oriented settings. The goals of treatment (e.g., abstinence or harm reduction) should correspond to the type of efficacy being assessed. They also caution that getting an accurate assessment of either type of efficacy may be difficult when individuals are in inpatient or residential settings where they have limited access to drinking or drug use behavior potentially inflating their sense of efficacy.

The current complete version of the AASE contains 40 items, but there are shorter versions used in different studies. Each item is rated separately on two 5-point scales (from not at all to extremely) to reflect first how tempted the person would be in that situation and in a separate scale how confident he or she would be in his or her ability to abstain in each of those situations. Other versions have been used to evaluate cutting down on drinking and for use in drug abuse treatment settings.

The AASE has been used in several treatment studies with alcohol-dependent individuals. Ito, Donovan, and Hall (1988) found that individuals involved following hospitalization in group-administered, relapse-prevention-focused aftercare showed a significant decrease in their level of temptation and an increased level of self-efficacy over the 8-week course. However, clients involved in an interpersonally based aftercare group therapy program demonstrated no significant changes in either temptation or confidence across the corresponding 8-week treatment phase. DiClemente and Hughes (1990) also found that clients entering outpatient treatment for an alcohol use disorder who were discouraged, less motivated, and less ready to engage in behavior change activities demonstrated the highest level of temptation and the lowest level of confidence. Finally, in a national study on alcoholism treatment (Project MATCH Research Group, 1997b), confidence scores from the AASE were prognostic of posttreatment drinking among outpatient clients: higher pretreatment confidence was associated with a greater percentage of days abstinent and fewer drinks per drinking day posttreatment. More intriguing was the finding that temptation relative to confidence (calculated as the temptation score on the AASE minus the confidence score) predicted drinking outcomes among outpatients and also among aftercare clients (those who participated in an aftercare treatment that followed a more intensive inpatient or day hospital treatment). For both populations of clients, the higher the temptation minus confidence score, the fewer the percentage of days abstinent during follow-up and the greater average number of drinks per drinking day (DiClemente, Carbonari, Daniels, et al., 2001). The relative differences between temptation and confidence appear to be critical in successful outcomes (Carbonari & DiClemente, 2000) and in predicting various dimensions of relapse (Holmgren & DiClemente, 2012).

The AASE scale is composed of four factors reflecting some of the key factors found in the IDS. The first is a negative affect factor, which includes intrapersonal (e.g., "When I am feeling depressed") and interpersonal (e.g., "When I feel like blowing up because of frustration") negative affect. Social situations (e.g., "When I am being offered a drink in a social situation") and the use of alcohol to enhance positive states (e.g., "When I am excited or celebrating with others") represent social/positive emotion items, the second factor. The third factor, physical and other concerns, consists of varied items representing physical discomfort or pain (e.g., "When I am experiencing some physical pain or injury"), concerns about others (e.g., "When I am concerned about someone"), and dreams about drinking (e.g., "When I dream about taking a drink"). The final factor, withdrawal and urges, represents withdrawal (e.g., "When I am in agony because of stopping or withdrawing from alcohol use"), craving (e.g., "When I am feeling a physical need or craving for alcohol"), and testing willpower (e.g., "When I want to test my willpower over drinking") items.

Assessment of Relapse Risk and Self-Efficacy

Some important cautions have been offered by Sobell and colleagues about assessing high-risk situations and evaluating relapse risks. Sobell et al. (1994) noted that one cannot presume a causal link between the types of situations endorsed, drinking behavior, and relapse probability. A number of other factors, such as coping skills deficits, may represent a common third factor that moderates this relationship. It is also important to explore in more depth the unique and personally relevant high-risk situations or areas in which the client lacks self-confidence in resisting drinking or drug use. One might choose to expand more fully on those situations associated with frequent substance use, high temptation ratings, or low levels of perceived confidence on the structured questionnaires. Sobell et al. (1994) also recommend that clinicians ask clients to describe in detail their three highest risk situations for substance use over the past year.

The latter recommendation is consistent with the recent development and use of semistructured, individualized approaches to the assessment of self-efficacy. Miller, McCrady, Abrams, and Labouvie (1994), for example, examined the usefulness of an individualized approach to the assessment of self-efficacy in an outpatient alcohol treatment program. An Individualized Self-Efficacy Survey (ISS) was developed for each client. This survey was derived by (1) administering the Drinking Patterns Questionnaire to identify important problem areas for the individual (e.g., work, children, marital problems) and specific drinking antecedents and (2) constructing a 15-item scale using each drinker's most important drinking cues. This method of having clients choose their own high-risk drinking cues appears to be clinically useful. Ratings on the ISS reflected changes in perceived efficacy over the course of treatment, and ISS scores at the end of treatment predicted subsequent relapse.

SUMMARY

• Assessment is the collection and use of information to obtain an understanding of an individual for purposes of planning treatment, modifying the treatment plan (as warranted) over time, and evaluating treatment progress and outcome. These methods can be formal measures, interview evaluations, or a combination of the two.

• Assessments for treatment planning differ from those that attempt to screen and should be tailored to the dimensions of the problem as well as the client's stage of change. Relevance and accuracy of the assessments can differ depending on problem severity and stage status.

• There are now several different methods of measuring stage of change. The methods most commonly reported in current literature are the staging algorithm and the University of Rhode Island Change Assessment (URICA) scale, although a few instruments specific to alcohol and drug use are becoming increasingly popular.

• Approaches for identifying a client's readiness to change are readily available, along with measures for determining the extent to which clients are engaged in a variety of experiential and behavioral processes of change that reflect coping activities related to stage-of-change tasks.

• A variety of measures are being used to identify and specify substance misuse. These assessments can be used to provide feedback to individuals on their substance use and its consequences (particularly to persons in the precontemplation and contemplation stages of change) and to identify factors associated with the maintenance of substance misuse.

• Several measures are available for assessing individuals in the preparation, action, and maintenance stages of change. Of particular relevance are measures to identify a client's vulnerability and self-efficacy in dealing with situations associated with risk for drinking or drug use.

4

Treatment Planning

The treatment plan, based on the information gathered during assessment, is one of the most important components of the treatment process. Developed in close collaboration with the client, the treatment plan is designed to address mutually agreed-upon treatment goals. The importance of the process of carefully and collaboratively developing the treatment plan cannot be overemphasized. The treatment plan organizes, integrates, and prioritizes the material collected during assessment and serves as the plan of action for pursuing the identified goals of treatment. As such, the plan serves a variety of important purposes, including prioritizing short-term and long-term goals, selecting the optimal interventions for specific goals, identifying barriers to the achievement of goals, and monitoring progress toward goals over time (see Donovan, 2003, in press; Kadden & Skerker, 1999). The therapist in significant part acts as a "broker" working to bring together treatment and client considerations in service of the change process endeavor (DiClemente & Scott, 1997).

This chapter opens with a description of the treatment plan. Following that is a section on developing treatment goals. An emphasis is placed on incorporating the collaboration of the client in this process. Then we discuss procedures for matching specific treatment activities to treatment goals, previewing in part some of the treatment techniques and strategies that are described in later chapters. Representative treatment plans are presented, the first dealing with an alcohol-dependent client in the contemplation stage and the second with a cocaine-dependent client in the action stage.

THE TREATMENT PLAN

The treatment plan is essentially the agenda that emerges from the assessment process. It is highlighted by a delineation of treatment goals and a corresponding set of clinical interventions designed to assist in the achievement of these goals. The treatment plan is unique to the individual because the presenting needs of clients vary considerably from person to person, as do their available strengths and resources for effecting change. Not surprisingly, the better and more precise the tailoring of the treatment plan to the client's needs and resources, the better the potential fit and the greater the likelihood of achieving the specified treatment goals.

The therapist and the client must develop a list of treatment goals and then prioritize those goals. In many cases the primary goal is a decrease in, or cessation of, substance use. Focusing on this goal may have an impact on other key goals, such as improving a family or employment situation. Secondary goals might include extending one's social support network, returning to school, and so on. Whatever the objectives are, it is important to prioritize them. While one obvious benefit of such prioritizing is that attention is focused on the most pressing problem areas, another advantage is that successes in these primary areas, such as cessation of substance use, often place the client in a much better position to subsequently address secondary goals.

As they identify and prioritize goals, the therapist and the client also need to specify which are short-term goals and which are long-term goals. Although there is no consensus about setting these terms, short-term goals often are identified as those that can be significantly addressed within 6 months (e.g., Lewis, Dana, & Blevins, 1988). Long-term goals are those more likely to be achieved over longer periods, although this would not preclude initial efforts to address such goals in the short term and over time. The distinction between short-term and long-term goals is important to highlight, as clients move through the stages of change at different times and at different paces.

A number of variables will influence the establishment of short-term and long-term goals. As identified by Miller and Mastria (1977), one of the key factors is the extent and seriousness of the problem. Any pretreatment evaluation of a substance will include assessment of severity of dependence and need for detoxification or some other form of medical management. By necessity, problems in this domain would require immediate attention.

Goal setting is influenced as well by the nature and extent of the client's motivation to invest in and pursue treatment goals. An assessment of the client's stage of change will yield information on his or her extent of readiness to embark on the change process, along with insights on which processes of change might be targeted. The client in contemplation will likely be vacillating between the advantages and disadvantages to making changes in his or her life. A client in the action stage will be more ready than one in an earlier stage to start the change process and much less likely to want to devote time and energy to deciding on whether to commit to change.

The determination that a client is in the contemplation or action stage of change does not preclude the full development of the treatment plan, but it has implications for how the treatment goals are established and operationalized. A possible short-term goal for the person in the contemplation stage would be evaluation of the pros and cons of making changes in substance use patterns, using principles of motivational counseling (DiClemente & Velasquez, 2002; Miller & Rollnick, 1991, 2002) and decisional balance exercises (Janis & Mann, 1977). Short-term goals for the client in the action stage could include, as examples, attendance at self-help groups and problem-solving alternatives to substance use, as such clients are going to be more ready to embark on such change efforts.

It is important to identify goals that are achievable, and where procedures can be established to allow the client to take small and progressive steps in gradually achieving these goals. There are two reasons for adhering to such a strategy. The first is that complex problems are not generally amenable to easy, one-step solutions, regardless of the person's level of motivation. Rather, breaking down the problem into its subcomponents and successively addressing these is both a more manageable and a more successful approach to the larger problem. Second, developing a step-wise plan for addressing problems sets the stage for the client to experience a series of small but meaningful successes in pursuit of his or her goals. This is particularly important when the client is not fully confident about his or her ability to succeed in the change process. Experiencing some initial successes lessens the likelihood of the discouragements clients often experience when their expectations or goals for treatment are too ambitious. Such discouragements are a major contributor to dropping out of treatment.

Miller and Mastria (1977) have identified several other factors that can influence the development of short-term and long-term treatment goals. These include the treatment setting, the availability of significant others, and the projected period of treatment involvement. In terms of setting, for example, short-term goals for clients in an inpatient unit will differ in certain ways from those established for outpatient clients. Outpatients have the benefit of trying out treatment strategies in their actual living environments but do not have the benefits of the more protective inpatient unit, which affords more opportunities for regrouping and consolidation. Availability of significant others and their investment in the client can influence the plans for achieving treatment goals. For example, spouses, other family members, and friends may be available to participate in treatment sessions or can be called upon by the client in other ways to support and contribute to his or her efforts to make changes.

Finally, the projected treatment period can markedly influence treatment planning. The treatment plan for a client allocated 3 months of outpatient treatment will differ from that developed for a client with the opportunity for a lengthier treatment intervention. Insurance policies can determine treatment periods, but clients themselves bring their own expectations about how long treatment should last—and such expectations need to be acknowledged and respected. For the client who expects treatment to be briefer than the therapist thinks advisable, negotiating a treatment plan that incorporates a compromise duration, at the end of which the plan and progress to date would be reviewed, may be possible.

It is important that the client and the therapist alike recognize the treatment plan as flexible and changeable. They should view the initial treatment plan, based on the pretreatment assessment and evaluation, as a working blueprint for change, and both should understand and acknowledge that changes can—and likely *will*—be made in it over time. As such, treatment planning actually is a continuous and dynamic component of the treatment process. There are several reasons for this (Sobell, Sobell, & Nirenberg, 1982). First, there may be some needs or problems that are not apparent during the pretreatment assessment. Second, progress on some treatment goals may need to await progress on other problem areas. In such cases, it may be necessary to rearrange treatment goal priorities. Third, some problems may take longer to address than other problems or than originally anticipated. Revisions of the treatment plan will help the client and the therapist to keep abreast of relative progress in the pursuit of treatment goals. Finally, it is not unusual for new problems to arise during treatment, problems that may require immediate incorporation into the treatment plan.

The most commonly identified components of a treatment plan are highlighted in Table 4.1 One important point listed in Table 4.1 that we have not yet discussed is the incorporation, as warranted, of interdisciplinary inputs. For example, each substance-abusing client should receive a physical exam and workup. In this context, the potential use of pharmacotherapy can be evaluated. Disulfiram, naltrexone, and acamprosate have been used with some benefits among alcoholics, and methadone and naltrexone have potential benefits in the treatment of opioid dependence. (The individual and combined uses of psychotherapy and pharmacotherapy are discussed in greater detail by Carroll, 1996a; Myrick & Wright, 2008; and O'Brien & Kampman, 2008.) Consultations with social workers, vocational counselors, and other

TABLE 4.1. Common Features of an Individualized Treatment Plan

- Developed as a result of a comprehensive assessment and modified over time as warranted.
- Reflects participation from appropriate disciplines (e.g., medicine, psychiatry, psychology, social work, vocational rehabilitation) as warranted.
- Reflects the client's presenting needs and specifies the person's strengths and limitations.
- Consists of specific goals that pertain to the attainment, maintenance, and/or reestablishment of physical and emotional health.
- Identifies specific objectives that relate directly to the treatment goals.
- Identifies the services and/or settings necessary for meeting the client's needs and goals.
- Specifies the frequency of treatment contacts.
- Includes provisions for periodic (and at other times, as indicated by changes in the client's life-functioning) reevaluations and revisions, as warranted, of the treatment plan.
- Identifies specific criteria for determining whether goals have been achieved and for terminating treatment.

Note. Data from Joint Commission on Accreditation of Healthcare Organizations (1994, pp. 22–23).

professionals who can assist in the client's transition to a substance-free lifestyle can also be useful.

DEVELOPING INDIVIDUALIZED TREATMENT GOALS

While the formulation of treatment goals on the surface may appear to be a fairly mechanical task, in fact it requires a dynamic and collaborative interplay between the client and the therapist on the identification of needs. Many of the assessment tools we identified in Chapter 3 are particularly relevant to this process.

In almost all cases, current substance use and its consequences are a primary concern. Treatment goals concerning substance abuse, as with all other treatment objectives, need to be clearly identified, since the absence of explicit goals would make it difficult for the therapist and especially the client to evaluate progress and success (Berg & Miller, 1992; Persons, 2008). Wherever possible, express treatment goals positively. As noted by Sobell et al. (1982), goals stated positively allow greater possibilities for producing behavior change. The positively stated goal of "achieve and maintain progressively longer periods of abstinence from crack" may hold more promise than the alternative goal of "stop getting high." Relatedly, it is often more effective to state goals in terms of increasing desired behaviors rather than focusing on decreasing unwanted behaviors.

An individual's substance abuse is almost always associated with various forms of life dysfunction, whether in the marital, family, vocational, health, or legal domains. Accordingly, treatment planning needs to give cognizance to all these areas, even though in many cases the initiation of abstinence or significant reductions in substance use will alleviate at least some of the more acute problems. In addition, substance use is often associated with other comorbid psychiatric disturbances, such as depression or anxiety (e.g., Kessler, 2004; Regier et al., 1990; Ross, 2008), and these issues require corresponding attention.

Regardless of the nature of the particular problem area, the same essential issues need to be kept in mind in developing the respective treatment goals. A listing of the key qualities of well-formed treatment goals, many of which have already been mentioned, is provided in Table 4.2.

TABLE 4.2. Some Qualities of Well-Formed Treatment Goals

- Salient and meaningful to the client
- Incremental and thus more manageable
- Concrete, specific, and behavior-focused
- Focused on increasing desired behaviors
- Include progressive steps for achieving goals
- Realistic and achievable
- Perceived as requiring work and effort
- Appropriate for the projected treatment period

Note. Adapted in part from Berg and Miller (1992).

Wherever possible, the goals of the treatment plan should reflect the client's goals, not the therapist's. Doing so affords the client a greater sense of ownership and potential responsibility for whatever treatment objectives emerge from the treatment planning process. Furthermore, clients more often than not decide for themselves, either before or after the initiation of treatment, the goals they consider primary. Clients by and large will decide and act upon their own substance abuse goals even if they are at variance with the treatment program goals (e.g., Sanchez-Craig, Annis, Bornet, & MacDonald, 1984; Miller, Leckman, Delaney, & Tinkcom, 1992a; Nordstrom & Berglund, 1987). Several studies have shown that better treatment outcomes are associated with treatment goals being consistent with the client's goal preference (Booth, Dale, & Ansari, 1984; Orford & Keddie, 1986).

Throughout the assessment and treatment planning process—indeed, from the point of initial contact—the therapist needs to engender a productive therapeutic alliance with the client and enhance the client's motivation to change. While some clients enter the treatment process highly motivated and ready for taking action, most present with reservations. Such clients are typically in the contemplation phase, and with these clients in particular therapists should key on strategies for increasing motivation to change and for keeping clients engaged in the processes surrounding development and implementation of the treatment plan.

The importance of establishing a positive therapeutic alliance cannot be overstated. Research summarized by Lebow, Kelly, Knobloch-Fedders, and Moos (2006) has documented that clients are more likely to further pursue treatment when a stronger alliance exists during the initial intake or assessment interview. Further, Lebow et al. found that stronger therapeutic alliances are associated with clients remaining longer in treatment, experiencing less distress and better mood states during treatment, and being more likely to be abstinent from alcohol and other substances during and after treatment.

Another useful approach to increasing the likelihood of sustained treatment involvement, beyond the establishment of a positive therapeutic alliance, is motivational enhancement. When used in the early stages of treatment, motivation-enhancing techniques can be helpful for reducing or preventing resistance, engaging the client in the treatment endeavor, and increasing cooperation with the treatment process. In almost all initial sessions, the therapist naturally would elicit from the client a description, in the client's own words, of the presenting problem and the factors contributing to his or her seeking treatment at this time. Using principles of motivational interviewing, the therapist would convey *empathy* through use of reflective listening techniques. At whatever point the therapist has accumulated sufficient information, the therapist would provide a summary of the concerns voiced by the client and *feedback* of indications garnered through the assessment process. This feedback could include topics such as the frequency, intensity, and duration of substance use; problems directly and indirectly associated with such use; other areas of functioning, such as mood; comparisons of indications from the assessment to norms from the general population and/or from treatment-seeking samples; and risk factors, such as family history or environmental factors, that might suggest an increased susceptibility to continued or worsening difficulties. The emphasis in these interactions should be on describing the client's functioning in terms that are meaningful to the client, as opposed to presenting a formal diagnosis. Often it is useful to provide the client with a written summary of the feedback to review later.

With the foregoing as foundation, the therapist is now in a position to help the client gauge for him- or herself the relative strength and importance of the costs and benefits of change. In doing so, the therapist would be attempting to move the client toward a greater commitment to change. The therapist makes clear to the client that the *responsibility* for deciding what, if anything, to do about his or her substance use is the client's. At the same time, the therapist provides clear *advice* to change. As part of the process of identifying strategies for addressing treatment goals, the therapist can provide a *menu* of options for change, ideally based on clinical research regarding effective treatments for substance misuse. Finally, the therapist engenders client *self-efficacy* by stressing that treatment is likely to be successful if the client is committed to making a change.

Throughout the intake and treatment planning sessions, the therapist can utilize a variety of strategies to move the client toward a determination that change is necessary, desirable, and achievable. These techniques, drawn from Miller, Zweben, DiClemente, and Rychtarik (1992), include the following:

- *Elicit self-motivational statements.* Self-motivational statements are those that reflect the client's openness to feedback on his or her substance use, an acknowledgment of problems associated to date with such use, and expressions of the need or willingness to make change. One of the most fruitful ways of eliciting such statements entails the use of open-ended questions.

- *Listen with empathy.* Sometimes called "reflection," or "active listening," this technique entails listening carefully to statements made by the client and then reflecting them back on the client. Such responses encourage the client to continue talking and are not likely to elicit resistance, both important advantages in early treatment sessions. Importantly, listening with empathy demonstrates the therapist's respect for and interest in the client, which contributes in turn to the development of a productive therapeutic alliance.

- *Ask open-ended questions.* Asking the client about his or her feelings, concerns, and plan is more productive than telling the client how he or she should feel or what he or she needs to do.

- *Affirm the client.* Affirming and complimenting the client in a way that acknowledges his or her serious consideration of and steps toward change can improve the treatment process.

- *Handle resistance.* One productive strategy for dealing with client resistance is to deflect it by simply reflecting the client's feelings or by shifting focus away from the problematic issue, rather than debating with or confronting the client.

- *Reframe.* The therapist can restate client perceptions in a form more likely to be conducive to and supportive of making change. In this fashion, new meanings and perspectives are provided to the client.

• *Summarize.* The therapist can consolidate the material presented by the client over the course of the session in a positive and realistic way. Summaries that reflect and repeat self-motivational statements made by the client are particularly helpful.

These clinical strategies are described in much greater detail elsewhere by Miller and his colleagues (Miller, 1995, 1999; Miller & Rollnick, 1991, 2002; Miller et al., 1992; Rollnick, Mason, & Butler, 1999). The use of these techniques, taken together, have great potential for engaging the client in a productive and well-planned treatment process.

APPLYING SPECIFIC TREATMENT ACTIVITIES TO TREATMENT GOALS

Once treatment goals have been identified, it becomes necessary to match them with treatment activities designed to accomplish them. Most treatment objectives are multifaceted, and even in their simplest forms there will be several treatment options potentially available for application. Accordingly, the therapist needs to evaluate treatment options in relation to the various treatment goals and determine which strategies to select, keeping in mind the client's unique strengths and resources. In addition, the client's current readiness to change will influence the nature of treatment options selected. For example, the use of action-focused techniques for abstaining from substance use may not be productive in the early stages of treatment with an individual who is only contemplating such change. Similarly, evaluating the pros and cons of making behavior change will not be particularly timely with the client who is already in the action stage of change.

While the fit between the individual's needs and capabilities and the treatment strategies is instrumental in fostering early progress in treatment, the treatment activities should not be viewed as etched in stone. Instead, the treatment activities associated with a particular goal can be modified as a function of progress toward that goal. In addition, it sometimes is necessary to utilize other treatment strategies if the client's circumstances change, such as when the severity of substance use increases beyond that presented at treatment entry. Flexibility in applying specific treatment activities is central to an individualized approach to a client's needs.

The range of treatment strategies potentially available for use in working with substance-abusing clients is wide, and in subsequent chapters we will discuss a variety of treatment activities, including strategies for use in individual treatment and group treatment formats. The case studies that follow pick up on those we presented in Chapter 2 and illustrate the development and implementation of individualized treatment plans.

REPRESENTATIVE TREATMENT PLANS

Case Example 1: Treatment Plan for an Alcohol-Dependent Client in the Contemplation Stage

As we discussed in Chapter 2, Maureen J is a 46-year-old divorced woman presenting at a community mental health center because she is drinking more than she would like and is thinking about quitting. Almost all of her drinking occurs with friends and other patrons in a local tavern that is close to where she works and lives. On Mondays she generally is abstinent. On Tuesdays, Wednesdays, and Thursdays she typically consumes three to five bottles of beer each day. On weekends she drinks more heavily, usually 10–12 beers a day. She acknowledges a variety of negative consequences of past drinking and is concerned about more potential consequences (especially in the context of driving after drinking at the tavern). Such consequences, taken together, have put her in a position of thinking more about her alcohol use and the possibility of quitting. This is countered, in her mind, by the fact she really has not been "burned" by her drinking and by her belief that important relationships with her friends will be negatively affected if she is not drinking and thus is not one of the gang. As such, she is unclear as to what she needs to do and about what she wants to do about her drinking. For that reason, she contacted the clinic.

Maureen and her counselor discussed her goals and developed the following treatment plan based on them.

Treatment Plan

Long-term goals

1. Sustained abstinence from alcohol as well as any other addictive substances
2. Acquisition and maintenance of meaningful and fulfilling social relationships
3. Acquisition and use of skills to recognize and deal with high-risk situations for relapse

Short-term objectives

Goal	Intervention
1. Identification of negative consequences of drinking	Conduct comprehensive alcohol and drug use history, via interview and questionnaire measures, to identify drinking consequences in life-functioning domains (e.g., work, family, social, physical, legal).
	Refer for physical examination and laboratory workup.
2. Evaluation of pros and cons of drinking	Provide objective feedback on drinking behaviors and pattern (especially since client evaluates drinking in context of how friends drink).
	Conduct decisional balance exercise to identify and weigh advantages of quitting drinking relative to disadvantages of quitting.
	Use motivational procedures specifically in this regard to maximize prospects for moving client beyond contemplation.
3. Implement plans to not drive after drinking and to reduce other alcohol-related risks	Develop plans to avoid driving after drinking, such as using a taxi.
	Identify and address other areas of potential risk similarly, as indicated.
4. Evaluate alternative environments for social ties	Investigate alternative environments for socializing, such as meeting friends in alcohol-free contexts.
	Explore avenues for meeting new friends and evaluate and address conversational skills, etc., as warranted.
5. Establish short-term abstinence	Initiate as warranted (i.e., as a function of client consent) an initial 30-day period of abstinence.
	Monitor cravings for alcohol and situational challenges to abstinence.
	Discuss techniques and strategies to deal with drinking situations (e.g., drink refusal training).
	Discuss alternatives to drinking (e.g., meeting friends in nondrinking situations).
	Attend self-help groups such as Alcoholics Anonymous during this period and evaluate with client benefits experienced.
	Discuss over time advantages and disadvantages of not drinking in context of decisional balance.

6. Further engage client in therapeutic endeavor	Provide support and encouragement for collaborative change effort.
	Foster confidence and efficacy on part of client by focusing on initially small steps toward change, thus providing early success experiences.

Comments

Treatment will entail weekly sessions for the first 6 months, with additional sessions during this period scheduled as warranted. Sessions for following 6 months will be tapered according to client status and needs. Treatment plan will be reviewed and updated accordingly at least every 3 months.

Case Example 2: Treatment Plan for a Cocaine-Dependent Client in the Action Stage

As described in Chapter 2, Paul J is a 34-year-old single man who reported using multiple substances in various combinations since junior high school. During the past 6 years his drug use entailed almost daily use of marijuana and alcohol and use of cocaine approximately four times a week. He noted that he occasionally would also use stimulants but that such use was infrequent (maybe once a month, he estimated). His drug use occurred with various combinations of acquaintances from a core group of around 15 persons. That is, he was part of a group of around 15 people who in different combinations would get together. Paul did not spend much time with these individuals beyond these specific drug use contexts.

Paul's drug use over the past decade had precluded the development of significant or long-term relationships with women (and often with friends more generally) and created difficulties maintaining gainful employment. In fact, he had spent most of the past 10 years either underemployed, on unemployment benefits, or on welfare support. The status that bothered him most was underemployment because he felt he was capable of working in more challenging positions. He noted, with some pride, that his drug use had not led to problems in his physical health (at least, as far as he was aware), accidents, or arrests. It was the absence of problems in these areas that he in the past had used as evidence that he did not have a problem with drug use.

At intake, Paul reported that he wanted to be abstinent from all substance use, including alcohol, and immediately wanted to start taking the steps necessary to achieve this goal. Although asserting the same in the past, he reported it was different this time because he "really" had decided to make changes. As proof of this commitment, he noted that he had not used any alcohol or drugs during the past 5 days, had attended his intake session, had begun to attend self-help group meetings, and had begun to spend time with acquaintances who did not use drugs.

Paul discussed his specific goals with his counselor, and together they drafted a treatment plan.

Treatment Plan

Long-term goals

1. Establish and maintain total abstinence from all addictive substances
2. Acquisition and maintenance of meaningful and fulfilling social relationships
3. Acquisition and use of skills to recognize and deal with high-risk situations for relapse
4. Stable employment consistent with his capabilities

Short-term objectives

Goal	Intervention
1. Identification of negative consequences of drug use	Conduct comprehensive drug use history, via interview and questionnaire measures, to identify drug use consequences in life-functioning domains (e.g., work, family, social, physical, legal). Refer for physical examination and laboratory workup.
2. Establish and maintain abstinence	Contract for continuation of the 5-day abstinent period client brought to intake. Monitor signs of withdrawal. Monitor cravings for drugs. Monitor contacts with drug-using friends. Apply strategies to deal with cravings (e.g., relaxation training, alternative activities) and invitations to use (e.g., refusal skills, assertiveness). Identify alternatives to drug use (e.g., preplanning evening activities with family or non-drug-using friends) to preclude getting together with drug-using friends. Attend self-help groups, such as Narcotics Anonymous or Cocaine Anonymous, at least three times per week.

3. Initiate vocational planning	Referral for vocational counseling to identify areas of strength.
	Review classified advertisements and other outlets to identify employment opportunities.
	Practice interviewing skills, including explanation for sporadic work history to date.
4. Expand scope of social contacts	Identify non-drug-using friends.
	Identify and attend functions not associated with drug use (e.g., seminars, classes).

Comments

Treatment will entail biweekly sessions for the first 3 months, with additional sessions added as needed. These sessions will focus primarily on short-term objectives 1 and 2. Assuming progress on objectives 1 and 2, attention will shift to objectives 3 and 4. Weekly sessions are planned for months 3–6; scheduling of subsequent sessions will be evaluated at that point in time. Treatment plan will be reviewed and updated accordingly at least every 3 months.

APPRECIATING THE DIVERSITY OF CLIENTS

The development of an individualized treatment plan requires a sensitivity to and appreciation of the wide diversity represented by the clients with whom we work. The factor most often taken into account is ethnic and racial background. However, as noted by Miller (1999), clients differ as well along the important dimensions of gender, age, education, socioeconomic status, sexual orientation, and psychological health. Accordingly, clinicians will need to be sensitive to these dimensions of diversity in their evaluation of assessment data, in the development of treatment goals, and in the application of interventions focused on behavior change.

SUMMARY

   • The treatment plan, developed in collaboration with the client, is intended to address treatment goals. It organizes, integrates, and prioritizes the information gathered during the assessment process.

   • The plan is highlighted by a delineation of treatment goals and a corresponding set of clinical interventions.

• Treatment objectives typically are prioritized and divided as well into short-term and long-term goals.

• The establishment of short-term and long-term goals is influenced by a variety of factors, including extent and seriousness of the substance use problem, client motivational readiness to change, the availability of significant others, and the projected period of treatment involvement.

• Treatment plans should be viewed as flexible and changeable.

• Qualities of well-formed treatment goals include being salient and meaningful to the client, manageable, specific, and appropriate for the projected treatment period.

• In developing the treatment plan, the therapist needs to attend as well to engendering a productive therapeutic alliance with the client and enhancing the client's motivation to change.

• Treatment plans need to reflect an appreciation of client diversity.

5

Individual Treatment

Individual treatment is uniquely suited to viewing change as a multidimensional, personal process that includes the stages of change. Moving forward through the journey of change requires individuals to address adequately the critical tasks and accompanying challenges presented by each of the stages (DiClemente, 2005a; DiClemente, Carbonari, & Velasquez, 1992). Tasks of a client in precontemplation who has little or no consideration of quitting cocaine use in the foreseeable future are much different from those that same person will face when he or she moves into the action stage and tries to implement a quit plan. The point at which an individual in contemplation resolves ambivalence and moves from decision making to creating and committing to an action plan depends both on individual effort and a variety of unique circumstances. In fact, each action plan is unique and has to be adapted to the skills and life circumstances of the individual substance abuser. The path to sobriety or risk reduction for each individual will differ greatly as he or she meets the various challenges along the path of intentional change. Although we can identify the overall shape of the path using the stages of change, how each substance abuser travels that path, becomes engaged in the recovery process, overcomes barriers along the way, and learns from his or her slips and relapses about how to "get it right" and be successful is unique.

Individual treatment is designed to assist each addicted individual to move forward in the process of change, to consolidate completion of critical tasks, and ultimately to achieve successful sustained change. The individual therapist is in a position to listen closely to the client, to provide assistance, to help access resources, and to offer support for multiple client needs so that he or she completes effectively and efficiently the key tasks of the various stages of recovery (see Table 5.1). There are two critical issues to consider when using individual treatment approaches to address the client's personal process of change. The first is the important distinction between a "treatment plan" and a "change plan." The former represents what the therapist and client develop and organize for the client, usually focused on what the therapist will provide and focus on in the treatment. The latter is the personal action plan that includes what the client incorporates, commits to, and completes as he or she works through the stages of change. The second issue is related to the first in that the "treatment plan" should be in the service of the "change plan." One of the advantages of individual treatment is that it can be flexible in addressing the diverse needs of the client. However, in practice many individual treatments are offered in a rigid format (a 50- or 60-minute session once a week) with a predetermined, modular content delivered in a rather inflexible sequence (12 specific CBT modules in 12 weeks). If the flexibility, adaptability, and personalization of individual treatment are lost or limited, its unique strength for facilitating individual change plans and the substance abuser's personal pathway to recovery is greatly weakened.

The first task of a therapist meeting the client in treatment is to assess not only the scope and severity of the problem but also where the individual stands in the process of changing his or her substance abuse behaviors. In the assessment chapter, we discussed ways that stage of change and related client change variables can be evaluated on entry to treatment. The ongoing assessment challenge involves the need to identify which key tasks have been or need to be accomplished and to

TABLE 5.1. Critical Tasks at Each Stage of Change

Stage	Critical tasks
Precontemplation	Generating concern, interest, and hope
Contemplation	Risk–reward analysis, resolving ambivalence, decision making
Preparation	Creating commitment, planning, prioritizing
Action	Implementing plan, overcoming obstacles, revising plan
Maintenance	Sustaining change, preventing relapse, integrating change into lifestyle, avoiding change fatigue

evaluate how engaged the client is in the coping activities or processes of change (e.g., consciousness raising, self-reevaluation, stimulus control, and/or counterconditioning). Only then can individualized interventions proceed.

Since stage status is viewed as a mutable state and not a static trait, it is productive to continue checking in often with the client to evaluate progress and how well he or she is accomplishing stage-related tasks. Substance abusers can move around in the stages from day to day or week to week, and sometimes during a single session. Stage status is a dynamic characteristic. Although some individuals can stay in the same stage for long periods of time spanning months or years (Carbonari, DiClemente, & Sewell, 1999), the potential for swift movement and sudden shifts in stage status is both understandable and well documented (DiClemente, 2006; Miller & C'de Baca, 2001; Wholey, 1984).

Recent criticisms of the stages have argued that a stage view is too linear and rational and that changes in smoking and other addictions can occur in a more chaotic and less planned fashion (West, 2008). Some retrospective reports of how the change happened seem to support a more "spontaneous" quick onset. When asked, individuals will say "I woke up and decided this was it," "One day someone in an AA meeting told my story," or "I quit cold turkey." However, often they fail to mention how many times in the past year they had tried to do this, how many years they had attended AA meetings, and that they had been gradually cutting back on smoking while making the decision to stop. On the other hand, if you follow individuals longitudinally over several time points, the process seems much more laborious, with individuals struggling with the various tasks of overcoming ambivalence, making a decision, creating and perfecting plans, and making repeated attempts (DiClemente & Scott, 1997; Marlatt & Donovan, 2005; Prochaska, DiClemente, Velicer, Ginpil, & Norcross, 1985; Prochaska et al., 1991).

The bottom line is that the experience of change is variable. Some individuals can get stuck in a stage or seem to therapists that they are spinning their wheels with multiple unsuccessful attempts to change. However, counselors also can see stage tasks being accomplished over a very short period of time. If one watches motivational interviewing training tapes, it is obvious that substantive work on stage tasks can happen within a single session. In one particular tape titled *The Rounder*, Dr. Theresa Moyers skillfully interviews an individual (Jim) who walks into the session pushed by his lawyer and believing that he did not need to be there or to change his drinking. By focusing on Jim's concerns and perspective, Dr. Moyers helped him reflect on and reevaluate his situation. By the end of that session he is considering that "maybe I need to do something about my drinking or I am going to be right back in this same place." At the end of this 20-minute interview Jim expresses a decisional balance tipped toward change as well as significant ambivalence about the prospect of making the change. This is a clear example of a client engaging in relevant processes of change (self- and environmental reevaluation, emotional arousal/dramatic relief, consciousness raising) that lead to beginning accomplishment of critical tasks of creating interest and concern and tipping decisional balance that lead to advancing stage status. As all clinicians recognize, it does not "always" happen this quickly. Although a leap of change that seems to take shortcuts around some of the tasks of the stages is possible, there is a lot of "work" that is accomplished on these tasks that is less obvious and not always fully recognized by clients or researchers (see discussion in Chapter 11).

The notion of stage as a state and not a trait implies that it is better to think about clients being "in precontemplation" rather than "being precontemplators." Stages should not be used as labels to sort people. Stage-specific tasks (see Table 5.1) offer direction as to the approach to be taken and strategies to employ, and even as to the type of interpersonal stance that may best promote change (DiClemente, 2003, 2005a; Prochaska & Norcross, 2007; DiClemente et al., 1992).

This chapter describes how to evaluate stage status and pursue the critical tasks of change during the course of treatment and suggests intervention techniques that could be used at each of the stages of change. Case examples will illustrate issues and strategies. Changing substance abuse behavior requires shifts in multiple areas of an individual's functioning and environment (DiClemente, 1999a). For each of the stages, we discuss what may need to occur in the functioning and in the environment of a client and highlight some strategies to help clients make the needed changes or shifts in thinking, experiencing, and behaving. There are some processes of change (client coping activities) that appear to be critical in making the transition from one stage to the next. We highlight these and offer some strategies for engaging these processes. The list of therapist strategies is never exhaustive, as clinicians search continually for new ways to influence clients or new techniques to promote movement through the stages. The search for new and unique ways to influence the process of change represents one of the most creative and dynamic aspects of therapy.

ASSESSING THE STAGES OF CHANGE IN A CLINICAL SETTING

As described in Chapter 3, there are a number of strategies to assess where individuals stand in the process of changing their substance use (Carey et al., 1999; DiClemente et al., 2009; DiClemente & Hughes, 1990; DiClemente, Schlundt, & Gemmell, 2004; Belding, Iguchi, & Lamb, 1996; Carney & Kivlahan, 1995; Isenhart, 1994; Napper et al., 2008). Each formal assessment strategy has advantages and disadvantages and only some of them can easily be used throughout the course of treatment. However, no matter what assessment is employed, a single intake assessment of stage status is completely inadequate to guide the entire course of treatment since individuals can move from one stage to the next and even slip back to an earlier stage from week to week, day to day, or even hour to hour. Consequently, ongoing clinical assessment of stage status and task completion is imperative. Even with an assignment to stage based on a measure administered at intake, a clinician must always check to be aware of precisely which stage tasks a client is facing.

It is important to view stage status as we do drinking or drug use status. For example, when clinicians want to be sure that a client is not using a drug, they ask the client and sometimes even collect a urine sample at some visits. The assumption is that drug use status can change at any point from one visit to the next. Failure to check substance use during the past week can provide some unwelcome surprises midway into a session. Similarly with stage of change, the client can move back and forth from one time point to the next. Accordingly, clinicians need to assess the client's stage of change frequently, ideally in a manner that is not obtrusive or burdensome and one that facilitates client self-understanding. Although more extensive paper-and-pencil assessments can be useful especially in research, a sensitive assessment and discussion of stage status by the therapist at the beginning and end of each session is an easy and efficient way to track stage for a particular client.

Clients can also be enlisted in the assessment process. In some cases, clients are taught the concept of stages and the processes of change at the beginning of treatment or are given the book *Changing for Good* (Prochaska, Norcross, & DiClemente, 1994). Then, during the course of therapy, they are asked to reflect and indicate where they think they are in the process (DiClemente, 2003; Prochaska, Norcross, & DiClemente, 1994; Velasquez et al., 2001).

In a recent consultation with a dual-diagnosis treatment program, one of us (DiClemente) interviewed a client who had returned to drinking and drug use in the past few days and was now back at the clinic. Staff thought of her as having relapsed and back in precontemplation for abstinence. However, the client believed that this was a slip and that she continued to be in action though sobered by the recent events and realizing that she needed to do something different. When this was shared with the staff and they approached the client consistent with her perspective, there seemed to be somewhat of a breakthrough and a mutual recognition of what needed to be done next.

Getting an accurate stage status assessment by interview requires an accurate understanding of client attitudes and behaviors. Predetermined or minimally informed judgments about the stage status of any particular client at any specific time can be erroneous. The staff of one treatment clinic erroneously assumed that almost all of the cocaine-addicted individuals entering treatment were in action simply because they had not used cocaine in the past 24 hours. However, these clients were merely resting between binges, seeking respite, and mostly not motivated to change. Clients and therapists often see things differently. Research has demonstrated that therapists' ratings of the therapeutic relationship were often different from those of their clients in responses to questions about important dimensions of the therapy relationship (e.g., Connors, Carroll, DiClemente, Longabough, & Donovan, 1997).

The difficulty in accurately assessing client motivation and stage of change is even more complicated in settings in which clients feel that they must give "right" answers or provide what programs want to hear. In these settings clients are less likely to make or share accurate self-appraisals. This is particularly relevant in criminal justice and legally mandated treatment settings. In any case, clinical judgments based on quick impressions, biased assumptions, or poor listening can contribute to inaccurate evaluations of clients. For accurate stage assessment, a therapist needs to allow the client to be open and listen carefully to what the client is experiencing, thinking, and doing with respect to the problem. The following vignettes represent second sessions with two different clients.

Armand M arrived about 5 minutes late for his therapy session, complaining about the traffic. He immediately began talking about his wife, Anne, and her hypercritical way of managing the children. He described in detail several incidents that illustrated his concerns, recounting several confrontations between his wife and their 10-year-old daughter, Amanda. One of these incidents happened the morning of the session and so was fresh in Armand's mind. When the discussion finally got back to talking about his drinking problem, Armand said that he had been "working on it." Contrary to his usual pattern, he declined an invitation to go out with his business associates on Friday evening. He was proud of this and felt that it proved that he had some control over his drinking. However, he had been drinking at home throughout the weekend. As he discussed his drinking, he mentioned that not drinking would present a real dilemma for him since he would have to change his business life-style. In addition, he acknowledged he would need to find other ways to manage his anger at Anne for her rigidity. Drinking helped him escape from his frustration at home.

Bill F arrived at his session on time and was accompanied by his wife, Barbara. At the beginning of the session he asked if Barbara could join in the session since she was concerned about the treatment and wanted to know more about his problem. He did drink a substantial amount of alcohol over the weekend and had been discussing the possibility of his being an "alcoholic" with Barbara. She was very disturbed by this revelation and the "alcoholic" characterization. Bill now believed he had a serious drinking problem and that it was time to do something. He had been thinking about how to solve the problem when he and his wife had this discussion about abstinence and about being an alcoholic. Barbara was very concerned that their social life would be threatened if he needed to be abstinent.

It is apparent that Armand and Bill are in different places with respect to changing their drinking. Although there are glimmers of insight and contemplation stage activity, Armand does not appear ready to move out of precontemplation. The focus on associated problems, such as his wife's child management skills and personal characteristics, provides a related but distinct sidebar and is a sign that he is not ready to focus on his drinking behavior. It would be a much different scenario if he were trying to problem-solve the child management issues in order to focus on his drinking. However, without discussing clearly how child management and his drinking were related, Armand is communicating that he is not ready to consider changing his drinking behavior at this time. Unwillingness to focus thought and energy onto consideration of the problem or change is a sign of precontemplation. Armand's acknowledgment that losing his drinking would have some serious other consequences is a beginning consideration but focuses on a reason not to change rather than a reason to change. Multiple problems in the life of a substance abuser are the norm. How the client and the therapist view these problems and their relationship with the drinking or drug use are critical to understanding stage status and the difference between target and contextual problems (DiClemente, 2003).

Bill, on the other hand, has moved through the contemplation stage and is entering preparation. The tasks that are a main focus of one particular stage often need continued attention throughout the entire process of change (DiClemente, 2003; DiClemente & Prochaska, 1998; Prochaska & DiClemente, 1984). Evaluating pros and cons, a primary task of the contemplation stage, continues into the preparation stage. In fact, Bill's wife, Barbara, raises concerns that Bill must now evaluate as potential cons for change. These considerations may encourage him to back off from making an action plan and become more ambivalent returning to the contemplation stage of change. However, Bill's acknowledgment that he has a serious problem with drinking and that something must be done is a sign of preparation stage activity. The plan is not yet developed, so additional work has to be accomplished to complete the preparation tasks well enough to move forward into action. Nevertheless, the tasks of preparation have begun. The therapist's challenge is to help Bill continue his movement forward and to neutralize the concerns of his wife so that they do not interfere with these efforts. Bill's opening remarks indicate that the involvement of his spouse would be an important addition to the treatment endeavor. In fact, both Armand and Bill and their respective spouses could potentially benefit from some couples intervention since the respective spouses seem to be presenting barriers to completing some change tasks. However, timing and the extent of spouse involvement should be different based on ongoing evaluations of how directly relevant and how supportive the spouse can be in the client's struggle with the tasks of change.

As becomes evident in this assessment of stage status, intervention strategies and topics are developed as the stage status and tasks unfold. There are key points to remember about assessing stage status clinically. The assessment should not focus on the labels of the stages but on understanding what current stage tasks clients are struggling with and where they are in the overall process of change. For example, assessing the client's level of interest and concern is critical for understanding how these are influencing the process of getting out of and staying out of precontemplation.

The following elements for a productive conversation about motivation and stage status are really part of every good interview. Not surprisingly, they overlap with the techniques presented in Chapter 4 in the context of moving clients toward a determination that change is necessary and achievable. The following techniques highlight why motivational interviewing (Miller & Rollnick, 1991, 2002) and the concept of stage status and tasks can be integrated so productively.

1. *Listen.* If the therapist begins by talking and asking too many questions, particularly questions that are closed-ended (ones that can be answered with a yes or no) or too leading (You are working on your plan, aren't you?), it will be difficult to assess stage accurately. To assess stage, therapists should listen specifically to reports about the target behavior (e.g., cocaine use, drinking, heroin use, gambling behavior) and any client thoughts, intentions, attitudes, and experiences related to that target behavior. Open questions such as "What concerns do you have about your cocaine use?" or "What, if anything, would you change about your drinking?" can elicit the client's thoughts about problems caused by substance use and ideas about change. The fact that a client drank or used drugs during the past week does not automatically indicate his or her stage as was illustrated above. Continuing abstinence is a good sign and often indicative of action or maintenance stage status unless the abstinence represents simply a normal hiatus in use (a cocaine user coming off a run and not using for a few days) or an imposed or coerced state (stopping drinking or drug use simply to prove that one does not have a problem or to satisfy some external demand). Answers to questions like "Did you drink?," "Would you like to stop?," and "Can you quit?" do not automatically or necessarily allow the therapist to assess stage. Listening carefully to the client's thought process and his or her attitudes, concerns, and intentions are the most productive ways to observe and assess client change process status and to promote movement (Rollnick et al., 1999).

2. *Ask probing, open-ended questions.* It is useful to seek additional information by focusing on the client's perspective and not those of wife, coworker, or probation officer. Stage assignment must be based

on the client's actions, attitudes, and views (DiClemente, 2003; DiClemente & Prochaska, 1998). The number of individuals who are nagging him or her does not measure client commitment to change nor does the number of consequences experienced. In fact, pressure to change can result in three very different responses from the client. On the positive side, sometimes pressure can provoke thoughtful consideration of the problem and the possibility of change. However, other times, pressure or confrontation brings with it feigned compliance and a hardening of resistance to change (Miller, Benefield, & Tonigan, 1993). Finally, pressure can provoke open resistance in a variety of displays (interrupting, denying, denigrating, ignoring). Only by asking open-ended questions and being open and understanding to all potential responses can a therapist gain access to client reactions. Thus, asking Armand about the good things and not-so-good things about his use of alcohol as a way of managing frustration with his wife, Anne, could engage a decision-making conversation and also give some view of the decisional balance.

3. *Check your perceptions.* One of the most useful motivational interviewing strategies for making an accurate assessment of stage status is summarizing (Miller & Rollnick, 1991, 2002). Summaries allow for periodically checking whether you, the therapist, have it right; asking if the client means this or that; repeating what you heard; and offering a summary in your own words of what you have heard from the client in terms of his or her stage status. Summaries also can acknowledge stage tasks and reflect what the client has accomplished or needs to accomplish. These strategies can assist therapists to understand client intentions and assess whether what the therapist sees as a pro or con for drinking or drug use has that same meaning for the client. These summaries and the ensuing conversation also support change talk and support Desire, Ability, Reasons, and Needs (DARN) language (Miller & Rollnick, 2002). Armed with accurate information from the client, the therapist can determine where the client is in the process of change and what current challenges he or she faces.

4. *Review stage status regularly.* If a client is moving forward through the stages, as Bill appears to be, the therapeutic work during a session helps clients engage in specific processes of change that produce movement. Reviewing stage status at the end of the session as well as at the beginning is another important strategy, again focusing on the tasks and not simply the labels. Clients generally make the transitions from one stage to the next on their own during the time between sessions.

After the session they have time to reflect and become engaged in relevant and specific process activity. While therapists sometimes may be able to observe clients move forward out of precontemplation and into contemplation or from contemplation to preparation during a session, this is not typical because such transitions often are difficult to capture and occur in the personal space of the client. In any case, it is important to check regularly on stage status so as to be able to determine when clients look like they are making or have made transitions from one stage to another.

It also is important to remember that regression is almost as likely as progression in the stages, so sensitivity to movement in either direction is warranted. Offering some type of process-of-change summary at the end of a session and checking it with the client can ensure a better understanding of his or her personal journey through the process. Establishing a clear understanding of stage status and tracking that status over time is at the heart of matching individual interventions to client stage of change. Respectful exploration of a client's stage status precedes development of the intervention plan. Of course, that plan also would need to be revised as needed based upon client movement or lack of movement through the stages of change.

MEETING THE CLIENT'S NEEDS AT EACH STAGE OF CHANGE

Precontemplation Stage

Individual therapy with a client in precontemplation allows the therapist to explore reasons why this person has come into treatment. A naïve observer might assume that no individual in a precontemplation stage would come to treatment. However, reports from clinical studies as well as descriptions from clinicians on the front lines indicate that many individuals come to treatment not seriously considering change and not prepared to change (Ryan, Plant, & O'Malley, 1995; Simpson & Joe, 1993; Simpson, Joe, Rowan-Szal, & Greener, 1995). Studies show that there is a wide range of scores on measures of motivation on entry to treatment depending on the treatment population (DiClemente & Hughes, 1990; DiClemente et al., 2009; Project MATCH Research Group, 1997a).

Many reasons for seeking treatment do not include changing substance use behaviors. The most obvious is a criminal justice referral to treatment. Judges, probation officers, and lawyers often tell an individual that they must go to treatment to satisfy a legal requirement or to impress those making sentencing judgments. Individuals in mandated treatment often attend and "cooperate" without any real intention to change their behavior permanently. The personal goal for these individuals is to satisfy the legal system and get out of trouble. For others the rationale is similar but the scenario different. Many clients simply want to satisfy a wife or husband who is threatening to leave, parents who have become fed up with the behavior, or employers who want something done to solve problems at work. Many clients openly admit that their primary motivation for seeking treatment is to satisfy an external demand. Other individuals in precontemplation may be seeking confirmation that they do *not* have a problem. Finally, some individuals come into treatment with a goal of changing others and not themselves. There are, of course, many variations on these themes. Unless programs are very selective, when therapists look closely at intakes and caseloads, they often discover that a number of treatment seekers are in precontemplation or contemplation for changing their substance use behavior even though they may be cooperating at a superficial level with program requirements (Isenhart, 1994; Donovan, 1999). Motivation for treatment is not necessarily the same as motivation for change (DiClemente, 1999b; Freyer-Adam et al., 2009).

Traditional approaches to meeting an individual who comes to treatment in precontemplation have included skepticism, advice, and a healthy dose of confrontation. Advice has often taken the form of labeling ("You are a drug addict" or "You are an alcoholic") in an attempt to convince the client in precontemplation that he or she has a serious problem (Johnson, 1986). This type of advice giving is likely to benefit only those clients who are in precontemplation by virtue of a lack of information or have been brought in by some dramatic event that undermines self- or social esteem, making them open to considering such a label.

Ignorance does not seen to be the reason most individuals remain in precontemplation. Many substance abusers stay in precontemplation by doing something to keep them there. They minimize risks, rationalize dangers and consequences, and/or resign themselves to their addiction (Daniels, 1998; DiClemente, 1991). Often there is an element of rebellion and resentment at being told that they have a problem. So confrontation and advice generally are met with resistance. However, resistance may well be a function of the approach that the therapist takes in conjunction with the client reluctance to seriously consider change.

Confrontation and telling people they are wrong or to do something they do not want to do usually elicit resistance behaviors from clients (Miller et al., 1993).

The introduction of motivational interviewing and enhancement strategies has moderated or eliminated to a large extent the use of these traditional approaches. Motivational enhancement approaches integrated with the stages-of-change model recognize lack of motivation as a part of the process of change and use motivational approaches to address the needs of the substance abuser in precontemplation (Miller, 1985, 1999; Miller & Rollnick, 1991, 2002; Rollnick, Miller, & Butler, 2008). Although motivation is a critical issue throughout the process of change, especially for addictions (Miller, 1999, 2006), it is particularly important for assisting individuals to progress who are dealing with precontemplation and contemplation tasks. Respect, careful and active listening, reflecting and summarizing, and highlighting discrepancies between goals and behaviors are all particularly useful parts of motivational enhancement approaches for early stage clients (Miller, 1985; Miller et al., 1992; Rollnick et al., 1999).

Motivational approaches have become standard in many substance abuse programs and organizations. Some have implemented intake procedures that include evaluating readiness to change and offering a brief motivational intervention to clients identified as the least ready—primarily those in precontemplation and early contemplation. Clients are reassessed at the end of these brief interventions. If they demonstrate sufficient readiness, they are given more intensive cognitive-behavioral or other types of interventions. Other programs offer a preintervention or brief motivational intervention that stimulates motivation prior to a more intensive treatment. The COMBINE study (Anton et al., 2006), for example, used a treatment that combined initial sessions of motivational approaches with a tailored series of cognitive-behavioral modules and self-help interventions. Whether programmatically or simply as part of clinical practice, therapists need to address the motivational needs of individuals entering treatment who are not really interested, concerned, or convinced of the need for change. If a client is not considering change, clearly it is contraindicated for a therapist to begin using intensive, action-oriented clinical interventions.

For clients who are actively discounting both the seriousness of their problem and the need to change, helping them to begin to consider change is not simple. However, within every substance-abusing client who does not want to consider that he or she has a drug use or drinking problem or needs to change, there lies a reservoir of doubt. The therapist has the task of encouraging and creating in the client thoughts that the problem perhaps is really larger than perceived by the client ("Maybe all these consequences are related to my use of cocaine," "Maybe my wife or husband is right"). The goal is to tap into that reservoir of doubt so that the doubt can be turned into serious consideration of change. Providing sensitive personal feedback, reflecting concerns, examining values, and exposing clients to convincing role models or to experiences that arouse emotions and awareness can be used to expose doubt and raise personal awareness. Leading someone in precontemplation on a path of discovery and realization requires a sensitive, empathic, but firm guide. Techniques that raise awareness without raising resistance obviously would be the most productive (DiClemente, 1991). Techniques highlighted in motivational interviewing approaches, such as double-sided reflection, objective feedback, and rolling with resistance (Miller & Rollnick, 1991; Bien, Miller, & Boroughs, 1993), along with basic relational elements such as empathy, genuineness, acceptance, and regard can also be effective in eliciting awareness (Prochaska & Norcross, 1999; Norcross, 2002).

The challenge for the individual therapist in each of the stages is to instigate the change processes that move the individual to complete the task and move to the next stage. For individuals in precontemplation, the processes of consciousness raising, self-reevaluation, environmental reevaluation, and emotional arounsal/dramatic relief are the most relevant. Table 5.2 provides a view of the strategies that could be used to engage the client in these processes, and the tasks to be accomplished as a result. These strategies can be done both in individual and group formats. For example, Velasquez and colleagues (2001) have created a stage-based group therapy manual that is infused with motivational enhancement strategies for early stage sessions. *PRIME for Life*, developed by the Prevention Research Institute (2009), is another example of blending motivational and personally relevant informational feedback strategies into a program for alcohol and drug users with driving offenses. These individuals often attend simply to fulfill requirements to get their licenses back with little or no interest in significantly changing their drinking.[1]

---

[1]Carlo C. DiClemente serves as a paid consultant to the Prevention Research Institute.

TABLE 5.2. Tasks and Strategies for Precontemplation Stage

Strategies	Tasks
Values clarification	Raising awareness of problem
Normative feedback	Realization of consequences and the impact of behavior on others
Visiting AA meetings	Peer influence and modeling
Couples meeting	Feedback from a significant other
Motivational interviewing	Contrast of current life and goals

There are also treatment strategies that are contraindicated for the client in precontemplation. Giving individuals in precontemplation action assignments would not be a good match of technique to client stage. Offering medications to curtail craving or create a negative physiological response to drinking would also be contraindicated. In fact, both medication compliance and the goal of medical management of drinking cues, craving, or consequences would be subverted without adequate motivation. There have been many examples of medication goals being thwarted by dedicated substance-abusing clients. Alcoholics have been known to learn how to drink even while taking disulfiram (Antabuse). Heroin addicts have been known to use cocaine, marijuana, and other drugs along with their methadone. Medicating a client in precontemplation for intentional change can be problematic at the very least. In addition, an individual who fails to change using a medication regime may come to believe that nothing can help. On the other hand, medications used properly and with behavior change strategies often can be very effective when the client is properly motivated (O'Brien, 1996).

Under threat of consequences, clients in precontemplation often will do what is required to fulfill the letter of the law. They may attend but not really participate in a change process and simply go through the motions. Nonetheless, access offers opportunity. Mandated and coerced presence offers a chance to find innovative ways to provoke self-reevaluation and to use the motivational strategies described above in order to engage the individual in activities that can increase interest and concern and foster serious consideration of change. Therapists need to use this leverage wisely and not lose it by telling the client that he or she can leave if he or she does not want to be there.

Contemplation Stage

Once an individual begins to seriously consider change, the focus turns to a personal evaluation of the pros and cons of the behavior and of the potential change and the need to resolve the ambivalence associated with the decisional process. This is not as straightforward a task as it might seem. Some therapists simply draw a line down a sheet of paper, write at the top "*Pros*" and "*Cons*," and then ask the client to list all of the pros and all of the cons that come to mind. It is seldom that easy. Many of the pros as well as the cons are rather ill-defined and not immediately accessible. Some are double-sided and have both positives and negatives within the same decisional consideration. When asked, substance-abusing clients often provide therapists with a long list of negative aspects of using. They believe that this is what the therapist wants to hear. Encouraging the client in contemplation to describe explicitly the good things about using drugs or drinking and how substance use has many functions for them is not easy. More importantly, this is not an intellectual exercise but a very personal risk versus reward analysis. Some of the reasons are very personal and require clients to admit how they rely on alcohol and/or other drugs to manage life. Assisting the client to explore these issues requires attentive listening and probing, open-ended questions as well as conveying a sense of caring and concern.

Completing contemplation tasks requires continued engagement in the processes of consciousness raising, self-reevaluation, and environmental reevaluation. Reevaluation involves values, and so it is critical to explore the current and core values of the clients. The objective is to tie reasons *for* change and *against* staying with the substance abuse status quo to important considerations and values of the client. Exploring values using a values card sort or some other type of values clarification activity is important for contemplation tasks. Instead of simply making the client aware of the consequences of the problem, the task of contemplation is a comparator one in which the individual evaluates the entire decisional matrix. What is critical is whether the considerations that foster change outweigh in importance and salience those that do not and lead to a firm decision. Figure 5.1 offers a schema for these considerations.

There are self-report measures that tap into these considerations and have clients rate their relative importance in service of assessing whether reasons supporting change outweigh reasons for resisting change. However, exploring this question is not simply an exercise in reasoning. Each

Supporting the status quo	Promoting change
Positives of the behavior	Negatives of the behavior
Negatives of the change	Positives of the change

FIGURE 5.1. Decisional balance worksheet.

reason has an affective valence or weight that is important to evaluate. There may be many moderately important reasons to change and one major reason not to change, or vice versa, that would influence the decision making. Similar types of considerations appear to be relevant for individuals with different substance abuse problems and for those in treatment as well as those who change without accessing formal treatment (DiClemente, 2006; Klingemann, 1991; Sobell, Sobell, Tonneato, & Leo, 1993; Tucker, Vuchinich, & Pukish, 1995).

Carl was a heavy drinker who had thought about his drinking and was well satisfied that there was little problem in his frequent drinking except that it led to nagging by his wife. One day while driving along a freeway, his 3-year-old son pointed to a billboard advertising a particular brand of liquor and stated that is what his daddy drank and that is what he was going to drink. This experience had such an impact on Carl's thinking and decisional balance that he moved to a decision to quit drinking and smoking. Rather quickly he stopped drinking almost entirely. His fear of his son imitating his pattern of drinking was a decisional consideration that clearly outweighed his many positive reasons for drinking.

Therapists and counselors would love to create such transformational moments but it is difficult to create them in a therapy session. But there are techniques that can foster the reevaluation and affective arousal processes that Carl experienced. Sometimes it is possible to have clients imagine past events that represent particularly painful or difficult consequences related to their substance abuse. For those clients with a family history, the therapist can help the client to recreate or reexperience some of the parental or familial events that were marred by drinking. The objective of these exercises is to have the client recognize and relive emotionally important experiences that may have been glossed over. In a similar way therapists can ask clients to imagine that they are functioning and interacting without the aid of the drug in order to trigger the discussion of the pros and cons of change. Psychodrama and exercises that were developed in gestalt therapy can also be used to make decisional considerations more vivid, affect-laden, and powerful. For example, role-playing a conversation with a parent, spouse, or boss where the client moves from one chair to another in the room and takes both parts of the conversation could elicit significant self-reevaluation. The ultimate goal of these exercises is to promote the reevaluation process and ultimately the creation of a firm decision to change.

Any strategies or techniques to promote decision making would be useful with the client in contemplation. Values clarification exercises in which the client is asked to explore hopes and dreams, to examine what values are represented by the current lifestyle, or to remember family values taught while growing up can set the stage for decision making. Few clients had as a goal in life to become a drug abuser. Most still have some ideas about what they would like from their lives. Accessing their aspirations and currently unrealized values can encourage a serious evaluation of "where I am" versus "where I want to be or hoped to be."

Many of the motivational interviewing strategies described by Miller and Rollnick (1991, 2002) are designed to address the ambivalence experienced in the contemplation stage and to promote decision making for change. Training in these strategies of amplification, double-sided reflection, and rolling with resistance can be very helpful for the therapist seeking to engender contemplation. There are also a number of books that discuss the social psychological phenomenon of persuasion (e.g., Cialdini, 1988). These outline strategies used in marketing and other professional settings where the objective is to have a consumer consider and ultimately purchase a product or choose a service. Adapting these strategies for use in the treatment of substance use would be particularly helpful in working with the client in contemplation. In many ways the therapist with a client in the contemplation stage must be a bit of a salesperson. The therapist needs to engender interest in and consideration of change and ultimately make change a product that is attractive to the consumer/client and one that is chosen (Backinger et al., 2010).

Preparation Stage

Making a decision and following through with appropriate action are not the same. Although the primary responsibility for taking action resides with the client, therapists can assist in helping the client prepare for action. A serious misconception held by some therapists is the belief that once a decision is made, the client moves automatically into action. Client statements like "I really am convinced that I should do something about my cocaine problem" or "I am going to quit drinking" are music to the ear of the therapist who has been working with a client in precontemplation or contemplation and represents important change and commitment language. However, the large numbers of clients who drop out of treatment early in therapy, often after making some of these statements, are a sobering reminder of the elusive nature of these decisions (Simpson & Joe, 1993; Smith, Subich, & Kalodner, 1995; Wickizer et al., 1994). The focus of treatment for the client in preparation is planning and commitment enhancement. It is the sufficiency of the plan and the strength of the commitment that will enable the client to begin to take appropriate actions and to follow through on the change plan.

From the stages-of-change perspective, as noted earlier in this chapter, the treatment plan should operate in service of the client's action plan. The action plan specifies what the client needs to do to change the drinking and drug use behavior. In the preparation stage, the therapist should help the client construct this action plan (DiClemente, 1991, 2003). There is some evidence from the smoking cessation literature that if there is some specificity to the action plan, such as setting a date when the action will begin, there is a greater probability of moving into the action stage (Agency for Health Care Policy and Research, 1996). Specificity and planning promote action.

The action plan should contain the specifics of what the client will do to quit or modify the behavior, how to handle the different days of the week, and how to manage the different opportunities to use that would be anticipated. The plan also should identify who could help and how and what could go wrong in order to build contingency plans. Figure 5.2 illustrates a change plan worksheet that was used in the motivational enhancement therapy developed for Project MATCH. How detailed a plan should be depends on the needs of the client and how much support needs to be provided in terms of treatment setting and intensity. A less detailed plan in a day treatment setting is less worrisome than the

The changes I want to make are: _____

_____

The most important reasons why I want to make these changes are: _____

_____

The steps I plan to take in changing are: _____

_____

The ways other people can help me are:

Person   Possible ways to help

_____   _____

_____   _____

I will know that my plan is working if: _____

_____

Some things that could interfere with my plan are: _____

_____

FIGURE 5.2. Change plan worksheet. From Miller, Zweben, DiClemente, and Rychtarik (1992).

same plan in regular, weekly outpatient treatment. Planning, however, is not ordinarily one of the strengths of the substance abuser. Instead, immediate gratification and what Albert Ellis calls "low frustration tolerance" (LFT; Ellis, McInerney, & DiGiuseppe, 1988) are characteristics of many substance abusers. The therapist needs to work diligently to overcome the reluctance to plan and identify planning as one of the important elements that promote successful change and differentiate the life of sobriety from that of abusing drugs and alcohol.

Planning should include both the identification of the strategies to move successfully into action as well as a checkup of the skills needed to implement these strategies. One of the most important contributions of the therapist to the client in preparation would be to provide an evaluation of the skills needed to implement the plan and attempt to remediate any skills deficits. For a client whose anger often triggers his or her drug use, a plan that does not include anger management training will be flawed from its inception.

The skills that are needed for change can be explored using several different techniques. The most extensive procedure is called a "functional analysis" of the various areas of the life of the drug abuser (Carroll, 1999; Sobell & Sobell, 1981, 1993). This analysis would cover all the major areas of life functioning in order to identify the factors that maintain the drug use behaviors. The objective would be to discover the problematic reinforcers and lack of appropriate reinforcers that influence the behavior of the individual. One approach that has emerged in response to the indications provided through a functional analysis of substance use is the community reinforcement approach, which involves setting up social events, employment groups, and other options to replace the problematic reinforcement system with a more adaptive one that is incompatible with drug use (DeLeon, Melnick, Kressel, & Jainchill, 1994; Mallams, Godley, Hall, & Meyers, 1982; Meyers & Smith, 1995).

The Addiction Severity Index (ASI) was created to obtain a more comprehensive view of the needs of drug abusers and examines multiple areas of functioning that can be problematic, including dimensions of substance use and associated medical, employment, legal, family/social, and psychological problems (McLellan et al., 1994). There are intriguing data indicating that the more services that are accessed to address the various needs of the drug- and alcohol-abusing population, the better the outcomes (McClellan et al., 1994). More comprehensive planning for addressing the varied needs of the clients appears to improve outcomes significantly.

If more extensive methods for assessment and planning are not available, the most productive way to explore problems that interfere with change would be to examine in depth the client's past attempts to change his or her drug and alcohol use behavior. Previous change attempts can be very instructive. What were the plans in the prior attempts? For how long did the client succeed? What were the circumstances of the return to using? Examine all the various tasks of the stages to see if they were completed adequately since often failure to make it through action and maintenance may be due to inadequate completing of earlier stage tasks and not simply the press of the environments or a weakness of self-efficacy. These are the same types of questions that are used to debrief a slip or relapse. The answers can offer a good view of the types of situations and challenges that the client found difficult or impossible to conquer. The skills and strategies to deal with these challenges should be addressed in the current change plan.

Darlene P was a 28-year-old cocaine addict who had a 10-year history of use that accelerated from snorting cocaine to smoking crack. The cocaine had destroyed her marriage and significantly impaired her ability to parent her 7-year-old son, who currently was being cared for by her mother. Darlene had completed high school and had held several jobs as a clerk in various retail stores. She had wanted to go to college but did not have the money and was unsure what she would do with a degree. She started using drugs in high school, and the problem escalated after she graduated and became involved with a man who was selling drugs. She had easy access to drugs for awhile, but after a breakup with this man, she became a prostitute as a way to support her habit. Her subsequent marriage was a bright spot, since she found a partner who wanted to take her away from her drug-abusing life and to have a family. But shortly after the birth of their son, she again began to use cocaine, which created severe marital problems. At the breakup of her marriage, she returned to her drug-abusing life. Currently she was living with a man who had a serious heroin problem. On the ASI, she indicated significant problems in the areas of family, employment, alcohol, drugs, and psychological functioning. She appeared to have a moderate depression that could have been present prior to the drug abuse. When she would try to stop using cocaine, she could stay clean only for a week or two. Some problem, often a frustrating interaction with her son, her mother, her ex-husband, or her boyfriend, would get her down, and she would seek escape in her cocaine and crack use. She had no female friends except for a couple of women she would meet up with when she would go on the streets as a sex worker. She had a sexually transmitted disease and was very concerned about contracting AIDS. She realized that this lifestyle was not working, and she came into the treatment center determined to change her life and get away from her cocaine habit.

Although one would need a more detailed exploration in each of these areas, it is clear from this thumbnail sketch that the action plan for Darlene should be multifaceted and comprehensive if it is to have a chance of success. Strategies and skills to deal with depression, relationships, employment, parenting, and family relations are pertinent to a viable action plan that will increase her ability to sustain abstinence beyond the 1 or 2 weeks that she had been able to achieve in the past. The action plan has to include where she will live, how she will handle her current relationship, who will support sobriety, alternative ways to manage frustration, and dealing with other drug-use related cues and problems. In addition, financial support, employment, and contacts between her and her mother and son would be important problem areas to address both in the action plan and in the treatment plan. If this appears to be an overwhelming task for the therapist, imagine what it looks and feels like to Darlene. Complexity complicates change as well as our attempts to provide realistic change plans.

Commitment is needed to negotiate the action plan, particularly in the early phases of action where the discomfort, sense of loss, disorientation, and physiological reactions are the strongest. It is also clearly needed to address multiple problems in the complicated contextual areas of the client's lifespace. Commitment enhancement is the other critical task of the preparation stage, although most addiction therapists are not given much training in this area. Motivation and willpower are the responsibility of the client and not the therapist. However, there are ways in which the therapist can support and enhance the client's commitment. Choice increases commitment (Prochaska & DiClemente, 1984). Making sure that the client makes choices among possible alternative elements in his or her action or treatment plan can increase a sense of commitment. Encouraging words about the client's ability to change as well as recalling past efforts that were successful can increase the sense of efficacy and choice (Bandura, 1997). Imagining success, as some of our world-class gymnasts and skaters do prior to a performance, can also enhance commitment. Denigrating ability or focusing on past failures would do the opposite. Encouraging positive self-talk can be helpful if based on realistic views of skills and problems. Posing potential barriers to change that enable the client to practice verbally how to overcome these barriers can also be used to create better prepared coping strategies. Helping the client remove any last vestiges of the ambivalence that interferes with action can also be viewed as commitment-enhancing.

Action Stage

Once the action plan is designed and the commitment to follow through with the plan shored up, individuals enter the action stage. The preceding sequence may sound idealistic since many clients move into action before a plan is completely formulated or move into action in fits and starts. What we are describing is an ideal path of movement through the stages of change. However, the tasks of each stage remain important regardless of how the action is begun. One way or another, the successful solution of these tasks is critical to effective action and long-term change.

The need for commitment in the early part of the action stage is paramount since there is much pain and no apparent gain in the first steps of breaking the addiction and removing the drug from the system physically and psychologically. Clients need hope of future relief and a strong desire to break the addiction in order to sustain the effort needed in the action stage. The action plan needs to be implemented, reviewed regularly, and revised as needed. It is the unusual planning process that does not encounter some unanticipated problems once the plan is undertaken. This is as true for building a house as it is for changing behaviors. Some expected support may not be forthcoming, drug-using networks may put more pressure than anticipated, or a drug-using spouse may be very threatened. All of these can create a crisis that requires additional problem solving and alternate strategies in the revision of the plan. Review and revision is an important task in early action that continues into the maintenance stage.

In some respects the therapist has less to do in the action stage when the client is working the agreed-upon plan. Like the coach who prepares the players for the game but can do little on the field once the game has begun, the therapist can offer encouragement and support and provide guidance and strategies along the way (DiClemente, 1991). It is up to the players to complete the plays. However, the coach who can help the players and the team adjust the best to on-field situations and at half time is the one whose team is usually successful. Shifting from more cognitive and experiential processes to the behavioral processes of counterconditioning, stimulus control, and reinforcement management seems to be a central task to be accomplished by the client (Perz, DiClemente, & Carbonari, 1996). These coping activities need to be used to promote abstinence and to cope with urges. The therapist should assist the client in building strategies that incorporate these processes. Creating alternative reinforcers and responses for cues to use; offering relaxation training, refusal skills training, assertiveness, and positive communication training; and helping the client avoid cues that cannot be tolerated are part of the action preparation that allows the client to succeed.

Orchestrating the elements in the action plan to mesh with the various types of treatments and interventions available to meet the needs of the client is a second important function for the individual therapist or counselor. The adage espoused by some self-help groups not to get involved in any other type of treatment or other stressful activities until the addict has 1 year of sobriety has an understandable basis. However, it is not a good rule for all and possibly not helpful for many clients (DiClemente, 2003; DiClemente et al., 1992). Some couples treatment, family therapy, anxiety and anger management, pharmacotherapy, job skills training, additional education, or other adjunctive interventions should be worked into the mix as the client moves through the action stage (Roth & Fonagy, 1996). The objective is to sustain successful action with regard to changing the alcohol- and drug-abusing behaviors for a long enough period of time to gain some stability so the client can move into the maintenance stage. Solving associated problems can assist in creating successful sustained action to continue to abstain from drugs for at least 3 to 6 months before the individual enters into the maintenance stage.

For some clients, pharmacotherapy is an important and valuable part of the action plan. A considerable amount of ongoing clinical research is focusing on developing medications to assist individuals to stop drinking and using drugs. These medications focus on replacing an abused substance with a safer one (e.g., methadone maintenance, nicotine replacement, suboxone), interfering with a drug's mechanism of action to dampen its effect or lessen the craving (naltrexone, acamprosate), or creating a reaction that would make taking the drug less attractive (disulfiram) (see Carroll, 1996a; Myrick & Wright, 2008; O'Brien & Kampman, 2008). Each of these types of medications can offer some assistance in breaking the habit pattern and allow the individual time to institute alternate patterns of behavior. However, it is important to note that these medications most often have been tested in combination with a behavioral or psychological treatment program. Engaging in the behavioral treatment in addition to taking the medication is usually the pattern that produces the significant effect. Note that most of these medications are not designed to be taken for extended periods. Ultimately the important behavioral tasks required to complete the action and maintenance stages successfully will need to be accomplished so that removal of the medication does not provoke relapse.

Maintenance Stage

Few clients remain in treatment as they enter the maintenance stage of change unless the focus of the individual therapy has shifted success-fully to encompass a broader spectrum of client problems beyond those related to the substance use. (Therapeutic communities are the signifi-cant exception to this rule since they usually require a stay of many months or even years.) This loss of contact during the maintenance stage is understandable. Once clients have successfully modified their substance abuse behavior, they reach a plateau of smoother road after the long climb up the mountain of the action stage of change. However, lack of contact during the maintenance stage is unfortunate since recov-ery from an addiction represents the stabilization of what generally had been a chronic condition. Stabilization takes time and requires effort and vigilance. For the most part this lack of follow-up contact is due to a failure on the part of both therapist and client to define the specific tasks of maintenance. Often expectations about how therapy can help during maintenance are unclear and/or limited.

Maintenance tasks are to sustain change over time and to integrate that change into the lifestyle of the individual so that the new behavior, abstinence from alcohol and/or drugs, becomes the preferred, habitual behavior. Sustaining change requires meeting successfully any challenge that arises to threaten the decision or any of the completed tasks on the path of change. Relapse after a long period of abstinence often follows one of several predictable paths (Marlatt & Gordon, 1985; Brownell et al., 1986). The first path begins when the client becomes somewhat overconfident in his or her ability to control drug use, is convinced that he or she will be able stop again without much trouble, and/or is still missing and fond of the recently changed drug-abusing behavior. The second involves the erosion of the commitment to quit using, often fueled by disillusionment with the sober life experienced after change. For this group often a decision either partially or well formed is made to return to the substance. In both cases the individuals decide to use or fail to avoid drinking or using drugs initially once or several times. This return to use compromises maintenance of abstinence and threatens to undermine previous progress toward sustained change. The problem for the individual therapist in this stage is to decide how and when to work with the client over the long haul in order to be able to help with the insidious processes and events that threaten change during this stage.

Individual treatment is ideal in the maintenance stage since it can be designed to occur at less frequent intervals and to include one or more associated goals beyond sobriety. Individual therapy can respond well to the multiple needs of clients in the maintenance stage if it remains flexible and broadly focused. Maintenance is the most productive time to work on the multiple problems that contributed to the development of the addiction or that remain as consequences of the years of abuse. Resolving marital conflicts, long-standing beliefs that undermine self-esteem and confidence, fears and anxieties, and past abuse or familial problems are important targets of longer term treatment of the substance abuser. Managed care's reluctance to support longer term care is short-sighted, since the resolution of these problems brings with it more stable change as well as healthier and more productive citizens (Finney, Moos, & Timko, 1999; McClellan et al., 1994; Moos, Finney, & Cronkite, 1990; Vaillant, 1995). For individuals who are doing well at resolving associated problems with minimal assistance, some type of office check-up schedule, similar to dental hygiene visits, may suffice. Follow-up visits would enable the therapist to meet once every 2 months with the client to see how things are going and whether there is any need for more assistance or access to resources. The function of the individual session in this case would be different. The check-up visit could consist of continuing to reinforce the decision and stage tasks needed on the path to sobriety, problem solving any remaining issues, and examining any threats to sobriety.

Medications for other psychiatric problems and adjunctive therapy or services often are useful to assist the client in making permanent the changes in drug and alcohol behavior. The individual therapist must avoid the problematic belief that he or she can help the client with every need or problem. Having an extensive list of resources where the client can obtain assistance in resume writing and job interviewing, be evaluated for medication for ongoing medical or psychological problems, receive family therapy, or seek Social Security and other benefits would be very important. Active referral with support is an important therapy skill during the maintenance stage. Finding out exactly what services the client can receive at a particular agency and how to access those resources is part of the therapist's responsibility. Helping the client realize the need for and the commitment to following through are also important elements in the treatment of clients in the maintenance stage. Finally, checking to see how the referral went and whether there is a need to reevaluate the referral represents another important task for the individual therapist with a client in maintenance.

Referral to self-help groups provides access to an important support system that individuals can use to help them successfully negotiate the maintenance stage (Longabaugh, Wirtz, Beattie, Noel, & Stout, 1995; Velasquez, Carbonari, & DiClemente, 1999). These groups (e.g., Alcoholics Anonymous, Smart Recovery, Women for Sobriety) can provide access to support when an individual needs an assist in meeting challenges and problems that threaten sobriety. There is an interesting new twist to these groups with the advent of technology. Access to self-help or mutual assistance groups through the Internet is becoming more popular and can provide a level of support that is even more accessible than the traditional meeting (Gainsbury & Blaszcynski, 2010; Lichtenstein, Zhu, & Tedeschi, 2010; Nowinski, 1999).

However, self-help and mutual support are not sufficient for some clients. This is particularly true for those who have associated psychopathology or who have serious skill deficits. More intensive individual and/or group treatments may be necessary to assist them to create a new lifestyle and to resolve related problems. In this case individual treatment or even individual case management becomes a primary vehicle for assisting the client in addressing psychological distress and symptoms, discovering and promoting alternative reinforcing activities and behaviors, developing and refining appropriate skills, and problem solving situations that pose dangers for sobriety and health.

Relapse and Recycling

The return to substance abuse is a discouraging event for both client and therapist. Even the single use of a substance after some period of abstinence can create a strain on the therapeutic relationship. To move forward in the process of change both the therapist and the client need to be invested in achieving successful, lasting change in the drinking and drug use behaviors. A slip or lapse raises many questions about the stability of the change and the dedication of the client. Suspicions, guilt, recriminations, and doubt are the normal responses to the violation of abstinence after a sustained period of change. If not checked, these feelings can create an atmosphere for a decrease in motivation and set the stage for a more robust return to the substance use (Brownell et al., 1986; Marlatt & Donovan, 2005). A relapse, or a more complete return to the substance-abusing behaviors, increases the intensity of the emotions and reactions described above. It is this insidious process that can undermine the therapeutic bond and create distance between therapist and client at precisely the time when they need to be working together to manage this threat to successful change. The therapist must set the stage for working together during this difficult time, while at the same time avoiding messages that predict or promote a relapse. This is a delicate and difficult task. We address the issue of relapse in considerable detail in Chapter 9. In this section, we highlight some of the most relevant clinical issues related to relapse, from a stage-of-change perspective, along with associated clinical responses.

If the therapist can create an atmosphere in which the client feels comfortable coming into the treatment setting to discuss the slip or relapse, the work of the individual therapy is clear. In this regard, the key tasks are to isolate and contain the substance use behavior, reinstate the commitment and decision to continue with the change, counter discouragement and depression, address the cognitive and behavioral triggers that are operating, and support reengagement in the process of change (Carroll, 1996b). For the individual who is slipping back and beginning to return to the former pattern of problem behavior, rapid action to help the client get back into action, to revise the action plan to address the slip, and to encourage and support the client are the most important tasks. Slips indicate that there is something wrong either in the prior tasks that have been completed or with the plan that is being implemented. In either case, problem solving should be used to address any loss of concern, decisional ambivalence, lack of commitment, interference from other problems that may be impacting prioritization, or plan deficiencies. If the slips have turned into a more significant relapse or collapse, the goals of the therapist's work with the client are to ensure that he or she becomes a recycler (DiClemente, 2003; DiClemente et al., 2010; Prochaska et al., 1992).

Normalizing the process of relapse without creating a relapse self-fulfilling prophecy is a significant challenge. Probably the most useful way to do this is to interpret relapse as an important step on the road to recovery and as part of the process of change. Race car drivers and their pit crews learn from every race how to improve the car, increase the speed, and develop strategies that make winning the race more probable. Talented basketball players continue to practice in order to raise the level of their game. The stories of Larry Bird and Michael Jordan or Kobe Bryant and Carmelo Anthony being the last ones to leave practice after having a subpar game or in preparation for a playoff game are interesting examples to give to clients who believe that they should be perfectly successful from the start.

Rather than dwelling on relapse when it occurs, the therapist would do better to focus on recycling. Most individuals have made multiple attempts and have continued to try to change (DiClemente et al., 2010). Learning from past attempts to change and then reevaluating where the individual is in the process of change are productive tasks for the client in relapse and his or her therapist. Some individuals are so discouraged and become so hopeless that they move back into precontemplation and refuse for the present to consider another change attempt. Others return to the ambivalence of the contemplation stage and consider the possibility of another attempt, but not immediately. Still others are like the rider who falls off the horse and wants to get back on as soon as possible. These individuals move back to preparation for another change attempt and are planning the next attempt. However, in our experience, movement from a relapse that either represents an almost complete return to the former habit pattern and precontemplation or recycling back into another quick attempt at action are less frequent than a return to contemplation. After a significant attempt to change a behavior that fails badly, the individual seems to need some time to regroup and get ready for another attempt. This is part of the reason that changing addictive behaviors takes such a long time both at an individual and at a population level. Forty percent or more of current smokers make a quit attempt each year with only 5–10% of those being able to sustain that change through 12 months (DiClemente et al., 2010).

Assessing where the individual has landed after the relapse is the first step to reorganizing the goals and strategies of treatment. In a relapse debriefing, the therapist needs to evaluate what went wrong both with the treatment plan and with the client's action plan (see Table 5.3). What were the elements of each of these plans that did not work? What ancillary treatments or resources were needed that were not provided? What unanticipated people, places, or things interfered with the plan? Was there a letdown in commitment, a deficit in skill, or some other problem that led to the collapse of the action plan? Problem solving at

TABLE 5.3. Therapist Problem Solving Questions for Slips and Relapses

Slips

- How can I isolate and contain the current substance use?
- Are the firm decision and commitment still there?
- How can I counter discouragement and keep attribution of slip situational?
- How can I help deal with the environment and triggers?
- Are there other important problems interfering with sustaining the change?

Relapses

- What went wrong in the various tasks of the stages of change: Was there a loss of interest in change, ambivalence in decision making, letdown in commitment, deficit in skills or planning?
- Is the client ready to make another attempt to change?
- What parts of the change plan did not work?
- What part of the treatment plan was not helpful?
- What unanticipated people, places, or things interfered with the plan?
- Did the anticipated support materialize?
- Where is the client with regard to considering or planning another serious attempt to change?

this point should look at the entire process of change and determine if there were tasks at various stages of change that were not sufficiently addressed or accomplished. For example, if the decisional balance was only slightly tilted toward action or the positive reasons for engaging in the substance abuse not countered adequately, work remains to be done with the client's decision making. The answer to the above questions can redirect the focus of the treatment to the appropriate stage tasks and strategies.

PLACING INDIVIDUAL THERAPY IN A PROCESS-OF-CHANGE PERSPECTIVE

The process of change is always more extensive than the formal interventions delivered by the therapist (DiClemente, 2003). In fact, multiple interventions and treatments often contribute to the process of successful change for any single substance abuser. In Project MATCH, almost 50% of outpatients and over 50% of the aftercare clients had had a previous inpatient treatment for substance abuse (Project MATCH Research

Group, 1997a). Prior treatment contributed in some way to the work of the Project MATCH therapists who saw the clients for 12 weeks of individual outpatient or aftercare treatment. This is an important reality to remember. In the best-case scenario, the therapist and the intervention contribute to the client's movement through the process of change or support the change the client is already making (Tucker et al., 1995). However, treatments or therapists are never completely responsible for the change in the substance abuse behavior. Most often therapists are not present to view the entire process of change for a particular client. Sometimes therapists are fortunate enough to be with a client long enough to see the ultimate positive outcome. For each therapist there are a few clients who have made significant and lasting changes and who either remain in treatment or return to therapy after a time to thank the therapist for changing their lives. However, many more drop out of treatment or leave treatment appearing not to have changed much. Precious little is known about their outcomes. When we look at the research evaluating long-term outcomes for substance abuse clients, it is clear that many who go to treatment programs do well (Moos et al., 1991; Finney et al., 1999; Vaillant, 1995; Project MATCH Research Group, 1998a). However, research also has demonstrated that even some of the dropouts from treatment are able to change and succeed in recovering from alcohol and drug problems (DiClemente & Scott, 1997). Ultimate client change may not necessarily occur within the context of a single dose of individual therapy and sometimes happens outside of treatment (Bischof, Rumpf, Hapke, Meyer, & John, 2001; DiClemente, 2006).

For most clients, the individual therapist assists them in moving along the path to change without ever seeing the ultimate outcome of the process of change. This is particularly true in individual therapy. Because of cost and the time involved in providing the individual focus, clients are often anxious to know when they can finish therapy. Some simply stop when they believe that they have had enough treatment. In the ideal world, it would be preferable if the client chose a single therapist and continued to work with that therapist until he or she reached successful, maintained change of the substance abuse problem, no matter how long that process took. Then the therapist could assist clients to move through the stages of change, help with relapse and recycling through these stages, and finally support the maintenance of change until the client reached sustained change of the substance abuse problem. However, with some few exceptions, this is not how treatment works. Most often treatment is episodic and delivered by a sequence of different programs and therapists. It is only when a single therapist or program has a vision of the entire process of change that they can see more clearly the role that they are playing for this particular client in this process of change. Each therapy experience can advance or hinder movement through the process of change. A therapist who has the opportunity to see a client for a single session or for a more substantial period of time has the responsibility to provide an experience that can foster client engagement in the process of change. For the therapist thoughtful, skillful, and respectful of this process, individual therapy can be the catalyst to move that individual through an important part of the journey through this process of change.

SUMMARY

• Individual treatment is uniquely suited to the concepts of the stages of change and their associated tasks.

• The initial challenge of individual treatment is assessing where the individual stands in the process of changing his or her substance use.

• It is important to assess the client's stage of change on an ongoing basis, as individuals can regress and progress from one stage to the next from week to week, or even day to day.

• Individual sessions with a client in precontemplation permit the therapist to explore the reasons why this individual entered treatment as well as ways to move him or her from precontemplation. An approach encouraged by the stages-of-change model has been to recognize lack of motivation as a part of the process of change and to use motivational approaches to address the needs of a substance abuser in precontemplation.

• When a client begins to seriously contemplate change, the focus becomes working with the client to elucidate the pros and cons of the problem behavior to help him or her make a risk–reward analysis of the behavior change. Strategies to promote decision making are useful in working with the client in contemplation.

• Clients do not necessarily move into action once a decision to change has been made. Instead, they often move into a stage of preparation, where the focus is on planning and commitment enhancement.

• Once the action plan is designed and the commitment to follow through with the plan developed, the individual enters the action stage where monitoring and revising the plan are needed.

• The tasks of maintenance are to sustain change over time and to integrate that change into the lifestyle of the individual so that the new behavior, abstinence from drugs, becomes the preferred, habitual behavior of the individual.

• Relapses, when they occur, can be discouraging events, for both the client and the therapist. It is important for the therapist to create an atmosphere in which the client feels comfortable coming into a session to discuss a slip or relapse.

6

Group Treatment

The group format is one of the most widely used modalities for treating substance use disorders, with a number of factors contributing to its popularity, including cost containment and efficiency of delivery (Rotgers, Morgenstern, & Walters, 2003; Weiss, Jaffe, de Menil, & Cogley, 2004). The terms "group treatment" and "group therapy" are often used interchangeably to describe a variety of therapeutic groups that include educational, didactic, process, support, motivational, and self-help groups. Approaches to these groups differ on a number of dimensions such as general philosophical orientation (e.g., disease or behavioral), treatment setting (e.g., outpatient or residential), and number of sessions. There are also different styles for facilitating groups. For example, some group leaders use treatment manuals with specific topics and exercises to guide group sessions, while others prefer a less structured, more process-oriented approach that focuses on interpersonal issues that arise in the course of the group (Ingersoll, Wagner, & Gharib, 2002). Five group models are common in substance abuse treatment: *psychoeducational* groups educate members about substance abuse; *skills development* groups help members learn skills needed to change their substance use; *cognitive-behavioral therapy* groups help members learn to alter thoughts and actions that lead to substance abuse; *support* groups provide a forum to share information about maintaining abstinence and managing day-to-day, chemical-free life; and *psychotherapeutic* groups provide an environment in which interpersonal processes are used to address major developmental issues that contribute to addiction or interfere with recovery (Center for Substance Abuse

146

Treatment, 2009a; Ingersoll et al., 2002). A sixth type of group, which can be described as a *motivational* group, is a relatively new model that is gaining in popularity. In this type of group the primary goal is to enhance members' intrinsic readiness to change their substance use by using a motivationally enhancing interpersonal style of group facilitation. These various group models can be used independently or they can be delivered in an integrated manner.

A number of studies suggest that group treatment can be as effective, and in some cases more effective, than individual treatment (Panas, Caspi, Fournier, & McCarty, 2003; Scheidlinger, 2000; Institute of Medicine, 1990; Weiss et al., 2004), and almost all major schools of individual psychotherapy have been adapted to group formats (Rounsaville & Carroll, 1997). In a comprehensive review, Weiss and colleagues (2004) compared group therapy for substance abuse to other treatment conditions, including (1) group therapy versus no group therapy; (2) group therapy versus individual therapy; (3) group therapy plus individual therapy versus group therapy alone; (4) group therapy plus individual therapy versus individual therapy alone; (5) group therapy versus another group therapy with different content or theoretical orientation; and (6) more group therapy versus less group therapy. Among the 24 studies reviewed, substance use outcomes for clients who received group treatment were similar to those who received individual therapies, and no single type of group therapy reliably demonstrated greater efficacy than others.

Despite the prevalent use of groups in substance abuse treatment settings, there has been a general lack of practical information for counselors about how to integrate theoretically and empirically based practices into their group-based services (Macgowan, 2008). Although recent efforts designed to bridge the gap between substance abuse research and practice have provided some much needed guidance for integrating best practices into "real-world" treatment settings (e.g., the National Institute on Drug Abuse Clinical Trials Network and the Substance Abuse and Mental Health Association's Addiction Technology Transfer Centers), in general, dissemination of evidence-based treatments has continued to focus on individual-based interventions. In this chapter, after a brief review of groups in substance abuse settings, we discuss recent developments in which individual psychotherapy approaches were adapted to a group format and the stages and processes of change were used as a guiding framework for structuring and facilitating groups. In addition, session examples from groups based on the stages-of-change model are provided.

INDIVIDUAL VERSUS GROUP TREATMENT

When compared to group therapy, individual therapy in general, and with substance abusers in particular, has a number of benefits (Rounsaville & Carroll, 1997), including (1) privacy and confidentiality may enable a discussion of more sensitive issues, (2) an individualized pace can offer more flexibility in addressing a client's problems as they arise over the course of therapy, (3) a greater percentage of time can be spent dedicated to a single individual's problem, and (4) an individual format may be more appropriate for addressing certain types of problems, such as relationship issues or personality disorders. At the same time, however, group treatment, compared to individual therapy, can have a number of advantages: (1) group members often provide positive peer support for each other, (2) feedback and modeling by peers may have more impact, in comparison to feedback and modeling from an "expert," (3) helping others can enhance members' sense of well-being and worth, and (4) groups can provide a meaningful social support system (Center for Substance Abuse Treatment, 2009a; Herkov, 2010). In addition, group treatment's cost effectiveness is often identified as the primary advantage of group-based interventions (Brook, 2008; Herkov, 2010; Miller & Hester, 1980). As Rounsaville and Carroll (1997) point out, most groups typically have at least six members and may have two therapists, thus leading to at least a tripling of the number of clients per therapy hour over individual therapy.

Research supports the importance of a number of these benefits from a client's perspective (Lovejoy et al., 1995). For example, methadone maintenance clients who completed a mandatory relapse prevention program were asked about helpful, curative factors. Over 70% of the clients rated their group therapy sessions as especially important because rather than feeling "alone" in dealing with their problems, they were able to talk openly—without feelings of shame—in a safe and supportive environment with others who had similar experiences. Similarly, Lovett and Lovett (1991) found that the most valued factors in the treatment group experience included assuming personal responsibility for one's behavior, overcoming isolation, increasing self-understanding, and experiencing a sense of group cohesiveness.

ADAPTING INDIVIDUAL PSYCHOTHERAPY APPROACHES TO GROUPS

Rounsaville and Carroll (1997) noted that almost all major schools of individual psychotherapy have been adapted to a group format. These adaptions include relapse prevention (Marlatt & Donovan, 2005; Marlatt & Gordon, 1985), contingency management (Higgins et al., 1993), and family systems approaches (Joanning, Thomas, Quinn, & Mullen, 1992), among others. More recently, motivational approaches such as Miller and Rollnick's (2002) motivational interviewing (MI) are also being modified for use in group settings (Ingersoll et al., 2002; Lincourt, Kuettel, & Bombardier, 2002; Sobell & Sobell, 2011; Van Horn & Bux, 2001; Velasquez, Stephens, & Ingersoll, 2006; Wagner & Ingersoll, 2013). MI is a collaborative, person-centered counseling style that enhances motivation for change by incorporating certain strategies that create opportunities for eliciting a client's "change talk." In turn, change talk, such as the desire, ability, and reasons for change as well as commitment language, predicts positive client outcomes (Amrhein, Miller, Yahne, Palmer, & Fulcher, 2003; Miller & Rose, 2009).

Because MI groups are a relatively new innovation and motivational-enhancing approaches are particularly important for individuals in the early stages of change, we will highlight the literature on MI in groups and some group treatments that attempt to use stages of MI groups. Although the evidence base to date has been somewhat limited, several recent articles have described the adaptation of MI for groups (D'Amico, Osilla, & Hunter, 2010; LaBrie et al., 2008; Velasquez et al., 2006; Velasquez et al., 2013). For example, Wagner and Ingersoll (2013) provide a foundation for designing and implementing MI groups and offer a four-phase motivational model that includes strategies for engaging the group, exploring group member perspectives, broadening member perspectives, and moving into action.

Stylistically, MI can be conducted in a relatively "pure" way in groups or integrated with other approaches. While there is relatively little research on the use of "pure" group MI, several studies of groups that incorporate MI with other methodologies have empirical support. For example, Sobell, Sobell, and Agrawal (2009), utilizing a "guided self-change" (GSC) intervention with cognitive-behavioral, self-management, and motivational components for mildly dependent alcohol and drug users, found sizeable and significant improvements in substance use that were comparable to those found with GSC in an individual format (Sobell & Sobell, 2011). The GSC model, described in the book *Group Therapy for Substance Use Disorders: A Motivational and Cognitive-Behavioral Approach* (Sobell & Sobell, 2011), provides a detailed framework for helping clients set and meet their treatment goals. Bailey, Baker, Webster, and Lewin (2004) also combined MI with cognitive-behavioral treatment in a group intervention that improved knowledge and attitudes about drinking among at-risk adolescents and, in comparison to a control group, also reduced the frequency of drinking. LaBrie and colleagues (2008) incorporated MI with cognitive-behavioral and relapse prevention into a group treatment for college-age women that significantly reduced drinks per week, peak alcohol consumption, and alcohol-related consequences when compared to an assessment-only control group.

A number of MI group interventions have tailored the approach to members' stages of change by using a motivational style with early stage clients and a more cognitive-behavioral approach with those in the later stages. For example, Annis, Schober, and Kelly (1996) developed an intervention with components of a structured relapse prevention model (e.g., assessment of high-risk drinking situations, MI, individual treatment plan, acquisition of relapse prevention skills, and maintenance counseling) targeted to a member's stage of change. Graham, Annis, Brett, and Venesoen (1996) also investigated the extent to which these types of targeted intervention strategies, which had been developed for individual therapy, could be generalized and successfully implemented in a group setting. In this study, Graham and colleagues compared a structured relapse prevention program delivered either as individual therapy or as group therapy with concurrent brief individual sessions. The two conditions resulted in similar levels of attendance and client satisfaction, and no differences were found in drinking-related outcome measures at a 12-month follow-up. Velasquez and colleagues (2009) conducted a randomized clinical trial to evaluate the efficacy of a stages-of-change-based intervention designed to reduce both alcohol use and incidence of unprotected sexual behaviors among HIV-positive men with alcohol use disorders. In this study, an integrated, manualized intervention that used both individual counseling and peer group education/support was compared to a control condition in which participants received resource referrals. The integrated intervention was based on the stages and processes of change and MI was used to enhance client readiness for change. Findings include significant treatment effects compared to control for reduction in number of drinks per 30-day period, number of heavy drinking days per 30-day period, and reduction in number of days on which both heavy drinking and unprotected sex occurred (Velasquez et al., 2009).

ADAPTING THE STAGES OF CHANGE FOR A GROUP FORMAT

As Miller (2001) points out, over the past two decades the stages-of-change model has provided a refreshing perspective and given rise to a very different way of thinking about motivation and the treatment of substance abuse. These developments are often reflected in changes in group facilitators' styles and strategies. Traditionally, substance abuse group treatment providers often viewed members as being helpless in regard to their substance use. In these types of groups, the atmosphere was highly confrontational as both leaders and members challenged other members' "denial" about their drug use. The stages of change shifted the perspective so that rather than blaming or dismissing group members who are not yet ready for change, clinicians now view motivation as a dynamic state—as opposed to a static trait—that can be influenced by strategically designed interventions. In this approach, group members are seen as individuals who have an inherent potential for change and are active agents in their own lives.

Before describing general stages-of-change group approaches, we will examine some of the logistical, practical, and conceptual issues that must be considered in developing a group treatment.

Open versus Closed Groups

A number of issues concerning the nature and composition of the group need to be taken into account when attempting to translate individual therapy principles into a group therapy format. The first is whether the group will be an "open" one in which new members are added on an ongoing basis or a "closed" one in which a single cohort of clients remains in the group throughout its duration. There are examples of each of these approaches in the stages-of-change literature for group therapy (e.g., Barrie, 1991; Center for Substance Abuse Treatment, 2009a; Yu & Watkins, 1996). The distinction between open and closed groups involves a number of logistical issues, such as the need to recruit a sufficient pool of clients to begin a cohort and develop a plan for clients on the wait list. Closed groups may benefit more from group-related curative factors, such as cohesion and the development of interpersonal trust, because of the ongoing involvement of the same clients across time. In contrast, in open groups members may be more frequently diverted from substantive issues as they work to assimilate the newer members. In addition, determining the optimal size of the group is essential because of the need to have a "critical mass" remaining if some members drop out.

Homogeneous versus Heterogeneous Groups

A second and somewhat related issue is whether the group should be homogeneous or heterogeneous with respect to a number of client characteristics, such as drug of choice and/or stage of readiness for change. N. S. Miller (1995) has argued for a heterogeneous group composition for substance users that includes clients who are in various stages of treatment and recovery, with different levels of motivation and treatment acceptance/resistance and diverse patterns and types of drug use. In these types of groups, members who are struggling to become alcohol- and drug-free participate with and learn from members who have been substance-free for longer periods of time and have developed a substance-free lifestyle. In advocating for heterogeneity with respect to levels of abstinence or stage of recovery, Vannicelli (1992) believes that hope and optimism can result when an individual sees that some members remain sober or drug-free for the life of the group while others, who relapse, do recover and remain in the group. Similarly, Washton (1992) has noted that heterogeneous groups have the potential of enhancing the richness of the group experience and making it possible for members to integrate more easily into a group in which they can identify readily with at least one other member. Thus, Vannicelli (1992) and N. S. Miller (1995) both suggest that the interactions between group members in different stages of treatment can be of therapeutic advantage to both. In this model of mixed-recovery groups, the group is not time-limited as members in early phases of recovery continue in the group as long as it is productive and therapeutic for them (Vannicelli, 1992). Other advantages of these types of groups are that clients who are new to treatment can learn from those more advanced in recovery that they are not alone or unique in their substance use, treatment can work, withdrawal symptoms can diminish over time, and self-help 12-step programs can be incorporated into an abstinent lifestyle (N. S. Miller, 1995).

In contrast to this position, others (Barrie, 1991; Levy, 1997) argue for homogeneous groups because of the importance of a common purpose, comparable goals, and similar characteristics for developing and maintaining a cohesive group experience. Advocating for a "hybrid" model, Washton (1992) suggested the principle of "maximum tolerable heterogeneity" as a general rule in that the composition of a group should be neither too heterogeneous nor too homogeneous. Consistent with this principle, Stinchfield, Owen, and Winters (1994) recommended that group therapists make decisions about accepting or retaining an individual in the group on the basis not only of the individual's needs or characteristics but also on the needs of the group as a whole.

Group Composition and the Stages of Change

The stages-of-change model provides a useful framework for developing, organizing, and delivering substance abuse groups. For example, considering a potential group member's stage of change at entry poses important considerations for group format (open vs. closed) and membership (heterogeneous vs. homogeneous) and allows for a number of possibilities. In groups for clients with similar levels of readiness to change their substance use, group leaders can specifically select exercises and content most appropriate for that group's needs. On the other hand, in more heterogeneous groups in terms of readiness, members in later stages can model behavior change for clients who are less motivated to change. In addition, clients who are in the earlier stages of change can provide opportunities for those in more advanced stages to reexamine and reaffirm their decisions for change. The first key decision, then, is how to structure the group in terms of members' stages of change.

There are several ways to compose stage-based groups, depending on the setting, resources, and participants. In the heterogeneous mixed-stage model, all participants, regardless of their stage of change at intake, attend a group that begins sessions focused on early stage tasks and processes and then progresses to sessions that address later stage tasks and needs. This approach assumes that the individuals who remain in group will be those who move forward through the stages of change. Another strategy involves two ongoing open groups that run concurrently (one an early stage-focused group and the other focused on later stage tasks and processes). In this scenario, new members are assigned to the group appropriate for their intake stage of change; then, as early stage members begin to take active steps to change, they transition into the later stage group. Conceivably, individuals who relapse and are struggling with the decision to change could move back to the early stages-focused group. In a third model, clients continue to participate in the same early or late stage group they were assigned based on their intake stage of change. This approach assumes that initial homogeneity of early or later stages status will be supportive and addresses the key deficits or barriers for which clients initially sought treatment.

When assigning group members based on the stages of change, our preference is that whenever possible, clients in earlier stages of pre-contemplation and contemplation be placed together and those in later stages of action and maintenance be in a separate group. In fact, there is some evidence to suggest that matching clients to groups in which the content is consistent with their stage yields better outcomes (Velasquez et al., 2011). This may be because later stage ("ready for action") clients' movements toward change are hindered in groups that focus primarily on building motivation, while earlier stage clients benefit less from developing change plans and completing other tasks that are more appropriate for action-oriented groups. Clients in preparation are closer to action and could be placed in the action and maintenance group as a general rule. However, depending on referral and treatment setting and whether individuals judged to be in preparation may not have completed early stage tasks well enough, they could be placed in the early stage group to ensure readiness for the action-oriented group. In short, assigning clients to groups that are consistent with their stage of change allows group leaders to focus on exercises that enhance processes of change specific to members' stage of change.

Incorporating the Processes of Change into Groups

As described in Chapter 2, the processes of change are thought to be the experiential and behavioral mechanisms that facilitate change (DiClemente, 1993; Prochaska & DiClemente, 1984; Prochaska, DiClemente, Velicer, & Rossi, 1993). These processes of change vary in intensity or frequency depending on the client's stage of change, as certain change processes "peak" during particular stages (Perz et al., 1996). Thus, the experiential processes are more typical in the early stages of change (precontemplation, contemplation, and preparation), and the behavioral, more action-oriented processes occur more often in the later stages of change (action and maintenance). Using the stages-of-change model, a group intervention described in *Group Therapy for Substance*

Abuse: A Stages-of-Change Treatment Manual (Velasquez et al., 2001) consists of 29 sessions designed to promote the use of one or more specific experiential or behavioral change processes. For instance, in the early change stage groups, exercises that help elicit experiential processes such as consciousness raising or self-reevaluation are emphasized, and later stage group activities engender behavioral processes such as stimulus control or self-liberation. Table 6.1 shows the various group strategies that can be utilized to promote process use. You will note that there is an important distinction between the processes of change and the techniques or strategies that can stimulate those processes. Many of these techniques will be familiar to the reader and are not unique to substance abuse treatment. However, the value of this intervention lies in applying strategies specific to a particular change process in a manner that is tailored to the client's stage of change.

Although the processes-of-change variables drive the design of the stages-of-change model group intervention by providing direction and structure, they are not "cast in stone," as clinicians can select sessions (that facilitate use of certain processes of change) that are most appropriate for a group's needs (e.g., members' stage of change, length of time in treatment). Once group leaders are familiar with all of the processes of change, they can recognize and incorporate other techniques—beyond those included in the stages-of-change model manual design—that correspond to and enhance process use and change movement. For example, MI strategies are particularly helpful in activating early stage processes such as self-reevaluation and environmental reevaluation.

A STAGES-OF-CHANGE APPROACH TO GROUPS

Motivation plays an important role in people's decision to change or to stay the same. As mentioned earlier, the stages-of-change model views motivation as something that can be influenced rather than as a stable personality characteristic or trait. In fact, increasing client motivation is a central part of a group leader's task, particularly when working with clients in the early stages of change. A motivational style of group facilitation should also be maintained as group members move into the later stages, even though the emphasis shifts to a more traditional cognitive-behavioral or relapse-prevention approach. We believe that an empathic, supportive, nonjudgmental counseling style is essential both for building motivation for early stage members and for promoting

TABLE 6.1. Techniques Useful in Enhancing Process Movement in Group Sessions

Process of change	Session topic(s)	Technique(s)
Consciousness raising	• Daily usage • Physiological effects • Expressions of concern	• Assessment/feedback • Psychoeducation • Cognitive recognition
Self-reevaluation	• Expectations of use • Values	• Cognitive recognition • Values clarification
Environmental reevaluation	• Relationships • Roles	• Cognitive recognition • Role clarification
Self-liberation	• Goals • Action plan • Recommitting after a slip	• Goal setting • Relapse prevention planning • Framing
Stimulus control	• Triggers	• Psychoeducation • Environmental restructuring
Counterconditioning	• Stress • Assertiveness • Refusal skills • Thought management	• Relaxation imagery • Assertion • Role play • Cognitive restructuring
Reinforcement management	• Rewarding success • Cravings and urges • Alternatives to using	• Reinforcement • Cognitive restructuring
Helping relationships	• Social supports	• Social skills enhancement • Communication skills
Social liberation	• Identifying needs and resources	• Needs clarification • Psychoeducation

Note. From Velasquez et al. (2001, p. 22). Copyright 2001 by The Guilford Press. Reprinted by permission.

self-efficacy and reinforcing accomplishments for those in the action and maintenance stages of change (DiClemente & Velasquez, 2002).

One predictor of positive client outcomes in individual treatment is the extent to which the client is engaged and does more talking in the session than the therapist (Miller & Rollnick, 2002). While this has not been studied extensively in groups, Cartwright (1987) indicates that an important consideration in group therapy is the extent to which the therapist/leader dominates the group, defines the group's activities, and specifies the group values, with all communication flowing through the leader. A number of authors have suggested, however, that such a style is not particularly well received or useful in substance abuse treatment groups. Rather, the ideal modality in these types of groups is one in which the focus is group-oriented rather than leader-determined and the leader acts as a facilitator of interpersonal process (Cartwright, 1987; Galanter, Castaneda, & Franco, 1991). In these types of open, more democratic and cohesive groups, members are more likely to disclose, explore, and begin to address their substance use problems. In sum, the maximum benefit to group members seems to be derived from their active participation and interaction with other members rather than being passive recipients of a leader's domineering and controlling efforts (Yu & Watkins, 1996).

Given that this type of collaborative group experience can be unfamiliar to many members, when facilitating these groups it can be helpful to provide a preview or introduction to it during the first group session. For example, instead of beginning with the usual introductions and discussion of group "rules" (e.g., not interrupting, avoiding monopolizing, arriving on time), the leader presents an overview of how the group will be conducted and explains that his or her goal as leader is to help members learn more about themselves and whether there are any changes they might like to make. In addition, the message that "if there is any changing to be done, the members will be the ones to do it" should be clearly communicated by emphasizing that because the responsibility for change is up to each member, the leader will not attempt to persuade or force any change. In informing members that they will each play an important role in helping other group members, the leader can explain that the group will use a motivational approach in which members help facilitate change in one another through supportive interactions. It can also be helpful to emphasize that because research shows that supportive, empathic conversations are much more effective than confrontational ones, this group will explicitly avoid confrontation and focus on attitudes of empathy, acceptance, and respect for individual differences. A leader may also want to tactfully note that because hostile or dominating speech is not part of the group's "style," he or she will help discourage disruptions and the possibility of one person's dominating the group. Before moving to the other topics, a few minutes may be set aside for members to talk about their reactions to this approach. Given that norms are established early in the course of a group and not easily changed (Yalom, 1995), we believe that these foundational precepts should be made explicit at the beginning of each session.

To capture these initial elements, some group leaders find it helpful to use the acronym "OPEN" in starting the group (Velasquez et al., 2006):

- Open with an overview of the group purpose: to learn more about members' thoughts, concerns, and choices.
- Personal choice is emphasized.
- Environment is one of respect and encouragement for all members.
- Nonconfrontational nature of the group.

GENERAL APPROACHES TO GROUPS AT DIFFERENT STAGES OF CHANGE

The following information, focusing on the several issues appropriate to groups at different stages of change, is derived from and integrates the work of Yu and Watkins (1996), Barrie (1991), and DiClemente and Velasquez (2002).

Precontemplation Stage

Many substance abusers in precontemplation come into contact with treatment agencies as a result of a legal mandate or pressure from family members or employers. They perceive the positive benefits of drinking or drug use and have not fully considered or accepted the negative consequences of their use. Given this position, a primary goal of a group working with individuals in precontemplation is to help raise their consciousness and increase their concern for and awareness of substance-related problems in order to move them toward a more comprehensive self-assessment in the contemplation stage, where hopefully they can begin to see a need for change. Such groups, whether they include only individuals in precontemplation or represent initial sessions of a closed-cohort group, are often conducted as psychoeducational alcohol or drug information groups. Participants are provided information about alcohol and drugs, the negative consequences associated with them, and the potential advantages to changing their alcohol or drug use patterns. However, these group sessions have to be motivational as well as educational, and group leaders should use methods such as empathic reflecting, asking for elaboration on statements that are consistent with the direction of the group, and validating personal choice and responsibility. If negative comments by one group member occur, the group leader selectively emphasizes the most positive part of the comment, reframes the comment, and/or affirms the member (e.g., for his or her concern, experience, energy, passion, pain). At times, the reframe or affirmation may be followed by a diplomatic, empathic reminder about the policies of the group (e.g., "We all have a lot of life experiences to share and sometimes it might be hard to remember that in this type of group we try not to tell someone else what to do because we know it is a matter of a personal choice—we each are the experts on our own life"). This can be followed by an open question designed to elicit change talk and move the group in a more positive direction. Also, "differential reinforcement" can be used by attending to positive, nonargumentative comments, or to highlight change talk. These selective reflections allow individual group members to be heard and reinforced for their constructive comments.

Ingersoll and colleagues (2002) warn that group leaders working with members in the early stages of change should assist members in seeing not only the negative consequences of their substance use, but also use consciousness raising, awareness exercises, and selective reflections to help members focus on the positive outcomes of making healthy change. If the group is facilitated in an empathic and skillful manner, client resistance to change is minimized and group members often become aware of their own reasons for change. It is important for group leaders to assure members that no one will try to make them change and that, while they may be offered information and maybe some advice, what they do with it is completely up to them. Informing potential clients that other members of their group will be similar in terms of their readiness to change can also be encouraging to those who are in the early stages. When approached in this way, clients in precontemplation are likely to be more receptive and open to participation in the group and more likely to increase appropriate interest and concern in changing substance use.

Contemplation Stage

Group members in the contemplation stage are thinking about change but often have ambivalent thoughts or feelings. They may have begun to consider that the benefits of continued drinking or drug use may be outweighed by the negative consequences and that they may need to change. They are likely to be ambivalent and not yet fully committed to making such changes. A goal of therapy with these individuals in contemplation is to tilt the decisional balance toward change and increase the strength of their decision to change. During this stage participants may be more receptive to information about alcohol and drugs and, on the basis of increased awareness, they may begin to change their view of their alcohol and drug use, noting a shift in the relative weighting of the positive and negative consequences of their use. In addition to focusing on the individual's problem areas, the group should also highlight positive experiences related to change and provide information about available treatment resources and self-help groups that group members may find helpful in implementing change if they choose to do so.

It is likely that groups with individuals in contemplation will at some point begin to shift away from a more psychoeducational orientation toward a discussion format associated with more traditional process-oriented group therapy. The therapist(s) must guide the process to have members openly discuss use patterns and their resultant implications for current life problems. Such discussions enable all to share their own personal experiences in a way that both supports the individual's shifting attitudes and beliefs and provides feedback to others. Yu and Watkins (1996) note that it is important for the therapist to try to maximize the input from each group member in such discussions while assuming a less active role, serving to shape the discussion, correct misinformation, and reinforce group members' contributions and self-disclosures. They suggest that members may have a greater investment in the group process if the ratio of participant-to-therapist input is high.

Preparation Stage

Individuals in the preparation stage have resolved the decision-making challenges faced during contemplation. It appears that the move from contemplation into the preparation stage follows a shift in attitude about and perception of continued substance use. The negative consequences of substance use are now perceived as clearly outweighing the positive benefits of continued alcohol or drug use. This attitudinal shift appears to contribute to the now-firm intention to implement behavioral changes. Clients have now committed themselves to a change plan that they intend to implement in the very near future. Many may have already begun engaging in a variety of experiential and behavioral change processes. The key tasks are to strengthen commitment and create an effective, acceptable, and accessible plan for making change.

As we discussed in Chapter 2, individuals in the preparation stage, in comparison to those in the precontemplation and contemplation stages, are stronger in their resolve to quit, more confident of their ability to change, already seeking out information about their problem and how it affects them and others, more likely to have sought out activities incompatible with substance use, more likely to have rearranged their lives and environment to avoid high-risk situations, and more likely to have developed personal and social networks that reward them for their decision to change. Thus, individuals in the preparation stage are high on key tasks and actions related to both the contemplation and action stages.

This stage, bridging the gap between contemplation and action, helps to determine a number of functions for the group. The major goal of the group in dealing with individuals in the preparation stage is to help them with commitment and planning and to provide them with the support necessary to put an action plan into place and to follow through on their intention to change. Although the level of ambivalence has been reduced, the initial steps that are taken during the preparation stage are vulnerable to reversal until they have been solidified through trial and error. The group needs to develop techniques that further enhance commitment and that help to initiate and sustain behavior change. In order for the individual to move forward in the change process, as opposed to falling back, the individual's efforts must be reinforced, both by the group and through the development of self-reward contingencies. As these initial steps are reinforced, the level of self-efficacy will increase; the individual will increasingly feel more confident that he or she can deal with potential problems that might jeopardize the original commitment. In addition to providing a source of reinforcement for behavior change, the group can also raise concerns if they see flaws in decisional considerations or weakening of commitment as the individual begins to regress to a previous stage. The group can also help identify high-risk situations that may need to be avoided early in the change process, suggest other ways to cope with stress and strong negative emotions rather than by drinking or taking drugs, and develop contingency contracts that will serve as special reinforcers when treatment-appropriate behaviors are engaged in and negative sanctions if substance-related behaviors are engaged in.

Action Stage

The primary goals for therapy groups dealing with clients in the action stage are to reinforce their commitment to change and help them develop, implement, and test out skills necessary for them to change their alcohol and drug use. Group facilitators should encourage any small steps members have taken toward change, acknowledge the difficulties and losses that are often involved in change, and help the group members identify access to services and social support (Center for Substance Abuse Treatment, 2009a). Barrie (1991) suggests that members should be taught general problem-solving skills in which they identify and explore the parameters of the problem, brainstorm possible solutions, choose the most feasible alternative, put it into practice, evaluate its effectiveness, and make changes as needed to improve its outcome. Such problem-solving approaches, which are common elements in many cognitive-behavioral interventions with substance abusers (e.g., Monti, Abrams, Kadden, & Cooney, 1989; Kadden et al., 1992), can be generalized to any problem area. Group members, based on their experiences, can contribute to the brainstorming process by suggesting possible ways of dealing with a problem. Sometimes change plans need to be revised in light of new information or problematic implementation. In addition to merely discussing these alternatives, it is possible to have members role-play situations or scenarios with other participants, with the therapist providing coaching and corrective feedback. The group may also serve as a source of support for the individual as he or she attempts to practice these new skills outside of the group session. Some group time should be set aside at the beginning of a session to review both successful and unsuccessful attempts at behavior change. Members who have been successful in their behavior change attempts serve as models for others who have been less successful.

The tasks for the therapist(s) in groups with clients in the action stage involve reinforcing the members' commitment to change, helping the group generate possible solutions to a member's problems, and reinforcing members' attempts at implementing the chosen strategies. In addition, the therapist(s) need to guide group exploration of the possible barriers to change among clients who are having difficulties implementing their change strategies. Rather than being critical and confrontive, group interactions with less successful clients must be supportive, empathic, constructive, and reinforcing of the individual's self-efficacy and sense of optimism that he or she will be successful in the future.

Maintenance Stage

In the maintenance stage, group members continue to maintain successful behavioral changes until they become permanent, solidified, and relatively automatic. It is also during this period that members are successful in avoiding temptations to return to their previous alcohol or drug use patterns, anticipating situations in which a relapse could occur, and preparing coping strategies to deal with it. Thus, group members are still involved in active problem-solving strategies and must remain vigilant concerning possible relapse situations. The function of the group in this case is to support the individual's ongoing efforts and to help the individual maintain a commitment to changing both substance use and lifestyle, maintain the therapeutic gains that have been made to date, and remain aware of personally relevant relapse triggers (e.g., Donovan, 1998). Barrie (1991) notes that there is a shift in the group's focus away from drinking and drug use per se to the broader issues of lifestyle change (e.g., creating new networks, resolving emotional or environmental problems, getting involved with work). As such, groups with clients in the maintenance stage are more likely to be open-ended as opposed to time-limited.

Relapse

A major focus during the maintenance stage is on the development of skills and problem solving for preventing relapse. However, many group members may struggle during the action and maintenance stages and may experience a lapse or return to alcohol or drug use. A goal here is to support and reinforce the members' ongoing use of their successful coping strategies, minimize the likelihood of a lapse, and manage lapses that do occur so that they do not become more full-blown relapses. (We will discuss relapse in greater detail in Chapter 9.) Continuing care during the maintenance stage is often more effective in minimizing the harm associated with relapse than in preventing lapses from occurring (Donovan, 1998). An important aspect of this process is that group members have learned during the action and maintenance stages that relapse is common in the course of recovery, that it can represent an important learning component of the process of change, and that many individuals, who ultimately achieve success do not necessarily do so without temporary setbacks—rather, they may cycle through the stages of change making repeated attempts several times before reaching successfully sustained maintenance. The hope is that the individual will not become so demoralized that he or she returns to the precontemplation stage but rather continues using the change strategies found most useful during the contemplation, preparation, and action stages. As discussed in the early chapters of this volume, successful change seems to represent successful completion of each of the critical stage tasks well enough to support sustained change of the substance use behaviors.

The therapy group plays a number of important roles during this stage. First, the group can be helpful in providing support for those individuals who are struggling and appear at particular risk for relapse during this time of increased vulnerability. It also serves as a source of support if a member does experience a lapse. Most individuals who experience a lapse feel angry at themselves, embarrassed, depressed, discouraged, and inclined to think of themselves as failures. The group must be willing to continue to work with and come to the aid of such individuals. Members who relapse, but have a positive attachment to the group, will be more likely to return to the group following a lapse. A group's history of providing comfort and aid to members who happen to relapse will also be a crucial factor. If those who relapse are spurned or confronted heavily by other group members, the end result may be a perception that the group "doesn't care" about the individual, is hostile and unsupportive, and increases the level of guilt experienced by the individual. It then becomes less likely that a member will want to return to the group if a lapse occurs. It is important for the group to remain objective, nonjudgmental, supportive, reflective, and empathic when dealing with a member who has lapsed. It is particularly important that the therapist(s) maintain this stance, model it for the group, and shape the discussion to engender this atmosphere. Also, having previously seen members who have lapsed return to the group, resume their therapy, reaffirm their commitment to change, examine the relapse situation to determine factors that may have served as triggers, develop plans to deal with these factors to solve similar problems in the future, take steps to make changes, and again achieve maintenance provides a sense of hope and optimism to anyone who lapses.

FACILITATING STAGE MOVEMENT AND PROCESS-OF-CHANGE USE

Teaching clients about the stages-of-change model can be a useful way to facilitate group discussion and to elicit group members' own reasons for change and goals for treatment (DiClemente & Velasquez, 2002; Velasquez et al., 2006). It can also be used to enhance "consciousness-raising." Using this approach, group leaders introduce the stages of change to members using simple illustrations, such as a stage diagram, and discuss vignettes about individuals who are in the various stages of change. The leaders then ask the members "Who would like to tell us about their stage of change for [the target behavior]?" or "How does this fit for you?" This typically elicits a great deal of discussion and creates an opportunity for members to share their own thoughts about change. These responses set the stage for leader-generated reflections and opportunities to reinforce clients' statements about potential change. This, in turn, builds rapport and strengthens the therapeutic alliance among members and between members and group leaders. We recommend teaching group members about the stages of change in early sessions because it provides both a shared vocabulary and helpful insight that promotes a positive group alliance. The discussion also serves to invite quieter group members into the conversation. In subsequent groups, clients often refer back to the discussion about stages of change and report changes in stage status.

Some examples from sessions based on the stages are presented here. In the first, the group facilitator reads a vignette about an individual who is thinking about quitting smoking during her pregnancy and then asks group members to determine the character's stage of change.

GROUP LEADER: Tanya wonders if her cigarette use is hurting her baby, but she is not sure that she can quit. She saw some babies at the hospital that were very small and she wondered if their low birthweight was related to their mothers' smoking. Her doctor has advised her to quit, but she is ambivalent about whether or not she'll follow his advice. She is worried that she'll gain too much weight if she quits smoking, yet she wants to do the best thing for her baby. What stage of change do you think Tanya is in?

GROUP MEMBER A: I think she's in the contemplation stage because she's giving the idea of change some consideration.

GROUP MEMBER B: Yeah, but she doesn't seem serious enough to me.

GROUP MEMBER C: She's in contemplation, though, because she's thinking about it and considering her baby. She's also worried that she'll gain weight.

GROUP LEADER: Yes, contemplation is when someone is thinking about both the pros and cons of making a change. Which of you has felt this way before? Who has felt two ways about making a change, like Tanya does about her smoking?

GROUP MEMBER C: I can really relate. Before I quit using cocaine, I didn't want to use and get my kids taken away, but at the same time I liked the feeling I got from the coke and it was what I did to have a good time with my friends.

GROUP LEADER: You were ambivalent. On the one hand, you wanted to do what is best for your kids, and on the other hand you liked the benefits you were getting from the drug use.

GROUP MEMBER C: Is that normal?

GROUP LEADER: Yes, it is a very natural part of the change process. People who are in contemplation often feel ambivalent about their use, and also about the benefits and costs of changing.

GROUP MEMBER A: Yeah, that would be contemplation. You were thinking about it but also not sure you were ready to quit, just like the lady in the example.

In the next scenario, the facilitator describes someone who is in the action stage of change and reads a related vignette.

GROUP LEADER: Ralph is thinking about quitting drinking, and his wife is very concerned about him when he drinks. Ralph's boss has also asked him to talk to the company's employee assistance counselor because he has smelled alcohol on Ralph's breath several times. Ralph also has trouble getting to work on time in the morning, due to his drinking. He doesn't want his wife to worry about him and he is concerned that if he doesn't change his drinking he will lose his job and his marriage. He reports that, on the one hand, he wants to quit drinking to preserve his marriage and his job; on the other hand, drinking helps him socialize and reduces his stress levels. Ralph has not had a drink in a week and he has made an appointment with the employee assistance counselor. He has also said "no" to his friends when they want him to go to the bar after work, and he has gone to the gym instead. What stage do you think Ralph is in?

GROUP MEMBER A: It's either preparation or action.

GROUP MEMBER B: I'd say action, because he hasn't had a drink in a week.

GROUP MEMBER C: But he's still thinking about it.

GROUP LEADER: Tell me more about why you picked action.

GROUP MEMBER D: It's action, because he has made the change. He is not just thinking about it anymore, he took action so he's not in contemplation. He's in action because he hasn't had a drink in a week.

GROUP LEADER: Yes, he's in action. That's the stage where someone has made a behavior change and adopts strategies to help prevent relapse. What strategies is Ralph using?

GROUP MEMBER B: Well, he made the appointment with the employee assistance counselor person.

GROUP MEMBER A: And he is going to the gym instead of to the bar.

GROUP MEMBER E: Yeah, I still think he needs the booze to stay calm, though. This is going to be hard for him.

GROUP LEADER: Yes, that might be right. People typically have to work hard, even after they have made a change and are in the action stage. Ralph's still doing some thinking about it, which can seem a little like contemplation. Although he has taken steps, he still needs to be sure he has committed himself to the change.

GROUP MEMBER C: He's pretty much at risk because he hasn't found other ways to reduce his stress. That means he should learn more about how to chill out or he'll continue to be tempted. He still seems a little unsure.

GROUP LEADER: It's normal for people to still have some ambivalence when they are in the action stage. It sometimes takes a very long time to resolve—and that's why people in action, and even maintenance, still need support after they've changed their behavior.

GROUP MEMBER F: I'm in action too and I need all the help I can get. I haven't had a drink in 32 days, but every day I'm tempted. The cravings are still there.

GROUP LEADER: You've made a really big change by not drinking in a whole month. You really took action once you made up your mind!

GROUP MEMBER D: Yeah, me too. I'm definitely in action for my drinking, but I'm still in contemplation about my pot smoking. As an artist, I'm not sure I'll ever give it up. It helps me be creative.

GROUP LEADER: You're not really sure if you want to quit smoking pot. You've been successful with your alcohol use, but pot is another thing. Yes, that is action for one behavior and contemplation for another.

GROUP MEMBER A: I used to be in precontemplation because I thought I didn't have a problem with my drinking. All my friends drank the same amount as me and I was proud that I could hold my liquor. I never did smoke pot, though. Is there a stage for never having done it at all? (laughter)

GROUP LEADER: You never thought your drinking was a problem.

GROUP MEMBER A: Yes, but it really was. I tried to drink socially but . . .

GROUP MEMBER C: And now you don't drink at all! You've quit!

GROUP MEMBER A: But it's not easy. I'm in that stage where I feel good about my change but still need support. That's action.

The next example describes an extended group interaction in which the group leader describes the stages of change and, rather than using vignettes to illustrate the various stages, she asks the group members to identify their own stage for the target substance. Note that the group leader is using a motivational style to elicit members' ideas about their own stages of change.

GROUP LEADER: (*Distributes a handout with a diagram depicting the stages of change.*) Let's look at a handout now that shows different stages somebody can be in when they are thinking about changing a behavior. You'll see that it shows someone going through the different stages of change. It could be for cocaine use, eating better, or drinking less. As you can see, when people are not really thinking about changing, see no reason to do so, they are in the stage we call "precontemplation." The next stage is one in which the person is thinking about change, kind of like a little idea that "Maybe I ought to do something different, I don't know for sure, but just maybe. . . ." We call that "contemplation"—just beginning to think about changing.

GROUP MEMBER A: That describes me!

GROUP LEADER: You're beginning to think about things being different, changing your alcohol use. The handout also shows somebody who is beginning to make some plans for changing, getting some ideas, and maybe finding resources that would help—this is called the "preparation" stage of change. The person is getting ready to change and planning how he or she might be most successful. Next, when people are actually making some changes, doing some things differently (like not drinking), we say they are in the "action" stage.

GROUP MEMBER B: Like coming here to group?

GROUP LEADER: That's right! That's an action to help change your drinking. So you are in action for coming to group and hoping the group will help you move through the stages to get you into action for changing your drinking. And finally, when the changes become kind of like a habit—take less effort to keep going, that's called the "maintenance" stage of change. The handout also shows that if a slip occurs, this doesn't mean the person has "failed." It just means that he or she had a temporary lapse. Many people reenter the change cycle after a slip, sometimes by coming right back into action or for others back to contemplation. So change is a process for us all – not an either-or state. What do you make of that? How does this idea fit for you?

GROUP MEMBER C: I'd say I'm in action, too. I quit using several weeks ago.

GROUP LEADER: You've taken some action. You have really made a major change in your life! Who else?

GROUP MEMBER D: Can you be in two places, two stages at one time?

GROUP LEADER: Tell us about that.

GROUP MEMBER D: Contemplation and preparation? See, I like smoking pot, although I know I probably should cut down. But alcohol's a different thing, I'm coming to this group, I also go to AA. . . . I'm planning on quitting my drinking. I haven't quit yet, but I *have* cut down, and I'm planning on more, on cutting down to nothing.

GROUP LEADER: Thank you for that excellent example. You are exactly right—a person can be, in fact often is—in different stages for two different behaviors. Sometimes we're really motivated to change one behavior, but less concerned about another behavior.

GROUP MEMBER E: I just keep bouncing back and forth. One day I want to quit and the next I'm not so sure. It's pretty confusing to tell you the truth. I don't know where I am.

GROUP LEADER: What you're describing is "ambivalence." That means feeling two ways about something. That's really common in the early stages where you think, "I know that this part is OK, but I'm not sure if this part is OK. I know I want to change this, and I'm not sure I can." There are also some really good things about staying the same. That is very normal and people typically go through that as they are going through the stages of change.

We have some themes in common here. Many of you are thinking about change, and some of you have already quit drinking or using. There are still some feelings about being unsure and maybe some ambivalence, yet at the same time many of you have taken steps toward change. As we meet together as a group, we can talk about these different stages. Some group members find it helpful to check in about the stage of change they're in from time to time during the group sessions and to support each other in making changes. How does that sound to all of you?

SUMMARY

• Group therapy is one of the most widely used approaches in substance abuse treatment. It has a number of advantages, as compared to other therapeutic measures, including the development of "curative factors" associated with the group process that may produce behavior change.

• A number of features of group therapy are thought to contribute to the process of behavioral change, including the realization that others share similar problems, aid in modeling appropriate behaviors, immediate peer feedback, and group support.

• A variety of logistical, practical, and conceptual issues need to be considered in developing a group approach. These include the use of an open versus a closed group, a homogeneous versus a heterogeneous group composition, and the phase of recovery that the clients are in.

• Use of the stages-of-change model and the associated emphasis on the processes of change has a number of practical implications for the group setting. It has been widely adopted in a number of countries and in many different cultures. Because of its wide appeal and evidence base, a growing number of providers are being trained in this model and many of them wish to use their skills in the group setting.

• Therapeutic tasks and goals for treatment groups vary as a function of each stage of readiness, with group interventions geared toward members' stages of change. For example, a group dealing with individuals in precontemplation would focus on increasing their awareness of their substance-related problems and move them toward contemplation. The primary goals for groups dealing with clients in the action stage are to reinforce their commitment to change and help them develop and apply skills needed for changing substance use.

• Group treatments can use the stages and processes of change to create types of groups, tailor treatment approaches, and develop treatments that promote successful completion of stages-of-change tasks and movement through the process of change.

7

Couple Treatment
and Family Involvement

Alcoholism and drug addiction have often been described as "family diseases" (Goodwin & Warnock, 1991). This phrase has both face validity and scientific backing. This depiction is most apparent when one does a search on the Internet, resulting in a long list of "hits" for popular literature, materials from self-help organizations, and infomercials from substance abuse treatment programs focusing on addiction as a family disease. The phrase has taken on a number of different meanings over time. One connotation suggests that alcohol and drug use disorders are familial in nature because of an apparent genetic predisposition toward substance abuse that runs within families and across generations (Agrawal & Lynskey, 2008; Dick & Bierut, 2006; Goodwin & Warnock, 1991). The risk of developing alcoholism is an estimated seven times greater among first-degree relatives of an alcoholic than in appropriate comparison groups, with this risk being particularly high among the sons of alcoholic fathers. Similarly, approximately half the brothers and a quarter of the sisters of an alcohol-dependent individual also had a lifetime diagnosis of alcohol dependence (Bierut et al., 1998). This apparent genetic predisposition has been more commonly found for alcohol problems than for other drugs of abuse (Bierut et al., 1998) and for the sons of alcoholics more than for their daughters (McGue, 1997; Muetzell, 1995). However, it is clear that there is also heritable risk and intergenerational transmission within families of dependence on drugs including opiates, cocaine, and cannabis (Bierut et al., 1998; Merikangas et al., 1998). This has been noted most recently for cannabis, the most commonly used drug of abuse (Agrawal & Lynskey, 2006). As an example, the odds of an adult sibling of an individual with a cannabis use disorder also having a lifetime diagnosis of a cannabis use disorder was over three and one half times greater than for siblings of an individual not having such a disorder, while the risk for adult offspring of an individual with a cannabis use disorder was nearly seven times greater (Merikangas et al., 2009). The fact that the spouses and adult siblings of cannabis abusers had comparable levels of risk of developing a cannabis use disorder suggests that both genetic and environmental factors contribute to the development of substance use disorders (Kendler, Schmitt, Aggen, & Prescott, 2008).

A second meaning of "family disease" relates to this environmental context within which an individual is raised. While genetic and/or other biological factors are important in the etiology of alcohol and drug abuse, such factors alone cannot account for the risk of developing substance abuse (Ellis, Zucker, & Fitzgerald, 1997; Kendler, Gardner, & Prescott, 2011; McGue, 1997). Rather, it appears that the most comprehensive models of substance use and substance use disorders reflect an interaction between genetic, family, temperamental, and social factors (Kendler et al., 2008, 2011). While genetic factors predispose potentially vulnerable individuals, substance abuse generally develops within a family context, often one that includes alcohol and drug use and abuse by parents and siblings (Heath & Stanton, 1998). In addition to providing an inappropriate model for substance use, the families of substance abusers are often characterized by other problems, including a high degree of conflict, chaos, unpredictability, and inconsistent messages to children about their worth. There is a breakdown of traditional rituals and rules that are found in more stable family systems (Hawkins, 1997; Hook, 2011; Sher, Gershuny, Peterson, & Raskin, 1997). Such environments are often associated with poor communications among family members (Cranford, Floyd, Schulenberg, & Zucker, 2011; Murphy & O'Farrell, 1997), high levels of perceived stress (Catanzaro & Laurent, 2004; Tempier, Boyer, Lambert, Mosier, & Duncan, 2006), domestic violence (Ritter, Stewart, Bernet, Coe, & Brown, 2002; Smith, Elwyn, Ireland, & Thornberry, 2010), child abuse or neglect (Huang et al., 2011; Magura & Laudet, 1996; Wells, 2009; Wilson & Widom, 2009), emotional and physical abuse (Magura & Laudet, 1996; Sheridan, 1995), and sexual abuse (Gil-Rivas, Fiorentine, & Anglin, 1996; Gil-Rivas, Fiorentine, Anglin, & Taylor, 1997; Pirard, Estee, Kang,

Angarita, & Gastfriend, 2005). Children who emerge from such settings have increased risks for adjustment problems, including poor school performance, criminal involvement, depression, suicidality, and the development of substance abuse (Johnson & Leff, 1999; Silverman & Schonberg, 2001). Many individuals raised in such substance-abusing environments continue to experience emotional problems into their adulthood, including depression, anxiety, and posttraumatic stress disorder as well as substance abuse (Gil-Rivas et al., 1996; Gil-Rivas et al., 1997; Langeland, Draijer, & van den Brink, 2004; Sher et al., 1997).

There is clear evidence that substance abuse has a negative impact on the psychological and physical health of not only the substance abusers but also nonusing family members (Copello & Orford, 2002; Copello, Velleman, & Templeton, 2005; Copello, Templeton, & Velleman, 2006; Hartera, 2000; Orford, Templeton, Velleman, & Copello, 2005; Templeton, Zohhadi, & Velleman, 2007; Velleman et al., 1993). Greater severity of alcohol dependence is related to a greater number of and more severe alcohol-related medical complications (Cook, Booth, Blow, Gogineni, & Bunn, 1992), and there is a higher level of medical burden among substance abusers in general than found in the general population (De Alba, Samet, & Saitz, 2004). Both the spouses and adult children of alcoholics have also been found to have higher levels of psychological symptomatology than comparison groups (Benishek, Kirby, & Dugosh, 2011; Hinkin & Kahn, 1995; Scharff, Broida, Conway, & Yue, 2004). Problems tended to be greater for concerned significant others who were women, partners of, or living with the substance abuser (Benishek et al., 2011). Family members of substance abusers appear to be significantly more likely to be diagnosed with substance use disorders, depression, and trauma than family members of individuals with other types of chronic disorders such as diabetes or asthma and their total health care costs are higher (Ray, Mertens, & Weisner, 2007, 2009). This is consistent with prior research findings indicating that families of individuals with alcoholism have increased use of health care services (Holder, 1998; Holder, Lennox, & Blose, 1992; Ray et al., 2007). In an early study of this issue, the health services utilization of members of intact nuclear families that included an alcoholic were compared with those of matched controls from families not including an alcoholic (Roberts & Brent, 1982). Members of the alcohol-involved family had significantly more physician visits and more medical diagnoses than did the comparison group. Of interest, this difference was found only for female family members; it may be that female spouses of alcoholic men are considerably more vulnerable to physical concerns or may see the family physician as a more acceptable resource than counseling or self-help support groups such as Al-Anon. The members of the alcohol-involved family tended to have a higher proportion of diagnoses of trauma and stress-related diseases, reflecting the difficult emotional environment of the family setting of substance abusers. Such findings concerning the negative physical and psychological consequences of substance abuse in the family have contributed to an increased focus on identifying and intervening with these family members in primary care settings as a means of increasing their coping skills and reducing stress and its associated psychological and medical burdens (Copello & Orford, 2002; Copello et al., 2009).

Lack of cohesion within substance abusers' families is related to both the severity of the individual's and the family's psychological problems and to poorer prognosis for substance abuse treatment (Costantini, Wermuth, Sorensen, & Lyons, 1992; Gruber & Taylor, 2006). If the physical and psychological problems of family members as well as those of the substance abuser are not addressed, the effectiveness of substance abuse treatment may be compromised (Copello et al., 2005; Copello et al., 2006; Gil-Rivas et al., 1997; Saatcioglu, Erim, & Cakmak, 2006). In addition to possibly enhancing treatment efficacy and family functioning, substance abuse treatment, whether provided through formal treatment programs or voluntary involvement with Alcoholics Anonymous, Narcotics Anonymous, or Cocaine Anonymous, also appears to have a positive effect of lowering the posttreatment utilization of health services by both the substance abuser and family members (Humphreys & Moos, 1996, 2001; Lennox, Scott-Lennox, & Bohlig, 1993; Lennox, Scott-Lennox, & Holder, 1992). As an example, family members of alcoholics who had not yet entered treatment had significantly more psychiatric and medical problems, as well as higher associated costs, compared to members of families not including an alcoholic (Weisner, Parthasarathy, Moore, & Mertens, 2010). However, the family members of alcoholics who had maintained abstinence for 1 year following treatment entry had medical costs comparable to the comparison families. The medical costs of those families whose alcoholic members were not abstinent at 1 year continued to be significantly higher than the comparison families and were on an increasing cost trajectory (Weisner et al., 2010). There is also evidence that treatment of the substance abuser may have a preventive effect, serving to reduce the risk of developing mental health and substance abuse problems among the children (O'Farrell & Feehan, 1999).

Despite the negative consequences to the substance user and his or her family, a relatively small percentage of those with substance use problems enter into treatment (Marlatt, Tucker, Donovan, & Vuchinich, 1997). An investigation of treatment seeking by individuals in the general population who had been identified as having diagnosed emotional problems found that while nearly half (47%) of the individuals with a major depressive episode sought help, only 16% of those with alcohol abuse or dependence sought help (Bland, Newman, & Orn, 1997). An early study similarly found that only 21% of the individuals identified as having an alcohol problem considered seeking help when they first identified the problem, and only 15% actually did seek treatment (Hingson, Mangione, Meyers, & Scotch, 1982). Of those who did not seek help, 84% said they did not believe their problem was serious and 96% believed they could handle it on their own. Over half acknowledged that they did not want to admit they needed help. In addition to the 15% who sought help initially, another 16% did so at a later time. Consistent with this pattern, a national survey in 2007 by the Substance Abuse and Mental Health Services Administration found that while 23.2 million individuals age 12 or older needed treatment for an illicit drug or alcohol use problem (defined as having met the DSM-IV diagnostic criteria for dependence on or abuse of alcohol or illicit drugs in the past 12 months), only 2.4 million (e.g., 10.4% of those meeting the criterion for "need") actually received treatment at a specialty facility (Substance Abuse and Mental Health Services Administration, 2008).

Given that most substance abusers may not choose to seek treatment on their own, the family plays an important role in initiating the treatment-seeking process. Despite the problems that substance abusers generate for themselves and their families, they maintain fairly frequent and ongoing contact with parents, siblings, and significant others (Stanton, 1997). It is through this contact that family members may serve an important role, increasing the individual's awareness of the problem, facilitating treatment entry, and helping to encourage and support behavior change and maintain recovery (Copello et al., 2005; Meyers, Miller, Smith, & Tonigan, 2002). Copello and colleagues (2005) suggest that family-involved interventions fall into three general categories: (1) working with family members and concerned others to facilitate the substance abuser's treatment entry and engagement, (2) family members' involvement in treatment that focuses primarily on the substance abuser, and (3) formal interventions or self-help group involvement to support and respond to family members independent of the substance abuser. Stanton (2004) has labeled the first of these as "Engagement-Primary" interventions, while those that combine engagement of the substance abuser into treatment with counseling for the concerned other family member(s) are described as "Dual-Purpose" interventions. These approaches cut across the stages of change, both for the family and the substance abuser, from precontemplation, through contemplation and taking action stages, to the maintenance of behavior change.

READINESS TO CHANGE IN THE FAMILIES OF SUBSTANCE ABUSERS: A PARALLEL PROCESS

There appear to be three broad approaches families have used in their attempt to cope with the problems of and generated by a substance abusing member (Orford et al., 1998). They can attempt to (1) tolerate the problem in a relatively inactive, accepting way, (2) withdraw from interacting with the user, or (3) engage in ways to try to change the user's behavior. This latter method of coping can be more or less confrontive, controlling, assertive, or supportive. The first two of these approaches are unlikely to promote change, while the more active engagement process may serve to initiate the change process for both the user and the family

A family member's decision to take action and do something to care for themselves and/or the substance abuser is often a difficult one. The family, in its response to the substance abuser's behavior, is likely to go through stages of readiness to change that parallel those of the substance abuser. Early on there is often a tendency to minimize or deny that a substance abuse problem exists either for the individual or the family. Family members may be described during this early stage as being "codependent" or "enabling" since they appear, based on the absence of active steps to change the situation, to be supportive of the individual's continued substance abuse (DuPont & McGovern, 1996; Rotunda, West, & O'Farrell, 2004; Thomas, Yoshioka, & Ager, 1996). This may also reflect their use of tolerance and withdrawal as familial coping strategies (Orford et al., 1998). A television commercial for private treatment programs has shown a family asking, "What do you mean, 'There's an elephant in the house'?" The elephant, representing the alcohol or drug abuse problem of one of the family members, is standing in the middle of the living room, having nearly destroyed the entire house in full view of the family—yet they are unable or unwilling to acknowledge a problem. Such a family is in the precontemplation stage.

Over time it is likely that members of the family begin to feel that something is wrong with both the substance abuser and the family. The negative consequences of the substance abuse, which likely persist and worsen, may clearly begin to be seen as outweighing the perceived benefits of maintaining the family and its dynamics as the status quo. A shift has taken place, with the family member, or the family as a whole, moving into the contemplation stage. There is continued evaluation of the situation. There is an evaluation of the family context, such as becoming aware that the children of the substance abuser have begun to have academic and disciplinary problems at school. There is also a more personal self-evaluation, in which the family member becomes increasingly aware that he or she is unhappy in the relationship with the substance abuser and more firmly determines that something must change in the family.

Moving from the contemplation to the preparation stage, family members have come to the point that they intend to do something in the near future and may have begun to take small steps toward change in the family system. They may seek out information about alcohol and drug abuse, attempting to raise their awareness of the impact of substance abuse on themselves, the family, and the substance abuser; experience emotional reactions to some substance-related event; and increase their awareness of alternatives to continued substance abuse within the family. One or more of the family members may become increasingly concerned and may begin to explore popular or professional literature, the local phone directories, Internet websites, substance abuse help-lines, as well as consulting friends, clergy, or health care professionals in an attempt to gain information to help them better understand substance use and dependence and to direct them toward possible treatment options.

At some point, now using more active engagement strategies, the family member will attempt to take more notable steps to induce change in the substance abuser and the family system. The specific actions taken by the family member will depend on a number of factors, but might include leaving the relationship or getting support and help through counseling or Al-Anon participation for him- or herself as a concerned significant other in a substance-abusing relationship. This action might also include attempts to encourage the substance abuser's entrance into treatment and/or an active involvement in family/couple counseling to help the substance abuser, the relationship, or the family. It is important that the family as a whole, and its individual members, receive the support and encouragement necessary to take and maintain such steps; otherwise, there is a risk that, in response to the potentially painful process of change and the resistance from the substance abuser, the family will fall back (or "relapse") into its previous patterns of behavior.

Once having made the decision and taken steps to change, there appears to be a relatively consistent sequence of steps that the substance abuser, concerned significant others, and the family go through in the treatment process (O'Farrell, 1993). These steps, which again parallel those found in the stages-of-change model, include initiating change and helping the family when the substance abuser is unwilling to seek help, stabilizing abstinence and relationships when the substance abuser seeks help, and maintaining long-term recovery and preventing relapse. Readers interested in more information related to many of the interventions associated with these stages are referred to O'Farrell (O'Farrell & Fals-Stewart, 2001), Stanton (2004), and Copello and colleagues (Copello et al., 2005, 2006).

MOTIVATING BEHAVIOR CHANGE AND ENGAGING THE SUBSTANCE ABUSER IN TREATMENT

Many, if not most, substance abusers seek treatment in response to some form of external pressure from their spouses or significant others, physicians, employers, and/or the legal system. Such external social pressures have been found to be highly related to help seeking in a population sample of current and former drinkers, especially among those who had high levels of alcohol dependence (Hasin, 1994). Krampen (1989) found a number of different reasons given for entry into alcoholism treatment. A subset of this sample was followed up for 1 year after completing treatment. One of the main reasons given by those who remained abstinent over the year was concern over the potential loss of one's marriage. However, drinking during the follow-up period was associated with already having had a spouse leave because of drinking. It may be possible to use such pressure and natural contingencies as a form of motivation to encourage treatment seeking by the substance abusers. In fact, next to legal coercion, pressure exerted by family and concerned significant others represents one of the most powerful routes to treatment entry and engagement (Marlowe, Merikle, Kirby, Festinger, & McLellan, 2001; Stanton, 1997, 2004).

A number of more specific interventions or approaches have been suggested for use in the motivation/engagement stage as family members begin to mobilize their energy and efforts. These approaches differ considerably in the degree of confrontation and coercion involved.

Johnson Institute Intervention

At the more coercive end of this continuum is what has become known as the Johnson Institute "intervention" (Faber & Keating-O'Connor, 1991; Johnson, 1986; Liepman, 1993). Once a contact has been made by a concerned family member, the treatment professional, known as an "interventionist," makes an initial assessment of the substance abuse problem; the strengths, composition, and structure of the family and social network; and determination of who among this network should be involved in the intervention. These family members and other concerned individuals (e.g., coworkers, friends, physicians) are brought together initially to meet with a trained counselor, forming an intervention team. The team members are provided an orientation to the intervention process, are educated about substance use, are asked to formulate their concerns and feelings about the substance abuser, and to determine what contingencies will be employed if the substance abuser does not comply with the intervention and continues to resist entering treatment.

Having practiced the delivery of their feedback, the intervention team members are brought together and the substance abuser is brought into their midst, often not knowing initially what is happening. Members then share their concerns and feelings with the individual, indicate that they hope the person will enter treatment, outline the consequences if the substance abuser refuses, and discuss the desired outcome of both the intervention and treatment. A referral to treatment is then made. In most cases arrangements have been made in advance with a treatment program so that, if the substance abuser agrees to follow through on the referral, he or she can be admitted directly with little loss in time and, presumably, in motivation. At a later date, members of the intervention team meet with the counselor to debrief their experiences and to lay out a change plan for the family to follow.

Liepman (1993) suggests that the Johnson Institute intervention is particularly useful in dealing with substance abusers who stubbornly resist entering treatment and who do not have any one person or institution that has sufficient authority or that can exert sufficient pressure to coerce the substance abuser into treatment. This approach is also more useful for those substance abusers who have a social network of individuals supportive of their recovery rather than those who have a limited social network or one that is composed of relatively superficial relationships.

Despite its availability and application in the field for nearly three decades, there has been relatively little research evaluating the effectiveness of the Johnson Institute intervention. Gentilello and colleagues (1988) employed the Johnson Institute intervention with the families of 17 individuals who had been admitted into an acute care trauma center and were assessed to be alcoholic. All of the 17 patients who received this intervention shortly before their scheduled discharge from the trauma center accepted the referral and entered directly into an inpatient treatment program. Loneck and colleagues (Loneck, Garrett, & Banks, 1996a, 1996b) found that alcoholics receiving the Johnson Institute intervention were more likely to enter treatment than were those who were referred through other means, both coercive and noncoercive. Those who entered treatment either through the Johnson Institute intervention or a coercive referral source (e.g., courts, legal pressure) were comparable with respect to treatment completion rates. It was subsequently found that those who received the Johnson Institute intervention had considerably higher relapse rates than those in other referral situations (Loneck et al., 1996b). Based on a meta-analysis of family-involved interventions in the treatment of alcohol dependence, O'Farrell and Fals-Stewart (2001) concluded that the Johnson Institute approach does not appear to be effective in promoting treatment entry. Clearly, while this approach appears to have potential benefits, it is in need of further evaluation.

A number of professional therapists and family members have chosen not to become involved in an intervention process (Faber & Keating-O'Connor, 1991; Miller, Meyers, & Tonigan, 1999). Liepman (1993) has discussed a number of ethical concerns that have been raised in response to the use of intervention procedures and that contribute to its not being a more widely used method of engaging individuals into treatment. The first has to do with issues of confidentiality about information that is revealed and discussed about the substance abuser, who has no say as to who will come to know of his or her substance-related problems (Faber & Keating-O'Connor, 1991). There is a related concern about the sense that the intervention, despite its presumably good intentions and focused goal of treatment entry, appears to be a "conspiracy" that may affect the substance abuser's personal freedom. Another concern has to do with the potential negative and harmful after-effects of an intervention, either for the substance abuser or for his or her family (particularly if treatment is rejected). A third concern is that there may be a perceived, if not real, potential for conflict of interest on the part of the counselor conducting the intervention—in that the treatment program to which the person is referred often is affiliated with the program that employs the counselor.

ARISE Program

Given such concerns about the Johnson Institute intervention approach, a modified, less confrontive, but progressively more intensive approach has been developed. This approach, A Relational Intervention Sequence for Engagement (ARISE) (Garrett, Landau-Stanton, Stanton, Stellato-Kabat, & Stellato-Kabat, 1997; Garrett et al., 1998; Landau et al., 2000), is based on a number of underlying assumptions. These include the following: (1) involving the substance abuser in the process, where possible, provides a sense of respect for that person and encourages openness in the family system; (2) intervention is a process that falls along a continuum of increasing intensity of therapeutic and family involvement; (3) providing alternatives for the substance abuser to choose from reduces resistance; (4) the intensity of family and therapeutic interventions should be matched to the degree of resistance presented by the substance abuser; (5) there is a bond of caring between the family and the substance abuser; (6) utilizing the strengths of a particular family or social network provides a sense of efficacy and the perception that it can overcome its problems; and (7) the family system benefits from and is strengthened by the intervention process even if the substance abuser does not enter treatment (Garrett et al., 1998).

The ARISE program is a graduated intervention that consists of three stages, each of which has greater family involvement, therapist direction, and possible coercion than the preceding stage. The first stage, described as an informal intervention without a therapist present, begins with a call by a concerned significant other to the treatment center seeking information about substance abuse and exploring treatment options when the substance abuser is resistant to the possibility of seeking treatment. Over the course of one or more phone sessions, in a manner similar to the Johnson Institute's intervention, the counselor assesses the nature of the abusers' alcohol or drug use, the circumstances surrounding it, and the social support network of the individual. A set of guidelines for counselors and treatment agencies has been developed to assist with and systematize the information collection process and how to respond to these concerned other calls to mobilize the family and support network in their attempt to engage the substance user in treatment (Garrett et al., 1999).

The network of concerned others plays an important role in motivating the substance abuser to seek treatment. The rationale is to involve these individuals in expressing their concerns to the substance abuser. The network group would be asked to attend at least an initial meeting at the clinic. They may be asked to attend one to two meetings per month over the first 3 months following the initial meeting as needed to facilitate the substance abuser's move toward treatment. Each meeting would consist of a number of components: eliciting a problem statement from each participant, reviewing efforts to engage the substance abuser, determining patterns of alliance among group members and with the substance abuser, discussing options to address the abuser's engagement problems, developing strategies to motivate engagement, and preparing to handle possible crises.

Up to this point, the effort on the counselor's part during the phone conversation(s) is to move the concerned significant other from the contemplation to the preparation or action stage, as well as mobilizing the social network in support of treatment. Commitments are made to have these individuals, as well as the substance abuser, invited to the clinic. The phone counseling also provides an opportunity for the concerned significant other to rehearse expressing his or her concerns.

While the counseling sessions over the phone can at times be sufficient to get the substance abuser to enter treatment, more often than not the process moves to the second stage, the informal intervention with a therapist present. Again, concerned others in the substance abuser's support network are invited to this meeting. This session (or several, if needed) is spent considering possible approaches that might be used to get the substance abuser into treatment. Emphasis is placed on expressing concern and caring for the individual, with the use of confrontation deemphasized. This is another feature that distinguishes the ARISE approach from the more confrontational style of the Johnson Institute intervention. Again, an attempt is made to have the substance abuser attend this meeting. If, after repeated attempts, the substance abuser is still resistant and unwilling to seek treatment, plans are made to use the more traditional Johnson Institute-like intervention, which represents the third stage in the intervention sequence. Again, the use of confrontation is minimized and an attempt is made to maintain a more positive atmosphere. The ARISE model attempts to use the least coercive steps early in the intervention and then moves to those involving greater counselor and family efforts only if these lower intensity steps do not succeed.

To date there has been limited evaluation of the ARISE program. A series of studies by Loneck and colleagues (Loneck, Garrett, & Banks, 1997; Loneck et al., 1996a) have compared the Johnson Institute intervention with methods of facilitating treatment entry that differed in terms of the type of referral (either coerced or noncoerced) and the intensity of the process (unrehearsed or unsupervised). The unrehearsed and unsupervised interventions are similar in nature to the initial phases of the ARISE program. It was found that individuals in the Johnson Institute intervention were more likely to enter into outpatient treatment, equal in the rate of treatment completion, and higher in their rate of relapse than those in the other conditions. From these findings it may be inferred that interventions that fall at the lower end of the continuum of coercion are helpful and, among those who enter treatment, have similar completion and lower relapse rates than among individuals involved in the more coercive, staff-intensive, and more costly Johnson Institute intervention.

More recently a pilot study has evaluated the outcomes from 110 consecutive concerned other calls, without exclusion, to two treatment programs employing the ARISE approach (Landau et al., 2004). The calls were primarily from family members about individuals using alcohol, cocaine, or other drugs. Using a dichotomous outcome measure (e.g., engaged in treatment/self-help or not), 83% of the substance abusers about whom the concerned other calls were made subsequently became engaged. The majority (66%) of those who became engaged did so during the first stage of the three-stage ARISE program; an additional 32% became engaged in the second stage. It took an average of 13.7 days between the concerned other's call and the substance abuser becoming involved in a treatment or self-help program. The larger the social network of family and friends involved in the process, the greater the likelihood of the substance abuser becoming engaged. The findings suggest that concerned other calls to treatment programs that adopt the ARISE approach can result in relatively rapid and successful treatment engagement without the intensity or confrontive style of the Johnson Institute intervention (Fernandez, Begley, & Marlatt, 2006; Landau et al., 2004).

Unilateral Family Therapy

Attempting to provide support and increase the well-being and functioning of individuals engaged in a relationship with a substance abuser is a primary goal of unilateral family therapy (Thomas & Ager, 1993; Thomas & Santa, 1982; Thomas, Santa, Bronson, & Oyserman, 1987). This approach (McCrady, 1991) attempts to influence the behavior of a resistant substance abuser indirectly by working directly with the concerned significant other. A primary goal is to increase the coping ability and overall functioning of the family by working directly with the concerned significant other. Changes made by the significant other may lead to modifications in the substance abuser's behavior, including the possibility of treatment entry.

Unilateral family therapy has three primary foci: (1) an individual focus that assists the concerned significant other by increasing coping skills and decreasing the emotional impact of substance abuse; (2) an interactional focus that assists the concerned significant other in mediating changes in family functioning by reducing nagging and other forms of negative communications, decreasing marital turmoil, and attempting to enhance the marital relationship; and (3) a focus on the significant other, attempting to help the individual develop more specific strategies to address the substance abuser's resistant behavior and facilitate treatment entry (Thomas & Ager, 1993; Yoshioka, Thomas, & Ager, 1992).

There are three main phases in unilateral family therapy with substance abusers, which takes place over the course of 4–6 months (Thomas, 1994; Thomas & Ager, 1993). The first phase focuses primarily on the concerned other, preparing him or her to assume a rehabilitative role toward the substance abuser. The second phase focuses on developing specific strategies that can be used to influence the substance abuser to consider, seek out, and enter treatment. The final phase is a maintenance phase that focuses on continuing to work on the treatment and behavioral goals established by and for both the substance abuser and the concerned significant other.

Unilateral family therapy has been classified as a promising but underutilized intervention (McCrady, 1991). Despite its apparent promise to increase the coping and emotional functioning of the concerned significant other and enhance the likelihood of treatment entry by the substance abuser, there are still insufficient empirical data to date to support its efficacy (Barber & Gilbertson, 1997).

Community Reinforcement and Family Training

An underlying assumption of behavioral approaches to family and couple's treatment of substance abusers is that the behavior of the substance abuser is governed by the principles of reinforcement. Therefore, shifts in the pattern of reinforcement and contingency management can be used to change the substance abuser's behavior. This principle is an integral component of what has been described as the Community Reinforcement Approach (CRA; Azrin, 1976; Hunt & Azrin, 1973). Sisson and Azrin (1993) indicate that, as they were implementing and evaluating a CRA program, they received a number of calls from concerned family members who were trying to enroll resistant substance abusers into treatment. Based upon the demand for services for dealing with such situations, they developed the Community Reinforcement and Family Training (CRAFT) program (Meyers, Dominguez, & Smith, 1996; Meyers, Miller, Hill, & Tonigan, 1998; Meyers & Smith, 1997; Meyers, Smith, & Lash, 2003; Meyers, Smith, & Miller, 1998; Smith, Meyers, & Waldorf, 1999).

The CRAFT program typically takes place over a number of sessions and has as its primary goals helping family members encourage the substance abuser to stop drinking and enter treatment. It also provides a focus on helping the concerned significant other learn how to take better care of him- or herself. The sessions focus on educating the concerned significant other about how to (1) reduce physical abuse and increase personal safety in the relationship, (2) encourage the goal of abstinence through contingencies that positively reinforce periods of prolonged abstinence and negative consequences for substance use that require the substance abuser to accept responsibility for the substance use and for making right the damage caused by this use, (3) encourage the substance abuser to seek professional treatment by identifying and attempting to capitalize on those moments when the abuser appears particularly motivated and potentially receptive to such a suggestion, and (4) empower the significant other to play an ongoing role in the treatment process through involvement in educational and therapy sessions.

If the training program is successful in getting the substance abuser to enter treatment, he or she is rapidly inducted into CRA (described more fully below). This will continue an active role of the concerned significant other in the treatment process through involvement in a family program used to provide ongoing monitoring of the use of disulfiram (Antabuse) and in reciprocity marriage counseling. In addition to taking disulfiram, or potentially other medications for the reduction of craving or use of drugs other than alcohol, the substance abuser would be involved in social skills training; job club and vocational skills training as needed; the development of social, recreational, and leisure activities that are intrinsically rewarding to the individual and incompatible with substance use; and the development of skills to deal with the urges to drink or use drugs. Many of the contingencies that were developed in CRAFT prior to treatment continue during this active treatment phase. The goal is to reshape the substance abuser's pattern of behavior through the application of positive and negative reinforcement.

There is considerable empirical support for CRAFT. Recent clinical trials have evaluated the effectiveness of CRAFT with the families of resistant alcoholics (Miller et al., 1999) as well as adult (Kirby, Marlowe, Festinger, Garvey, & LaMonaca, 1999; Meyers et al., 2002) and adolescent drug abusers (Waldron, Kern-Jones, Turner, Peterson, & Ozechowski, 2007). Miller et al. (1999) compared three different types of significant other involvement. The first was a traditional Johnson Institute intervention, with concerned others developing an intervention plan and confronting the resistant alcoholic. The second was an approach that attempted to encourage involvement in Al-Anon, a self-help program for spouses and significant others in relationships with substance abusers (Cermak, 1989). Al-Anon provides support and change in self-perception of the significant other. There is no attempt to get the substance abuser into treatment; rather, there is the suggestion that one should detach from the substance abuser. The third approach was CRAFT, which combined elements of unilateral family therapy with those of CRA. Through the use of behavioral contracts and contingency management, the focus is on changing the pattern and contingencies of the substance abuser's social reinforcement, providing the concerned significant other with improved communication skills, and developing more effective coping and conflict resolution strategies. Each of these approaches was delivered as individual counseling sessions. The therapists in each condition used the particular approach as their primary mode of trying to get a resistant alcoholic into treatment; thus, they delivered therapies in which they believed and had considerable clinical experience. All the therapies were manual-guided.

The primary outcome of this study was the rate of entry into treatment by the alcoholic. Involvement of the significant other in the CRAFT therapy had the highest overall treatment entry rate (64%), compared to 30% for the Johnson Institute intervention, and 13% for the Al-Anon facilitation therapy. The vast majority (70%) of families involved in the Johnson Institute intervention chose not to follow through with the confrontation. However, completion of the confrontation was associated with a high rate of treatment entry (75%), versus a treatment entry rate of only 11% among those alcoholics whose families did not follow through with the intervention. A secondary outcome was the emotional adjustment of the concerned significant others in these three approaches. All three groups demonstrated significant reductions in their levels of depression, anxiety, anger, and family conflict and significant improvements of perceived family cohesion and relationship happiness. The improvements in these areas of function were comparable, with no significant differences across the three approaches.

Kirby et al. (1999) compared a unilateral community reinforcement training (CRT) approach with a 12-step self-help approach based on the principles of Nar-Anon. The primary outcomes of interest were attendance at and completion of the 14-session program, entry of the drug abuser into treatment, reductions of the drug abuser's drug use, and reduction of family problems. Secondary outcomes included mood states, self-esteem, social functioning of the significant other, and functioning of the family. At a 10-week posttreatment follow-up, the unilateral CRT was found to be significantly better than the self-help program on three of the four primary outcomes. Compared to significant others in the self-help condition, those in the CRT attended more sessions (8.6 weeks vs. 5.2 weeks of attendance), were more likely to complete the entire program (85.7% vs. 38.8% of scheduled sessions), and had higher rates of treatment entry by the drug abusers (64% vs. 17% treatment entry). Both groups demonstrated significant improvement, but did not differ from one another, on the reduction of drug use by the abusers, presenting problems, mood states, self-esteem, significant other social function, or family function.

In the most recent randomized trial, the concerned others of illicit drug users were assigned to CRAFT, CRAFT plus aftercare, or a condition facilitating involvement in Al-Anon and Nar-Anon (Meyers et al., 2002). Each group received 12 weeks of its respective manualized treatment. The two CRAFT conditions were significantly more effective than the 12-step-oriented support group in engaging the unmotivated substance abuser into treatment, with the CRAFT plus aftercare condition having the highest overall rate of treatment entry. Rate of treatment entry for the CRAFT group (59%) was double that of the Al-Anon/Nar-Anon condition (29%), while CRAFT plus aftercare (77%) demonstrated an incremental benefit over and above CRAFT alone. Although not compared against another condition, a CRAFT intervention working with the parents of resistant adolescent substance users was highly successful in engaging the adolescents in treatment (71%). Parents also reported considerably better psychological function and reduced negative emotional symptoms regardless of whether or not their child entered treatment.

A recent meta-analysis (Roozen, de Waart, & van der Kroft, 2010) indicated that CRAFT produced three times more patient engagement than Al-Anon/Nar-Anon and twice the engagement of the Johnson Institute intervention, with an overall treatment-entry rate of approximately two-thirds. It concluded that CRAFT was superior to more traditional methods of attempting to get resistant substance abusers to engage in treatment, a conclusion similar to that reached by Stanton (2004), who indicated that CRAFT was the best available clinical option for the dual purposes of helping the concerned other cope more effectively and engaging either adult alcohol or drug abusers into treatment.

ACTION AND TAKING STEPS

The goal of the interventions described in the preceding section was to encourage and support the substance abuser's entry into treatment. Once there, the treatment may have varying degrees of spouse or family involvement, ranging from little involvement as a collateral informant to active and primary involvement in couple counseling. Regardless of the specific orientation or type of treatment, involving available family and significant others in the treatment and aftercare process appears to improve outcome. For example, involving patients' families or friends in the assessment and treatment planning process has been found to result in fewer readmissions in the year following discharge from inpatient care when compared to those who had no involvement by concerned significant others (Peterson, Swindle, Phibbs, Recine, & Moos, 1994). Two therapeutic approaches to incorporate a spouse or significant other into the ongoing treatment are behavioral marital therapy and CRA.

Behavioral Marital Therapy

As previously noted, substance abuse affects marital relationships in a variety of ways, including miscommunication, conflict, nagging, poor sexual relations, and domestic violence. Behavioral marital therapy (BMT; McCrady, 1991) directly targets both the client's substance use and the marital relationship. Although previously considered a promising but underutilized approach (McCrady, 1991), BMT has developed a solid and extensive empirical basis. Originally developed and evaluated by both O'Farrell (O'Farrell & Cutter, 1984; O'Farrell, 1989, 1994; O'Farrell, Cutter, Choquette, Floyd, & Bayog, 1992; O'Farrell, Choquette, Cutter, Brown, & McCourt, 1993), and McCrady (McCrady et al., 1986; McCrady, Stout, Noel, Abrams, & Nelson, 1991), BMT can serve as an adjunct to or a component of more intensive substance abuse treatment or as a stand-alone outpatient intervention.

The initial step in BMT is a thorough behavioral assessment of the parameters of the client's drinking or drug use behavior; the environmental and interpersonal situations (particularly those in the family and marital relationship) that trigger and maintain drinking and drug use; the nature and stability of the marital relationship; current communication, conflict resolution, and problem-solving abilities; the history and current risk of domestic violence; and other substance-related crises that may require immediate attention. The goal of the assessment is to target changes necessary to reduce or stop substance use and to improve the quality and satisfaction of the relationship. It also provides the context in which the couple can negotiate individual and couple goals that will be worked toward over the course of 10 to 15 sessions.

A number of specific behavioral interventions are used in BMT.

Those focusing on reducing substance use directly might include goal setting for achieving either a reduction in hazardous drinking or abstinence, the development of behavioral contracts that define desired behaviors and the positive and negative consequences for either making or not making the desired changes in these targeted behaviors, the use of monitored disulfiram or other anticraving or use-blocking medications, the development of a hierarchy of both interpersonal and intrapersonal high-risk drinking or substance-using situations, and the development of specific coping responses for both the client and the spouse to address these situations. Interventions targeting the relationship might include communication, conflict resolution, and problem-solving skills training; the development of behavior change and contingency management contracts; and exercises to increase pleasing behaviors, positive interactions, and shared leisure and recreational activities (also see Rychtarik, 1990, for a discussion of coping skills for the spouses of alcoholics). The overall goal of these relationship-targeted interventions is to decrease the level of conflict and discord in the relationship, increase the positive feelings and goodwill between client and spouse, and strengthen the commitment both have for their relationship.

There is considerable empirical support for behavioral marital therapy (Epstein & McCrady, 1998; Powers, Vedel, & Emmelkamp, 2008). A recent meta-analysis of 12 randomized clinical trials of BMT for married or cohabiting individuals who had sought help for alcohol or drug dependence (Powers et al., 2008) concluded that compared to other individual-based treatments, BMT demonstrated a clear advantage across a number of domains, including the frequency of alcohol or drug use, negative substance-related consequences, and relationship satisfaction. As an example, McCrady and colleagues (McCrady et al., 1986, 1991) compared three treatment conditions: minimal spouse involvement, alcohol-focused involvement, and alcohol-focused involvement plus BMT. Clients in all three groups showed a reduction in drinking and increased life satisfaction over a 6-month follow-up period. However, those who received BMT had a more rapid decrease in their drinking, had a longer period of time before relapsing, and maintained marital satisfaction better. A number of these initial gains persisted through an 18-month follow-up. While those who received BMT showed gradual improvement in the proportion of abstinent days, clients in the other two groups showed gradual deterioration in the proportion of abstinent days and light drinking days. Also, those who received BMT reported better marital satisfaction and well-being and had fewer marital separations.

Community Reinforcement Approach

CRA (Meyers et al., 2003; Smith et al., 2001; Smith et al., 1999) is a comprehensive treatment that also has been identified as promising but underutilized (McCrady, 1991). The underlying principle of CRA is to provide the substance abuser access to valued reinforcers contingent on his or her remaining alcohol- and drug-free; the intent is to develop a lifestyle in which these other sources of reinforcement become more salient and rewarding than drinking or using drugs. Detected use of alcohol or drugs would lead to removing access to these potential positive reinforcers and possibly having them replaced with aversive consequences. This contingency management takes place in the context of a number of other therapeutic components such as vocational job skills training, interpersonal and communications skills training, alcohol- and drug-free social clubs, and social support. As noted previously, the spouse or concerned significant other plays an integral role in the CRA, together with the substance abuser and counselor negotiating the behavioral contingencies, determining reinforcers, and establishing treatment contracts.

Contingency Management

An important component found in both CRA and BMT is the use of behavioral contracting and contingency management. In contingency management, an active attempt is made to change those environmental contingencies that may influence substance use behavior (Higgins, 1999; Higgins, Tidey, & Stitzer, 1998). The goal is to decrease or stop alcohol or drug use and to increase behaviors that are incompatible with use. In particular, those contingencies that are found through a functional analysis to promote as well as reinforce substance use are weakened by associating evidence of alcohol or drug use (e.g., positive blood alcohol concentration or drug-positive urine screen) with some form of negative consequence or punishment. Contingencies that promote and reinforce behaviors that are incompatible with substance use and that promote abstinence are strengthened by associating them with positive reinforcers. Contingency management approaches have been found to be among the most effective interventions for initiating and maintaining abstinence as well as increasing the attainment of other meaningful personal and treatment goals among individuals who are dependent on alcohol and a variety of other drugs of abuse (Carroll & Onken, 2005; Prendergast, Podus, Finney, Greenwell, & Roll, 2006; Stanger & Budney, 2010; Stitzer & Petry, 2006; Stitzer & Vandrey, 2008). Of particular relevance to families of substance abusers is the finding that cocaine abusers involved in a contingency management program who engaged in three or more family activities over the 12-week intervention, consistent with one of their goals, remained in treatment longer, had longer drug-free periods, and had a greater reduction in family conflict than those who did not engage in family activities (Lewis & Petry, 2005).

There is an increasing attempt to incorporate real-world reinforcers and contingencies into such programs (Higgins, 1999). Clearly, programs can build contingencies such as take-home medication or increased clinic privileges into the structure of their programs. An early example of a more real-life contingency management system is found in the work of Mark (1988). Approximately one-third of a group of substance abusers who were referred to treatment by a referral source (e.g., family, job, court, welfare, or child protective agencies) that had the ability to withhold anticipated rewards (e.g., welfare checks, return to job and a source of income, return to family) maintained continuous abstinence and treatment involvement over a 6-month period. In contrast, less than one-fifth of those substance abusers referred by noncoercive agents (e.g., self, friend, social agency, medical facility) met these same outcome criteria. A more recent example of such real-world contingencies is provided by Milby and colleagues (Milby et al., 1996, 1998, 2005, 2010). Homeless substance abusers were enrolled in an intensive outpatient day treatment program. In addition, a group of these clients was also involved in a contingent work therapy and housing program. As long as the clients remained substance-free, they were able to remain in the job-training/work program and remain in the therapeutic housing; if they were found to be drinking or using drugs, they were dropped from the housing and work settings. Clients involved in the abstinence-contingent program had fewer cocaine-positive urine samples, fewer days of drinking, fewer days of homelessness, and more days of employment during the follow-up period than did those in the standard treatment. Krampen (1989) has suggested the potential utility of other naturalistic contingencies. Threatened loss of job, spouse, or driver's license was positively related to treatment outcome among alcoholics. However, the prognosis was considerably less favorable in those clients who had already experienced a loss in one of those areas (e.g., the contingency no longer existed) (Mark, 1988).

Behavioral Contracting

Higgins et al. (1998) note that often, but not necessarily always, written contracts can be used to help implement a contingency management program. The contract specifies clearly, often using the client's own words, the target behavior to be changed, the contingencies surrounding either making the desired behavior change or not, and the time frame in which the desired behavior change is to occur. The act of composing and signing a contract is a small but potentially important public ritual signifying the client's commitment to the proposed change. In the contract, the client may include contingencies, especially rewards or positive incentives that reinforce target behaviors (e.g., attending treatment sessions, getting to 12-step meetings, avoiding stimuli associated with substance use). Goals should be clearly defined, divided into small steps that occur frequently, and revised as treatment progresses; contingencies should occur quickly after success or failure.

An example of a behavioral contract is the "sobriety contract" that is frequently used as a component of CRA or BMT (O'Farrell & Fals-Stewart, 2002). The negotiated contract involves the substance abuser on a daily basis affirming his or her commitment to not drink or use drugs; this intent is reinforced by the spouse/partner, who expresses support for this stated goal of abstinence. For those individuals taking some form of medication such as disulfiram as part of their treatment, the contract also involves an agreement that the spouse/partner will monitor/witness the taking of the medication and reinforce the substance abuser for doing so (Allen & Litten, 1992; Krampe & Ehrenreich, 2010). The process involved in behavioral contracting is found in the descriptive report of O'Farrell and Bayog (1986). In working with couples having an alcoholic member, O'Farrell and Bayog developed a disulfiram contract procedure. The procedure has three primary goals: (1) to increase the alcoholic's compliance in taking disulfiram, (2) to decrease the number of alcohol-related interactions and arguments between the alcoholic and spouse (which represent a source of stress and a potential relapse precipitant), and (3) to increase the likelihood of the alcoholic maintaining abstinence. As outlined above, the alcoholic agrees to take the disulfiram daily while being observed by the spouse and to refill the disulfiram prescription before it expires. The spouse agrees to maintain a record on a calendar of the dates on which the alcoholic was observed taking the medication and to remind him or her to refill the prescription before it expires. Together, the alcoholic and spouse agree not to discuss the alcoholic's past or possible future drinking (e.g., decrease nagging and drinking control efforts); to thank each other after the observed disulfiram use for being helpful toward one another and for doing something positive about the drinking problem; to contact the therapist if two consecutive days go by without observed use of the medication; and to agree on a time frame for the contract and on their willingness to discuss renewing or modifying the contract at that point in time.

While promising, the effectiveness of this disulfiram-contracting procedure, as well as other behavioral contracting with substance abusers, has not been evaluated adequately. However, such behavioral medication contracts and the supervised/monitored taking of medication are associated with increased adherence and the clinical effectiveness of disulfiram as a component part of the treatment of alcohol dependence (Allen & Litten, 1992; Krampe & Ehrenreich, 2010). Most often, behavioral contracts and contingency management procedures are embedded in a more comprehensive treatment program. Contracts targeting goals supportive of recovery (e.g., improving vocational behavior, saving money, being prompt and regular for counseling and medication) are generally more likely to be achieved and may lead to better outcomes than those more directly related to substance use (e.g., clean urine samples). Iguchi, Belding, Morral, Lamb, and Husband (1997), for instance, found that receiving vouchers contingent on completing objective, individually tailored goals related to one's overall treatment plan was more effective in reducing drug use than either a voucher system specifically targeting drug-free urine samples or the standard treatment without either of these contingency contracts added.

MAINTENANCE OF BEHAVIOR CHANGE

While having a substance-abusing family member enter and complete treatment is an important step, it is equally important (possibly even more so) to maintain the therapeutic gains made during treatment once the individual has returned home (Marlatt & Donovan, 2005). For instance, while considerable positive changes might be found in substance use and marital adjustment of both male and female clients who were involved with their spouse/partner in BMT, some of the drug use and relationship adjustment differences can begin to dissipate over the course of the months following treatment. A component of the continuum of treatment targeting this phase of the recovery process is aftercare or continuing care (Donovan, 1998; McKay, 2001, 2005, 2006, 2009). In addition to involvement during treatment, involving available family and significant others to facilitate the entry of the substance abuser into as well as actively participating in continuing care during the maintenance stage also appears to lead to improved outcomes (O'Farrell, Murphy, Alter, & Fals-Stewart, 2008). Two primary approaches of family involvement in continuing care are through behavioral contracts and relapse prevention approaches.

Behavioral Continuing Care Contracts

In addition to the behavioral contract to take and monitor disulfiram or other anticraving or relapse-risk-reducing medications as described above, behavioral contracts have also been used to try to increase attendance at continuing care meetings following an initial more intensive treatment. A relatively easy-to-implement behavioral contracting procedure was initially described by Ossip-Klein and colleagues (Ossip-Klein & Rychtarik, 1993; Ossip-Klein, Vanlandingham, Prue, & Rychtarik, 1984). The contract is negotiated as the client is approaching the transition from an intensive treatment (e.g., inpatient, day hospital, or intensive outpatient) to a less intensive continuing care. The counselor presents the client an appointment calendar for continuing care sessions and assists in negotiating an attendance contract between client and spouse. The contract involves the client's agreeing to post the appointment calendar in a prominent location at home, attend all scheduled aftercare sessions, and call to reschedule if an appointment must be missed. In exchange for adhering to these behaviors, the spouse agrees to provide a mutually negotiated incentive within 1 week of the appointment. The contract is then referred to at each subsequent continuing care session.

This straightforward contracting procedure, relative to clients receiving standard care, resulted in significantly greater continuing care attendance, especially at the first continuing care session (72% vs. 36% for contracting and treatment as usual patients respectively), a greater likelihood of being abstinent at 3-, 6-, and 12-month follow-up points, greater rates of employment (46.7% vs. 13.3%) at the 1-year follow-up, and a greater likelihood to be considered treatment successes (77.8% vs. 38.9%, based on abstinence and reduced drinking) (Ossip-Klein et al., 1984). More recently, Lash and colleagues (Lash, Burden, Monteleone, & Lehmann, 2004; Lash et al., 2005; Lash, Petersen, O'Connor, & Lehmann, 2001; Lash et al., 2007) have incorporated social reinforcement along with prompting and contracting procedures in an approach called Contracting, Prompting, and Reinforcing (CPR). In addition to the contract and prompts, the counselor provides social reinforcement (e.g., handwritten letters, certificates, medallions) for reaching specific aftercare group and individual therapy attendance landmarks. In a randomized trial comparing CPR to standard continuing care arrangements, individuals receiving CPR were more likely to complete 3 months of aftercare, remain in treatment longer, and have higher rates of abstinence at the 1-year follow-up (Lash et al., 2007). Although the contracting in CPR was done with a counselor prior to discharge from inpatient treatment, it could easily be adapted to include the involvement of a spouse, partner, or concerned other in the process.

Couple Relapse Prevention

Another avenue of family involvement during the maintenance stage is through relapse prevention programs that are integrated into couple counseling (McCrady, 1989, 1993; McCrady, Epstein, & Hirsch, 1999; McCrady, Epstein, & Kahler, 2004; O'Farrell, Choquette, & Cutter, 1998; O'Farrell, 1993; O'Farrell et al., 1993). There are three main components of the relapse prevention process (O'Farrell, 1993). The first is to help the substance user, the significant other, and their relationship to maintain the positive gains they have made during couple therapy. To this end, they are encouraged to continue with the contracted monitoring of disulfiram or other medications, relationship-enhancing shared activities, and attendance at self-help support groups such as AA and Al-Anon. The second is to deal with unresolved or emergent relationship problems utilizing therapist input and the communication, conflict resolution, and problem-solving skills gained in couple counseling. The third is to develop and try out a relapse prevention plan. This would include the identification of high-risk relapse situations and the early warning signs for relapse, and the development and practice of cognitive and behavioral coping skills to deal with these situations, and a specific plan of dealing with relapse if it occurs.

O'Farrell and colleagues (O'Farrell et al., 1998; O'Farrell et al., 1993) examined the benefit of adding a couple relapse prevention component as continuing care during the year following 5 months of weekly behavioral marital therapy. Alcoholic husbands and their wives/partners were randomly assigned either to a condition that received no further treatment or to one involving 15 additional sessions of conjoint therapy focusing specifically on relapse prevention spread with decreasing frequency across a 1-year period. An initial analysis of outcomes (O'Farrell et al., 1993) indicated that both groups demonstrated significant improvements as a result of their participation in the initial behavioral marital therapy. However, those who received the subsequent conjoint relapse prevention sessions had more days abstinent, fewer drinking days, and improved relationships with spouses longer than those who received no further treatment beyond the behavioral marital therapy. A subsequent follow-up 3 years after the original initiation of treatment (O'Farrell et al., 1998) affirmed the incremental benefit of the added relapse prevention component with respect to both marital and drinking outcomes, particularly for those individuals who initially presented with more severe alcohol and marital problems

Working with alcoholic men and their spouses/partners, McCrady and colleagues compared alcohol behavioral couple therapy (ABCT) alone to ABCT with either relapse prevention or involvement in Alcoholics Anonymous (AA). At a 6-month follow-up (McCrady et al., 1999) all three groups demonstrated significant, but not differential, reductions in heavy drinking days and alcohol-related consequences as well as increased abstinent days. However, compared to the ABCT plus AA condition, those who received ABCT alone had a longer time before relapse to heavy drinking and those who received ABCT plus relapse prevention had shorter drinking episodes. It was concluded based on these results that there was no added benefit from combining AA with behavioral couple therapy. This conclusion was modified by longer term outcomes at an 18-month follow-up (McCrady et al., 2004). For those with sufficient data across the 18-month period (73% of the original sample), there were no differences between the three groups with respect to marital happiness or drinking outcomes. Attendance at AA meetings, both for the group receiving ABCT plus encouragement to attend AA and for the sample as a whole, was positively related to abstinence.

Self-Help Involvement

Dealing with the substance abuse of a family member is a stressful process. The concerned significant other and other family members may need ongoing support over and above that which they might receive from involvement in the substance abuser's treatment. This is one of the main roles of family-oriented self-help groups such as Al-Anon, Nar-Anon, and Alateen (Nowinski, 1999; Schulz & Chappel, 1998). These groups represent one of the most readily available, widely utilized, and least costly resources for family members of substance abusers (Fernandez et al., 2006); it is estimated that there are over 15,000 Al-Anon groups in the United States and Canada (Schulz & Chappel, 1998), which are based generally on the 12 steps and 12 traditions of AA. A major tenet of these self-help/mutual-support groups is that, even if the substance abuser continues to drink or use drugs, family members are able to get help for themselves through their involvement. Two primary ideas are conveyed and reinforced in these groups (Schulz & Chappel, 1998). The first is that alcoholism or drug dependence is a disease and that the substance abuser, rather than the concerned significant other, is responsible for his or her behavior and recovery. There is an emphasis on detachment from and letting go of the substance abuser, not being involved as an enabler of continued use. This may represent an active rather than a passive form of withdrawal as a coping strategy (Orford et al., 1998). It is important to allow substance abusers to experience the natural consequences of their substance use. Group members provide support to the significant other as he or she tries to accomplish this difficult task. The second tenet is that the particular program is for the concerned significant other, not the substance abuser. The significant other has an opportunity and obligation to focus on his or her own emotional needs and self-esteem.

The studies by Miller et al. (1999) and Kirby et al. (1999) found that concerned significant others' involvement in 12-step self-help facilitation was less successful than CRAFT in getting resistant alcoholic and drug abusers to enter treatment. However, the concerned significant others who became involved in these mutual-help groups demonstrated a considerable change in a number of areas of psychosocial functioning consistent with the goal of working on one's own needs. These studies found significant reductions in levels of depression, anger, anxiety, family conflict, and other presenting problems; significant improvements were also noted in family cohesion and function, and relationship happiness. The significant others in the mutual-help groups did not differ from those in the CRAFT with respect to these improvements. Of note is that the changes in the significant others' emotional functioning was independent of the substance abusers' drinking or drug use status, consistent with the view that the support of and benefit from these self-help groups is for the significant other.

SUMMARY

• Substance abuse is a family disorder, due to both the genetic predisposition toward developing substance abuse problems among family members and to the negative impact on the family, its function, and its members.

• Substance abuse treatment that includes family members or significant others is effective in reducing drinking or drug use, decreasing psychological and physical problems among family members, reducing health care utilization, and improving personal and familial functioning.

• The family and its members go through a series of stages in their attempt to deal with a family member having a substance abuse problem that parallel those through which substance abusers move in their process of change.

• Having come to the point of action, the family then must work to motivate the substance abuser to enter treatment.

• A number of interventions meant to encourage treatment entry have been used and evaluated. These range along a continuum of coercion from the Johnson Institute intervention through the ARISE program to unilateral family therapy and the Community Reinforcement and Family Training (CRAFT) program. A large number of families never come to the point of implementing the Johnson Institute intervention, but when this approach is used it may be successful in facilitating treatment entry but is less effective than other approaches. There is limited research evaluating unilateral family therapy and the ARISE program. The CRAFT program is quite successful in getting resistant substance abusers to enter treatment and to change their behavior and has been described as a "best bet" clinical option among the "engagement-primary" approaches.

- Family involvement in the active phase of treatment appears to increase outcome success as well as family functioning.

- Both behavioral marital therapy (BMT) and the community reinforcement approach (CRA) are effective treatments. Contingency management and behavioral contracting, components of both BMT and CRA, have demonstrated empirical support.

- Continued family involvement during the maintenance stage contributes to further improvement over and above that achieved during the active intervention stage.

- Couple relapse prevention appears to be an effective component of BMT, leading to decreased substance use and improved relationship function. It is also a very cost-effective intervention.

- Mutual-support groups such as Al-Anon and Nar-Anon, which are based on the 12 steps and 12 traditions of AA, represent a readily available source of support for family members who are dealing with a substance abuser. While not being particularly effective in getting substance abusers into treatment, involvement in these groups appears to lead to positive benefits such as reduced anger, depression, and anxiety and increased self-esteem among those who attend.

- Given the positive effects of family involvement, treatment programs should attempt to include family members whenever possible.

8

Populations with Special Needs
The Cases of Women and DUI Offenders

Substance abusers represent a heterogeneous group of individuals, with a variety of subtypes of alcohol- and drug-dependent individuals having significant implications for etiology, treatment, and recovery (Basu, Ball, Feinn, Gelernter, & Kranzler, 2004; Hesselbrock & Hesselbrock, 2006; Moss, Chen, & Yi, 2010). Among the clinically meaningful dimensions across which they vary include race/ethnicity (Blume, Morera, & Garcia de la Cruz, 2005), gender (Greenfield, Back, Lawson, & Brady, 2010; Tuchman, 2010), age (Roe, Beynon, Pickering, & Duffy, 2010), and the presence of co-occurring psychiatric (Brady, Verduin, & Tolliver, 2007) or medical problems (De Alba et al., 2004), including HIV/AIDS (Metzger, Woody, & O'Brien, 2010). In addition to differing with respect to demographic characteristics, substance abusers also differ in the severity and nature of presenting problems, motivations for seeking treatment, perceived barriers that delay or prevent their seeking and entering treatment, and needs to be addressed in treatment (e.g., Caldeira et al., 2009; Carise, Gurel, McLellan, Dugosh, & Kendig, 2005; Cunningham, Sobell, Sobell, Agrawal, & Toneatto, 1993; Cunningham, Sobell, Sobell, & Gaskin, 1994; Freyer et al., 2007; Gayman, Cuddeback, & Morrissey, 2011; Tucker, 2001). Many of these subgroups also have limited access to and are commonly underrepresented in and underserved by the substance abuse treatment system, representing a prominent form of health care disparity (Blume, Resor, & Kantin, 2009; Lowman & Le Fauve, 2003). This view is consistent with an early definition of "special populations" as populations or groups sharing common social, psychological, or legal characteristics that have encountered barriers in obtaining appropriate treatment (Gomberg, 2003; Institute of Medicine, 1990). The constraints that make treatment entry difficult may be cultural, financial, and/or programmatic in nature.

Among the many possible special populations, important subtypes that have relatively unique concerns and may require targeted interventions include women, minority ethnic groups, age groups (adolescent and elderly) (Gomberg, 2003; Stasiewicz & Smith, 2002), and those with comorbid psychiatric disorders in addition to their substance abuse or dependence (Brady et al., 2007). Another group in which motivation for behavior change and treatment engagement may be of particular issue are individuals mandated to treatment for offenses such as driving under the influence of alcohol or drugs (DUI) (Dill & Wells-Parker, 2006; Wells-Parker, Williams, Dill, & Kenne, 1998).

Given the apparent difficulties in engaging and retaining such subgroups in treatment, the individual's stage of readiness to change may need to be taken into account and stage-targeted motivationally oriented interventions employed. Such approaches need to take individual difference, environmental, and cultural factors into account. The purpose of the present chapter is to provide a brief overview of a variety of clinical issues related to the stages of readiness to change in two such populations, namely, women substance abusers and DUI offenders. These were chosen because they represent exemplars of populations with special needs and have received attention from the stages-of-change perspective. (In addition, approaches designed specifically for pregnant women are discussed in Chapter 10.)

WOMEN SUBSTANCE ABUSERS

The majority of research conducted in the area of substance abuse has been based largely on studies with men. A concern has been that this information may not generalize to women, who have a number of specific issues that may be overlooked by this focus on men. There has been an increased awareness of these issues, and women have become the focus of increased attention in clinical research and practice (Greenfield et al., 2010; Hecksher & Hesse, 2009; Tuchman, 2010). If left unaddressed, these factors may reduce the effectiveness of treatment (Hagan, Finnegan, & Nelson-Zlupko, 1994). Despite this increased attention, women are often underrepresented and underserved in substance abuse treatment (Green, 2006; Ramlow, White, Watson, & Leukefeld, 1997). Women, compared to men, face multiple barriers to accessing specialty alcohol or drug treatment, are less likely to seek treatment, and if they do, are more likely to seek care in mental health or primary care settings rather than in addiction treatment programs (Green, 2006). However, if women enter specialty substance abuse treatment, gender does not appear to be a predictor of treatment retention, completion, or outcome (Greenfield et al., 2010; Greenfield, Brooks, et al., 2007) and women may actually have better outcomes than men (Green, 2006). This suggests that efforts are needed to reduce the barriers to treatment entry and to facilitate treatment engagement for women.

Reasons for Substance Use

Men and women substance abusers have been compared on a number of dimensions that may bear on the unique needs of women in treatment. One area of difference is in the apparent reasons for drinking and using drugs. Men and women report different reasons for maintaining the use of the substances. In comparison to men, women have been found to misuse alcohol in response to stresses related to current circumstances or life events. This may be even truer for middle-age women since a number of significant life events occur during midlife (e.g., divorce, bereavement, departure of children from home) (Allan & Cooke, 1985), and women who are heavy drinkers experience more health-related stressful events (King, Bernardy, & Hauner, 2003). Women also have a significantly higher prevalence of comorbid psychiatric (particularly mood and anxiety), eating, and posttraumatic stress disorders than do men, and these disorders often predate the onset of substance-abuse problems (Brady & Randall, 1999; Greenfield et al., 2010). Additionally, women are often the victims of sexual, psychological, and/or physical abuse that contribute to the experience of trauma and mood disorders (Brady & Randall, 1999; Greenfield et al., 2010; Hecksher & Hesse, 2009). Consistent with this, depression has been found to be a major trigger for relapse in women with alcohol and drug problems (Snow & Anderson, 2000), and women appear more likely than men to report heavy drinking in response to negative emotional states and interpersonal conflict with others (Annis & Graham, 1995). Within this context, it has been hypothesized that alcohol and drug use may be relied on more heavily to self-medicate mood disturbances among women than among men. However, results from a series of recent epidemiological studies in nationally representative nonclinical samples argue against this idea, finding, in fact, that men are more likely than women to drink or use drugs to self-medicate (Bolton, Robinson, & Sareen, 2009; Leeies, Pagura, Sareen, & Bolton, 2010; Robinson, Sareen, Cox, & Bolton, 2009). Regardless of whether it is viewed as self-medicating or not, the high rates of relapse associated with co-occurring depression, anxiety, trauma, and PTSD suggest that these disorders represent important targets for intervention in women substance abusers.

Consequences of Use

Negative consequences associated with substance abuse are different for men and women. Women substance abusers are at greater risk and are more vulnerable to a wide variety of health problems and may develop medical side effects to their abuse of alcohol, tobacco, stimulants, and opioids more rapidly than their male counterparts (Hernandez-Avila, Rounsaville, & Kranzler, 2004; Johnson, Richter, Kleber, McLellan, & Carise, 2005; Kay, Taylor, Barthwell, Wichelecki, & Leopold, 2010). This more rapid progression of negative consequences among women is called the "telescoping phenomenon" (Piazza, Vrbka, & Yeager, 1989). Early research that identified this phenomenon found women to start drinking later, get drunk regularly, experience their first drinking problems, and exhibit loss of control over their drinking at later average ages than men (Brady & Randall, 1999; Randall et al., 1999). Despite this later onset of drinking, women were found to progress faster than men between first getting drunk regularly and experiencing their first drinking problems and between first loss of drinking control and onset of worst drinking problems. Women also exhibited shorter average progression times between first getting drunk regularly and first seeking treatment, as well as entering treatment earlier in the course of their substance use problem than men (Brady & Randall, 1999; Greenfield et al., 2007a, 2010; Johnson et al., 2005). However, this pattern has not been found consistently (Keyes, Martins, Blanco, & Hasin, 2010b; Schuckit, Anthenelli, Bucholz, Hesselbrock, & Tipp, 1995).

More recent research has shown that this gap between men and women has narrowed considerably and that the previously noted differential rates of symptom development and progression are minimal and may no longer be found. The sequence of occurrence of alcohol- or drug-related problems appears to be comparable across men and women (Keyes et al., 2010b; Schuckit et al., 1995; Schuckit, Daeppen, Tipp, Hesselbrock, & Bucholz, 1998); this appears to be particularly true among younger cohorts of individuals (Johnson et al., 2005; Keyes et al., 2010b). It has been suggested that the narrowing of this gap may be related to changes in the patterns and the increased prevalence of alcohol and drug use among women over recent years (Schuckit et al., 1998; Zilberman, Tavares, & el-Guebaly, 2003). It has also been found that, in addition to the influence of age, there are marked differences in the onset and course of substance use as a function of race/ethnicity that may be as important, if not more so, as gender (Alvanzo et al., 2011; Johnson et al., 2005). These latter findings suggest that differences in onset and patterns of use as well as symptom progression may be more attributable to sociocultural factors rather than gender-based biological factors (Johnson et al., 2005). However, both gender and racial/ethnic issues and factors need to be taken into account in understanding the etiology and maintenance of substance use disorders and to inform appropriately tailored prevention and treatment programs to meet the needs of these differing subgroups (Alvanzo et al., 2011; Greenfield et al., 2007a, 2010; Lowman & Le Fauve, 2003).

Reasons for and Barriers to Treatment Seeking: From Contemplation to Action

It typically takes some time before a substance abuser seeks formal treatment for his or her disorder (Gayman et al., 2011; Tucker, 2001), often choosing to seek treatment only after significant negative consequences are experienced (Cunningham et al., 1994). Experiencing negative physical, social, interpersonal, and psychological consequences plays a major role in the decision to seek help.

There are both internal and external barriers that lead individuals to delay or to not seek treatment (Cunningham et al., 1993; Rapp et al., 2006; Xu, Rapp, Wang, & Carlson, 2008; Xu, Wang, Rapp, & Carlson, 2007). Prominent internal barriers include the belief that one does not have an alcohol or drug problem, negative or lack of social support for seeking treatment, fear of treatment, privacy concerns, and committed lifestyle (e.g., drug use is an important component of life and is not easy to give up) (Xu et al., 2007). Common external barriers include having difficulties and conflicts in scheduling time for treatment, treatment accessibility, treatment entry difficulty (e.g., wait lists), and financial problems (e.g., inability to pay for treatment or lack of insurance coverage) (Xu et al., 2008). While men and women both experience somewhat similar internal and external barriers, there also appear to be some differences in their reasons for seeking treatment (Green, Polen, Dickinson, Lynch, & Bennett, 2002; Thom, 1987). In one of the earliest and most extensive examinations of gender differences in substance abuse help seeking, Thom (1987) found that while both men and women report serious health problems as a major reason, men also indicated that marital disruption was also important. Job loss, debts, legal problems, and homelessness were also important factors in the decision to seek treatment (Green et al., 2002). Positive reasons, such as forming a new relationship, were also given (Thom, 1987). Women often express greater levels of negative social support for their seeking treatment and more financial concerns as deterrents to treatment seeking than do men (Xu et al., 2008; Xu et al., 2007).

Thom (1987) found that women substance abusers were more often seeking treatment in an attempt to alleviate problems other than their substance abuse. Few patients accepted referral primarily to change their drinking behavior. Women reported problems with children (fear of losing a child, recent loss of a child) significantly more often than men; men reported difficulties with aggression significantly more often than women. Among alcoholics who reported sobriety of 1 year or more, women more frequently cited relationships while men more often noted their legal difficulties and status in the community as motivational influences on their decisions to become abstinent (Lutz, 1991).

Women appear to experience more barriers, both internal and external, and to be less likely to enter specialty substance abuse treatment compared to men (Gordon, 2007; Green, 2006; Greenfield, Brooks, et al., 2007; Tuchman, 2010). The greater the number of barriers experienced, the less likely it is that women will seek or enter specialty treatment (Rosen, Tolman, & Warner, 2004). If women do seek treatment, it is more likely to be in the context of primary care or mental health services than in a substance abuse program (Green, 2006). Barriers that lead women to delay or not to seek substance abuse treatment or self-help group involvement represent intrapersonal (e.g., personal characteristics and beliefs of the substance user, health problems, psychological issues, cognitive functioning, motivational status, treatment readiness), interpersonal (e.g., relationships, family dynamics, support systems), sociocultural (e.g., cultural differences, perceived stigma and bias, societal attitudes, health disparities), and structural (program characteristics, treatment focus and treatment process, availability of wrap-around services for co-occurring disorders and child care) factors (Center for Substance Abuse Treatment, 2009b; Gordon, 2007).

One internal personal barrier that may reduce motivation for change or treatment is a form of denial, in which the individual minimizes the severity of her substance abuse problem. This may, in part, be based on a lack of understanding of the behaviors and consequences that constitute alcohol or drug abuse, the severity of one's use, or the perceived need for assistance in changing one's drinking or drug use behaviors (Gordon, 2007). Framing this phenomenon as lack of awareness or lack of problem recognition (Rapp et al., 2008b), which is a more acceptable and malleable factor than the defensive trait of denial, is more consistent with motivational enhancement approaches (Miller & Rollnick, 1991).

Even if there is an awareness of a developing problem, there is often a reluctance to acknowledge it publicly and to seek treatment. The higher the level of treatment reluctance, the less likely one is to recognize one's substance use as problematic and the lower the levels of desire to change and readiness for treatment (Rapp et al., 2008b). It is important to note that readiness to change and readiness to seek treatment are two related but different components of motivation (Freyer et al., 2004; Freyer et al., 2005). Among other factors, often this reluctance is related to fear of being stigmatized as a substance abuser (Schober & Annis, 1996). Women substance abusers appear to be more stigmatized than their male counterparts, often being viewed more negatively by others. This is particularly true for those who have children, where there is fear of being labeled as "bad mothers" with the additional potential risk of possible loss of child custody. This stigma, whether held internally by the woman or perceived by her as how she feels she is viewed by others, contributes to a sense of shame and guilt that reduces her willingness to step forward, acknowledge (at least more publicly) that she has a substance use problem, and seek help (Center for Substance Abuse Treatment, 2009b). Fears about losing one's privacy, being labeled as an alcoholic or drug addict, and the stigmatizing effects of current treatments may be more powerful disincentives to seek treatment than denial of having a problem or structural factors such as treatment cost and accessibility (Keyes et al., 2010a; Luoma et al., 2007; Marlatt et al., 1997; Myers, Fakier, & Louw, 2009).

Lack of or negative social support for treatment is another major factor in delaying treatment (Gordon, 2007; Rapp et al., 2006; Xu et al., 2007). The response to a woman's possibly entering treatment is often quite negative, even more so than for men (Xu et al., 2007). Spouses, relatives, and significant others often deny that the woman has an alcohol or drug problem and sometimes even actively oppose seeking treatment. Women in a treatment sample reported greater opposition from family or friends as compared to men (Beckman, 1984, 1994; Beckman & Amaro, 1986). As such, significant others' opposition to treatment is a key factor in outreach attempts to bring alcoholic women into treatment (Beckman, 1994).

Another family issue that influences the decision about seeking treatment has to do with child care responsibilities (Gordon, 2007; Wilsnack, 1991). It has often been thought that having children, and wanting to be able to keep them, served as a motivator for substance-abusing women to enter treatment. However, this is not always the case, and in many instances children may represent a disincentive for seeking treatment (Wilke, Kamata, & Cash, 2005). There are at least two aspects of this. The first is having to find someone to care for the children while receiving treatment. Child care responsibilities fall more heavily on women substance abusers than on their male counterparts, which restricts their ability to enter treatment, especially residential care, unless the program has some form of child care available (Stewart, Gossop, & Trakada, 2007). If parenting women in fact do enter treatment, the provision of child care is associated with their remaining in treatment for longer durations (Campbell, Alexander, & Lemak, 2009). The second aspect is the fear of being perceived as an unfit mother due to substance use, with the real threat of losing custody of one's children (Wilke et al., 2005). Community leaders, social agency staff, and substance abuse treatment professionals are in agreement that child care accommodations at treatment programs are the most needed resource for women (Gordon, 2007; Wilsnack, 1991) and it appears that there has been an increase in such services over time (Grella & Greenwell, 2004).

In addition to these personal barriers, a number of factors related to the dominant treatment model and aspects of the treatment process have led women to be reluctant about entering treatment (Wilke, 1994). A primary concern is that the most prevalent treatment model, which was developed to a large degree to address men, may not provide appropriate strategies to meet women's needs (Jordan & Oei, 1989;

Ramlow et al., 1997). A major reason women do not enter treatment is because many treatment programs are not structured in ways that meet women's needs, nor do they provide gender-sensitive treatment services (Beckman, 1984; Wilsnack, 1991; Nelson-Zlupko, Dore, Kauffman, & Kaltenbach, 1996). It has been argued that in order to address many of the unique concerns of women, it is necessary to provide gender-specific support services such as aftercare, child care, treatment for children, and women's halfway houses and all-female self-help groups (Ashley, Marsden, & Brady, 2003; Greenfield & Grella, 2009). There has been an increasing consensus among treatment professionals, social agency representatives, and community leaders for the need for gender-responsive or female-specific treatment services (Grella, 2008). Also, there needs to be sufficient financial support for women to be able to afford the service, since inability to pay or lack of insurance coverage continue to be major external barriers for women (Xu et al., 2008).

From Contemplation to Action

Given these reasons for and barriers to substance abuse treatment for women, a number of possible points of intervention can be found to try to move them along the stages of change. The first would be to focus on primary care settings to identify women with substance abuse problems and increase their motivation to seek treatment. This is a more likely venue for women than specialty substance abuse treatment programs (Cyr & McGarry, 2002; Green, 2006). Often, and particularly for women, treatment entry is preceded by discussion of substance-related problems with a health care professional (Room, 1989; Price, Cottler, & Robins, 1991; Bucholz, Homan, & Helzer, 1992; Marlatt et al., 1997). However, female problem drinkers and substance abusers are less likely than males to be identified in the primary care setting (Chang, Behr, Goetz, Hiley, & Bigby, 1997). It is necessary to utilize screening measures that have been developed and validated with women and are sensitive in the identification of substance use problems among women (Bradley, Boyd-Wickizer, Powell, & Burman, 1998; Burns, Gray, & Smith, 2010). However, even with validated measures or reviews of medical records, many women who drink at a hazardous level with a variety of medical problems go unidentified (Chang, Fisher, Hornstein, Jones, & Orav, 2010). Primary medical care settings may provide early contact points for problem identification and possible referral for substance abusers (Green, 2006). Expanding the involvement of primary care medical providers may facilitate appropriate help seeking and may reach substance abusers who otherwise would avoid traditional intensive treatments (Thom, 1987; Copeland & Hall, 1992; Marlatt et al., 1997). A similar identification and referral process should also be conducted in other medical and social service agencies that have ongoing contact with women, especially those settings (e.g., family practice, OBGYN clinic, pediatric services, emergency room, trauma center, welfare office) having high rates of substance abusers in its clientele.

Women who perceive barriers associated with treatment are less likely to purse treatment entry. Beckman and Amaro (1986) found that nearly half of the women, but fewer than 20% of the men, in a sample having entered into alcoholism treatment experienced one or more costs (e.g., problems with family, money, or friends) because of entering treatment. In order to increase the likelihood of treatment entry and retention, these barriers must be minimized or there needs to be a way in which they can be addressed effectively.

Women do frequently enter substance abuse programs despite the fact that they view problems other than their substance abuse as their primary reason for seeking treatment and despite concerns that the program may not be particularly relevant to these other primary problems. Given that most patients experience such ambivalence about treatment even after entering it, and since this ambivalence may turn women away from treatment in the absence of services thought to be important and effective, it is particularly important to maintain or increase women's motivation to stick with treatment. It is possible to use a number of techniques, such as a decisional balance exercise in which the pros and cons of continued use and of treatment entry are weighed, as a means of increasing the motivation for and commitment to treatment. While such approaches derived from motivational interviewing may be of use, given the extent of the problems and barriers encountered by substance-abusing women, they may be less likely in and of themselves to facilitate treatment entry and engagement than case management approaches that are better able to provide ongoing support and address the multiple needs of these individuals (Morgenstern et al., 2006; Morgenstern et al., 2009; Rapp, Otto, et al., 2008).

Another important approach to moving from contemplation to action is based on the family's reaction to the woman's substance use and the attempt to seek treatment. As noted above, women encounter lack of support or opposition to treatment from family and friends significantly more often than men (Gordon, 2007; Xu et al., 2007). Overcoming the opposition of significant others to treatment is a critically important feature in outreach attempts to bring alcoholic women into treatment. This suggests that involving the significant others in the treatment process, either as a member of a positive support network or more formally in couple or family therapy, is critical when resistance is encountered (see Chapter 7 for information about engaging significant others).

Female-Only versus Mixed-Gender Treatment: Action and Maintenance

Based on these concerns about the increasing prevalence of alcohol and drug use among women, coupled with the multiple barriers to treatment and the "male-as-norm" orientation of many treatment programs, there has been an increased focus on and development of gender-responsive and women-focused substance abuse treatment services (Green, 2006; Greenfield & Grella, 2009; Grella, 2008; Grella & Greenwell, 2004; Tang, Claus, Orwin, Kissin, & Arieira, 2012; Wilke, 1994). This shift in focus, which includes an increased number of women-only programs as well as an expansion of gender-specific components in mixed-gender programs, is consistent with recommendations made over two decades ago by the Institute of Medicine in discussing appropriate treatments for alcohol abuse (Institute of Medicine, 1990). It indicated that the evidence up to that point supported the contention that treatment programs that deal specifically with the multiple problems more frequently faced by women would lead to better outcomes (Institute of Medicine, 1990). They also listed those gender-specific features that they felt would enhance treatment outcomes for women: These include "(1) child care; (2) assessments of psychiatric disorders and treatment for depression, when indicated, (3) methods of building self-esteem, perhaps through skills training, (4) support offered to and education of family and friends, (5) assessments of accompanying medical disorders, (6) availability of staff to work with families, and (7) teaching of coping skills for dealing with stress and other negative emotional states" (Institute of Medicine, 1990, p. 358). Also, as noted previously, in order to integrate the treatment necessary to address the broad range of presenting problems, case management can be used in conjunction with the primary intervention in order to enhance treatment outcome for women in alcohol and drug treatment (Morgenstern et al., 2006; Morgenstern et al., 2009; Rapp, Otto, et al., 2008; Sullivan, 1994). However, the Institute of Medicine also indicated that further research was needed to determine the effectiveness of these treatment components for women (vs. men) and the characteristics of women for whom treatment is differentially effective.

Women who present to women-only programs differ from those seeking treatment in mixed-gender programs (Copeland & Hall, 1992; Copeland, Hall, Didcott, & Biggs, 1993; Niv & Hser, 2007). Those in the women-only program were significantly more likely to have dependent children, be lesbian, have a maternal history for drug or alcohol problems, and have suffered sexual abuse in childhood (Copeland & Hall, 1992). Those in women-only programs are more likely to have a recent history of having been physically abused and to have more severe alcohol, drug, family, and psychiatric problems than those entering mixed-gender programs, and as a result have typically utilized more treatment services (Hser & Niv, 2006; Niv & Hser, 2007). In comparing the beliefs and perceptions of women in women-only versus those in mixed-gender programs, the women in the women-only programs felt that these problems and related issues (such as low self- esteem, being victims of physical and sexual abuse, sexual orientation, and sex-role conflict) could be met better in the gender-specific rather than in mixed-gender programs (Beckman, 1984; Kauffman, Dore, & Nelson-Zlupko, 1995).

It appears that women's-only programs such as the Women's Recovery Group (Greenfield, Trucco, McHugh, Lincoln, & Gallop, 2007) may be particularly beneficial for those with high levels of psychiatric severity (Greenfield et al., 2008) and those with low levels of self-efficacy at treatment entry, which often is associated with increased severity of substance dependence and psychosocial problems (Cummings, Gallop, & Greenfield, 2010). Also, women who were able to have their children in treatment with them were found to have significantly better retention rates than those who were in treatment without their children (Szuster, Rich, Chung, & Bisconer, 1996). This latter point is of note, since length of stay in treatment for women is associated with subsequent substance use outcomes, and women-only programs appear to have better retention rates than do mixed-gender programs (Greenfield et al., 2004; Zilberman, Tavares, Andrade, & El-Guebaly, 2003). Further, it appears that women with children who are involved in women-only treatment have significantly higher rates of continuing care following residential care than do those whose initial treatment was in mixed-gender programs (Claus et al., 2007).

Despite the strong advocacy for gender-specific women's programs, the results from studies evaluating treatment outcome of such programs versus mixed-gender programs have been equivocal. One of the first evaluations of this issue compared the outcomes of 80 women treated in a gender-specific women's program to those of 80 women recruited from two mixed-gender programs (Copeland et al., 1993). Both programs were based on the traditional disease model and the 12-step philosophy; however, the gender-specific program had only female staff and provided residential child care. Six months following treatment there were no significant differences in any measure of treatment outcome between the two treatment groups. The results suggested that simply providing women-only treatment and child care does not substantially improve treatment outcome without changing treatment content. A similar result of no differences in outcomes was found in a study comparing women-only versus mixed-gender programs (Kaskutas, Zhang, French, & Witbrodt, 2005). Other studies have found somewhat more mixed results. One found that women treated in both women-only and mixed-gender outpatient programs reported improvements across four primary outcome domains; however those in the women's-only programs reported significantly less substance use and criminal activities but no differences in arrests or employment status at the 1-year follow-up (Prendergast, Messina, Hall, & Warda, 2011). On the other hand, despite having more severe substance-related and psychosocial problems and utilizing more services, women in women's-only programs appear to have had better substance use and legal outcomes than those treated in mixed-gender programs (Niv & Hser, 2007). These differential benefits of women-only programs, which occur early on in the recovery process, may not be sustained long term (Hser, Evans, Huang, & Messina, 2011).

While the issue of whether service is provided in gender-specific or mixed-gender programs is unresolved and in need of further evaluation, the importance of gender-responsive approaches and services that address the unique and multiple needs of women substance abusers is clear. Particular attention should be paid to engaging and retaining women in treatment, assuring adequate lengths of care, and bridging the transition from residential or intensive outpatient care (Greenfield

& Grella, 2009; Grella, 2008; Grella & Greenwell, 2004; Niv & Hser, 2007).

Maintenance and Relapse

While women may be less likely than men to enter substance abuse treatment, it appears overall that treatment retention, completion, and outcomes are comparable across gender (Center for Substance Abuse Treatment, 2009b; Greenfield, Brooks, et al., 2007a). Women, however, appear somewhat more likely than men to engage in continuing care following the completion of a more intensive phase of treatment (Carter et al., 2008; Center for Substance Abuse Treatment, 2009b; Claus et al., 2007). While the rates of relapse also are comparable across gender, the precipitants or relapse "triggers" appear to differ for men and women (Connors, Maisto, & Zywiak, 1998; Heffner, Blom, & Anthenelli, 2011; Rubin, Stout, & Longabaugh, 1996; Saunders, Baily, Phillips, & Allsop, 1993; Walitzer & Dearing, 2006). The Center for Substance Abuse Treatment (2009b), in its Treatment Improvement Protocol on the treatment needs of substance abusing women (TIP 51), have summarized the relapse risks identified in prior research that are unique to or more common among women. These include interpersonal problems and conflicts; low self-esteem and self-worth, especially related to intimate relationships; severe untreated childhood trauma as well as current trauma and PTSD; strong negative affect; more symptoms of depression; greater difficulty disengaging from other people; failure to establish a new network of friends, especially those supportive of recovery; and a lack of relapse prevention coping skills. Women are also more likely to relapse in the presence of others, particularly other female friends or a significant other. Additionally, the TIP suggests that women differ from men in their response to a relapse, both negatively and positively, if one does occur. On the negative side, following a relapse women typically are more likely to report depressed moods and to escalate their drinking or drug use following a relapse associated with unresolved trauma. On the positive side, compared to men, women often experience somewhat shorter relapse episodes and are more likely to seek help following a relapse (Center for Substance Abuse Treatment, 2009b).

Based on these findings, women may need the greatest support, skill building, and relapse prevention training in dealing with negative emotional states, such as depression, anger deriving from interpersonal conflicts, loneliness, low self-esteem, and trauma-related experiences.

Mutual support/self-help groups represent one potential source of support, particularly in light of the finding concerning the difficulty women substance abusers have in developing a network of new friends. Findings concerning the involvement of women in Alcoholics Anonymous (AA) have been mixed. Women who reported long periods of abstinence following treatment reported having been involved in a fellowship of recovering alcoholics (Gillet et al., 1991). Similarly, women have been found to be more likely than men to become involved in AA and to benefit more, with respect to both alcohol-related and general psychosocial outcomes, from their continued involvement in AA (Moos, Moos, & Timko, 2006). Further, women also were found to have greater reductions in depression and avoidance coping, with these reductions being associated with an increased likelihood of remission. One factor that may contribute to this level of engagement and benefit is the perceived level of social support derived by women from their involvement in AA, especially for those who have a sponsor (Rush, 2002).

This pattern of results has not been found consistently, with women having been found to benefit less from AA involvement than men (Tonigan & Hiller-Sturmhofel, 1994). This has led to the development of alternative self-help groups, such as Women for Sobriety (WFS), that are not based on the underlying philosophy and principles of more traditional 12-step programs (Kaskutas, 1996a, 1996b). WFS represents a self-help option that is oriented toward positive thinking and behavior modification. The belief that behavior is dependent on one's thoughts serves as the underlying premise of WFS. This leads to a cognitive-behavioral approach in which members are taught that maintaining sobriety is based on believing that one can control negative thoughts and emotions and how well one copes with these negative emotions. The goals of WFS include abstinence, improved self-esteem, and spiritual and emotional growth (Kaskutas, 1996a, 1996b). As is true of many self-help and mutual support groups dealing with addictions, WFS is in need of further research into its therapeutic process and outcome.

Summary

Although there has been increased sensitivity to the needs and issues that face women with substance abuse problems, this continues to be an understudied and underserved population (Gomberg, 2003; Greenfield et al., 2010; Greenfield et al., 2007a). Women, representing one of a number of populations having unique needs, are confronted by multiple real and perceived barriers that make it difficult for them to seek out and remain in substance abuse treatment. These barriers are more likely to negatively affect the likelihood of treatment seeking of women rather than men. To effectively address the needs of women, special efforts must be made to attract women into treatment settings and retain them. The interventions chosen should take into account the stage of readiness for change that a woman is in as she approaches treatment, engages in the treatment process, and maintains the gains made during treatment. Interventions need to be focused on the transitions from contemplation to preparation, from preparation to action, and from action to maintenance and relapse prevention.

While there is a continued need to look at factors that impede or facilitate treatment entry, many of the barriers confronting women who are seeking treatment are being addressed in various treatment settings, including using family and couple therapy as standard therapeutic interventions (Brady & Randall, 1999; Green, 2006; Greenfield et al., 2010; Greenfield & Grella, 2009). It is hoped that such gender-sensitive treatment services will encourage more women to seek treatment, especially those who otherwise might not have done so (Greenfield & Grella, 2009; Grella, 2008).

MOTIVATIONAL ISSUES IN INDIVIDUALS MANDATED TO TREATMENT

Scope of the Problem

Driving while intoxicated (DWI) or while under the influence of alcohol or drugs (DUI) represents a major concern from a public safety and a public health perspective. From a public safety perspective, drinking and driving is a frequent occurrence. A survey conducted in 2008 found that one in five (20%) of the U.S. population age 16 and older had driven within 2 hours of drinking alcohol during the past year, with the percentage of males (27%) nearly doubling the rate for females (14%) (National Highway Traffic Safety Administration, 2010a); it was further estimated that this group had 85.5 million past-month drinking–driving trips. Drinking drivers are responsible for a large number of accidents annually. These accidents are more likely to involve injury and death than accidents in which alcohol is not involved (Hingson & Winter, 2003). In 2009 there were 10,839 individuals killed in accidents in which a driver had a blood alcohol concentration (BAC) of 0.08 or above (the legal level for alcohol-impaired driving) (National Highway Traffic Safety Administration, 2010b). However, there is an extremely low probability of arrest for impaired driving; in the early 2000s it was estimated that there were 82 million occasions of individuals driving with a blood alcohol level of 0.08 or above, but only 1.5 million individuals were arrested for DWI (Hingson & Winter, 2003). The preponderance of alcohol- or drug-impaired arrestees have been men, but the gender gap has been narrowing over the past two decades, with an increase in the rates of women arrested and convicted of DUI (Robertson, Liew, & Gardner, 2011; Schwartz, 2008). Additionally, the rates of recidivism to driving while impaired are relatively high (Nochajski & Stasiewicz, 2006).

Public Safety Issues and Approaches

Individuals who are arrested, charged, and convicted of DWI typically face a number of potential sanctions, which may involve fines, jail time, ongoing monitoring, and the requirement to use an ignition interlock device that prevents one from starting his or her car if one has alcohol-positive breath (Elder et al., 2011; Voas, DuPont, Talpins, & Shea, 2011). Despite the effectiveness of ignition interlocks in reducing recidivism, their use has not been widespread due to the relatively small proportion of arrestees who have used them (Elder et al., 2011). This has led to a number of approaches to increase arrestees' motivation to utilize these devices, such as court-imposed penalties (e.g., jail time or electronically monitored house arrest) for those choosing not to install an ignition interlock; such motivational incentives do in fact increase the rates of the devices' use with a resultant reduction in recidivism (Roth, Marques, & Voas, 2009; Voas, Blackman, Tippetts, & Marques, 2002).

Coerced Treatment and Motivation to Change

Increasingly the oversight of interventions with alcohol- or drug-impaired drivers has been assumed by DUI courts that take the offender out of the criminal justice system and instead shift the focus more to therapeutic and public health issues that emphasize more of a public safety approach (Fell, Tippetts, & Ciccel, 2011; MacDonald, Morral, Raymond, & Eibner, 2007). This process consists of increased coordination with and interaction between the treatment and judicial systems, with treatment being seen as an alternative to legal sanctions. This often results in what many view as coerced treatment involvement, a topic that has been questioned with respect to ethical concerns and to its efficacy (Sullivan et al., 2008; Urbanoski, 2010).

Individuals who are mandated or coerced into treatment represent a population often considered to have low levels of intrinsic motivation to change alcohol or drug use behaviors. While there is typically some form of social or interpersonal pressure that contributes to the decision to seek treatment (DiClemente, Doyle, & Donovan, 2009; Wild, Cunningham, & Ryan, 2006; Wild, Newton-Taylor, & Alletto, 1998), those who are required to enter treatment under legal duress may minimize their need for such care. Perceived institutional pressure to enter treatment, including that exerted on the individual by the criminal justice system, is often viewed as being coercive and is associated with low motivation to change compared to pressures exerted by family or friends (Polcin & Beattie, 2007). This includes individuals such as those having been arrested for and mandated to treatment because of driving under the influence of alcohol or drugs (Dill & Wells-Parker, 2006; Wells-Parker, 1995).

However, the presence of legal referral and/or social network pressures to quit, cut down, and/or enter treatment does not appear to necessarily affect client engagement at treatment entry (Wild et al., 2006). While those mandated to treatment may perceive greater pressure to be in treatment than those who enter voluntarily, this does not necessarily lead to differences between these two groups with respect to their motivation to engage in treatment once having entered (Stevens et al., 2006). It has been found that legal pressure and readiness to change are relatively independent constructs, exerting independent influence on treatment retention; however, motivational readiness appears to be more highly related to improvements in retention and therapeutic engagement than is legal pressure (Knight, Hiller, Broome, & Simpson, 2000). Although not always consistent, evidence suggests that individuals who are coerced into substance abuse treatment under legal duress may have less severe substance use and psychosocial (other than legal) problems, are less likely to drop out of treatment, and have outcomes comparable to or better than those who are "volunteers" who enter treatment without such legal pressures (Burke & Gregoire, 2007; Perron & Bright, 2008; Polcin & Beattie, 2007; Schaub et al., 2010).

The apparent therapeutic benefit derived from legally mandated treatment raises a question about the relationship between perceived coercion and readiness to change and to engage in treatment. However, relatively little is known about DUI offenders' readiness to change their drinking or drinking–driving behaviors, and the findings in regard to this relationship have been mixed (Nochajski & Stasiewicz, 2005). On the one hand, among a group of individuals entering a 4-week-long court-mandated program for impaired drivers, the majority were classified as in the action stage on the Readiness to Change Questionnaire (RTCQ) and measures assessing efficacy and readiness to change drinking and driving, with the fewest categorized as being in precontemplation (Wells-Parker, Kenne, Spratke, & Williams, 2000; Wells-Parker et al., 1998). On the other hand, nearly two-thirds (62%) of a large sample of DWI offenders recruited from a special drinking and driving offenders program, probation, and the courts were found to be in the precontemplation stage as assessed by the University of Rhode Island Change Assessment (URICA) (Wieczorek, Callahan, & Morales, 1997). In a sample of nearly 600 individuals convicted of DWI and referred for court-mandated substance abuse evaluation, 31% were in the precontemplation stage, 24% in contemplation, 31% in action, and 1% in maintenance (Nochajski & Stasiewicz, 2005). Using the Stages of Change Readiness and Treatment Eagerness Scale (SOCRATES) with this same sample, 60% were in the ambivalent stage, 3.5% were in the recognition stage, and 34% were in the taking steps stage. There was only a moderate degree of agreement in the classification of stages by these two different measures, and in conjunction with the studies by Wells-Parker, the stage of readiness to change may vary based on the measure one uses to assess this construct (Nochajski & Stasiewicz, 2005).

Despite this methods variance, there was cross-study consistency with respect to the relationship between the stage of readiness and alcohol consumption and drinking-related problems. Individuals in the precontemplation stage based on the URICA or the ambivalent stage based on the SOCRATES had the lowest levels of alcohol consumption and drinking-related problems, with the highest levels most often found among individuals in the contemplation stage on the URICA or the SOCRATES recognition stage. Individuals in the action or taking steps stage had use patterns and problems that fell intermediate to the other two stages. Thus, the interpretation of low levels of motivation among DWI offenders, as reflected by precontemplation or ambivalence stages, may more accurately reflect a lower level of problem severity than an apparent attempt to minimize or deny their problems (Wells-Parker et al., 1998). Classification in the action stage, with respect to initiating change in both drinking and drinking and driving behaviors, was associated with the lowest rates of recidivism, while contemplation was associated with the highest recidivism rates (Wells-Parker et al., 2000; Wells-Parker et al., 1998).

Treatment to Increase Motivation and Treatment Engagement

There are a number of clinical implications associated with the pattern in these findings. First, many individuals mandated into special programs for drinking drivers may be more motivated than is often thought and may have already begun to make changes in their drinking and/or drinking and driving behaviors. It should be noted that these two sets of behaviors, while related, represent separate constructs, and as such also represent potential targets for intervention (Wells-Parker et al., 2000; Wells-Parker et al., 1998). Second, although there is the possibility of purposeful minimization of drinking and related problems (Chang & Lapham, 1996; Lapham, C'de Baca, McMillan, & Hunt, 2004; Nochajski & Stasiewicz, 2005), individuals classified as being in precontemplation may require less intensive treatment than those in contemplation or those who are ambivalent, whose problems seem more severe. These individuals in precontemplation may be social drinkers with minimal problems, a number of whom may be prompted to change their behavior as a result of the negative consequences associated with their arrest (Wells-Parker et al., 2000). While having negative opinions about a number of court-mandated sanctions is common, the negative emotional reactions to many of these sanctions has been found to be a deterrent to subsequent drinking–driving (Lapham & England-Kennedy, 2012). Also, among these individuals, most of whom are required to undergo an evaluation of their alcohol use and psychological status as part of court-mandated interventions, many may benefit from the therapeutic aspects of the assessment process (Lapham, 2004–2005; Schrimsher & Filtz, 2011). Similarly, this group may be an appropriate target for brief interventions (Dill & Wells-Parker, 2006; Lapham, 2004–2005; Wells-Parker & Williams, 2002). Third, individuals in the contemplation or recognition stages, with more serious problems and higher risk for recidivism, may benefit from multicomponent approaches that combine more intensive court-mandated sanctions (e.g., license revocation, ignition interlocks, house arrest, electronic home monitoring, vehicle impound) and increased court monitoring with alcohol education and specialty substance abuse treatment, which by themselves have a limited impact on recidivism (Dill & Wells-Parker, 2006; Voas et al., 2011; Voas & Fisher, 2001). In addition, for repeat offenders/chronic recidivists, often described as "hard-core" drinking driver offenders (Voas & Marques, 2004), the use of anticraving medications, such as extended release naltrexone, may also be of benefit (Lapham & McMillan, 2011).

As noted, alcohol education programs, often a key component in court-mandated approaches to the management of DUI arrestees, are often of limited effectiveness in preventing or reducing recidivism (Dill & Wells-Parker, 2006). There have been a number of approaches that recently have attempted to improve these outcomes by incorporating components that target readiness to change, drinking behavior, and/or drinking and driving among DWI first-offenders and recidivists (Brown et al., 2010; Rider et al., 2006; Rider, Voas, Kelley-Baker, Grosz, & Murphy, 2007; Robertson, Gardner, Xu, & Costello, 2009; Wells-Parker & Williams, 2002; Woodall, Delaney, Kunitz, Westerberg, & Zhao, 2007). This has been done primarily by integrating components of brief motivational interventions, including individualized feedback from screening and/or more comprehensive evaluations, brief advice, and counseling strategies specially adapted for a relatively small number of short sessions, into standard DUI-focused education and treatment programs (Dill & Wells-Parker, 2006; Lapham, 2004–2005).

The Mississippi Alcohol Safety Education Program (MASEP) was one of the first programs to integrate motivational interviewing into a DUI alcohol safety program (Wells-Parker & Williams, 2002). The MASEP program, which all first-time DWI offenders in Mississippi are mandated to attend, has adapted its curriculum over time based on empirical data. Since its inception in 1972 as a purely educational approach it has evolved into one that is multicomponent and more therapeutic/psychoeducational. In its most recent iteration in 2000, it is 12 hours in duration and has incorporated elements of motivational interviewing into the curriculum. For instance, prior to this, participants, at the discretion of the counselor, were provided with a written feedback report that included their blood alcohol level at arrest, their scores on an alcohol-screening test, and a brief interpretation of these results. In the updated curriculum, counselors are required to distribute and discuss the feedback with participants by the third session of the program, with an increased focus on the connection between indicators of alcohol use patterns and problems to the risk of drinking and driving and DUI recidivism. Participants also developed and revised DUI avoidance plans over the course of the four sessions, tailoring them to their own needs and circumstances as they became more aware of the nature and extent of their problems and were provided with group feedback. Finally, and most significantly, all the counselors were trained in the principles of motivational interviewing and the techniques of motivational enhancement therapy (Miller et al., 1992b) and were instructed to use these in group and individual counseling sessions. These principles include incorporating a nonconfrontational style that involves expressing empathy, developing discrepancy, avoiding arguments, rolling with resistance, and supporting self-efficacy. The incorporation of these principles and techniques was meant to enhance motivation for change with the goal of reducing subsequent DUI recidivism.

An evaluation of the MASEP program compared the 3-year recidivism rates of first-time DUI offenders who completed, enrolled but failed to complete, or failed to enroll in the program (Robertson et al., 2009). Additionally, changes in recidivism rates of those enrolled in the program prior to and following the incorporation of the motivational enhancement components were examined. Program completion was associated with a decreased likelihood of DUI recidivism (21.1%) compared to those who did not enroll (29.5%), and those who enrolled but did not complete the program (35.8%). Those who were enrolled in the program following the more recent curriculum adaptation also had lower rates of recidivism than those who had been involved in the previous version; however, the difference in rates was relatively small (23.8% for the new program; 26.5% for the older program). Clearly, engaging and retaining participants is critical, and adding motivational enhancement components to a court-mandated program may improve its effectiveness.

An interesting and important finding in an earlier evaluation of the MASEP program is its differential effectiveness for DUI first-offenders who are depressed (Wells-Parker et al., 2009; Wells-Parker, Dill, Williams, & Stoduto, 2006; Wells-Parker & Williams, 2002). Particiants were randomized to either a 4-session group intervention or an enhanced version of this program to which were added two brief 20-minute individual sessions that again incorporated more tailored and individualized feedback based on an initial assessment and the use of motivational enhancement principles; those randomized to the enhanced program were also offered the availability of a supportive follow-up counseling session 4 - 6 months after completion of the main program. The outcomes of these two interventions were examined across four subgroups previously identified as at increased likelihood of recidivism: young minorities, problem drinkers, women, and depressed offenders. No differential treatment effects were found based on age, minority status, or gender; nor was an effect found for problem drinking status once the level of depression was controlled (problem drinkers had higher rates of depression). However, a significant interaction was found between program type and the presence or absence of depression. Participants who were depressed and received the enhanced program were 35% less likely to have a subsequent DUI arrest than those in the standard program; no differences in recidivism were found across program type for participants who had low levels of depression. In a subsequent series of studies using a variety of indicators of depressed mood (Wells-Parker et al., 2006), DUI offenders who were classified as depressed were found to be more receptive and less resistant to counseling than those who were not depressed.

This finding is particularly important since depression is one of the most common comorbid psychiatric conditions found among both first-time and repeat DUI offenders (Lapham, C'de Baca, McMillan, & Lapidus, 2006; Palmer, Ball, Rounsaville, & O'Malley, 2007). Motivationally focused interventions also appear to contribute positively and incrementally to the outcomes of jail-based DUI programs, especially for arrestees with antisocial personality disorder, another comorbid psychiatric condition with higher prevalence among drinking and driver offenders than found in the general population (Woodall et al., 2007).

A second recent intervention approach, the Preventing Alcohol-Related Convictions (PARC) program (Rider et al., 2006; Rider et al., 2007), differs in its focus from that of many other alcohol education and treatment programs for DUI offenders. It is based on prior research that suggested that despite initial resolve not to drive after drinking, once having driven to a drinking event, the likelihood of drinking is high, with a resultant increased risk of driving after drinking despite the initial resolve not to do so. It is assumed that it is easier to plan for alternative transportation in advance and while not being under the influence of alcohol than once one has begun drinking at an event to which he or she has driven. Rather than the more traditional focus on reducing drinking or alcohol abstinence, PARC aims instead to reduce recidivism by teaching participants about making a decision before leaving home not to drive to a drinking event, thus reducing the risk of driving after drinking. The focus of the prevention curriculum is thus on controlling driving rather than controlling drinking. The intervention is a 2-hour module that can be added to or substituted for a session in a standard DUI alcohol education program. While PARC's primary focus is on separating driving from drinking, the more comprehensive program into which it is integrated may encourage examination of and changes in drinking behavior.

As part of an interim evaluation of the program (Rider et al., 2006), an adapted stages-of-change measure was developed that mapped onto either the more traditional approach to reducing drinking or the PARC focus on choosing not to drive to drinking events. The content of precontemplation and contemplation stage items are the same for each approach, while that for the preparation and action stage items differ and are specific to each approach. As an example, items from the traditional preparation and action stage scales, respectively, focus on drinking behavior: "I plan to just have soft drinks when I am at a party away from home" and "I am not just thinking about controlling my drinking, I am drinking less." In contrast, the items adapted to be specific to the PARC approach focus on not driving: "I have a plan for reducing my driving after drinking" (preparation) and "I have told my buddies that I do not intend to drive to the ball games any more" (action). Individuals randomized to either the traditional alcohol education program or the intervention into which the PARC module had been integrated demonstrated comparable decreases in precontemplation and increases in contemplation scores, which was expected since the first sessions were comparable across interventions and focused more generally on behavior change. The PARC intervention differentially influenced the planning and action stages, with an increased adoption of plans to control driving rather than drinking behavior relative to participants in the traditional program. A subsequent evaluation (Rider et al., 2007) found that participants randomized to the PARC intervention had significantly lower 1- and 2-year DUI recidivism rates compared to those in the traditional alcohol education program. This suggests that approaches such as PARC that attempt to increase the motivation to change driving habits and patterns either separate from or in conjunction with a focus on drinking may have benefit over and above those approaches that only focus on drinking behaviors.

The MASEP and PARC interventions represent ones in which individuals are mandated to participate by the courts, and clearly, those who enroll and complete them appear to reduce their risk of subsequent DUI (Robertson et al., 2009). However, despite such mandates, some first or repeat offenders, choose not to follow through and enroll in the court-ordered programs. As an example, 35% of first offenders mandated by the courts failed to enroll in the MASEP program, while another 17% enrolled but failed to complete the program (Robertson et al., 2009). A recent study evaluated the impact of a brief 30-minute motivational intervention on readiness to change and drinking among a group of repeat DUI offenders who had alcohol problems but were not participating in a DUI program (Brown et al., 2010). Individuals were recruited through a number of techniques to be involved in a study of "different methods of sharing information on the risks of alcohol use." Participants had at least two prior DUI convictions and had evidence of alcohol problems within the past 6 months. They were randomized to either a brief motivational intervention, based on the principles of motivational interviewing (e.g., empathic interviewing style that acknowledges, examines, and attempts to resolve patient ambivalence to facilitate behavior change; individualized feedback if deemed tactically appropriate to provoke greater problem recognition and cognitive reappraisal) or to a control condition of comparable length that instead provided more general information about the risks of drinking and driving and nonspecific advice about alcohol misuse. Although there were no differences between groups with respect to changes in their readiness-to-change scores, those in the brief motivational intervention appeared to have greater subsequent reductions on a number of measures of problematic alcohol use than were found for those in the control condition. The authors conclude that such brief motivational interventions warrant further investigation for use outside the more traditional clinical context of court-mandated treatment programs.

Summary

There has been a long-standing perception that individuals mandated to treatment by the legal system may evidence less readiness to change their behavior around alcohol and drug use than those entering treatment voluntarily. While those mandated to treatment view this as coercive, the findings concerning their stage-of-change readiness is equivocal and to some extent may depend on the measure of readiness being used. It is the case that mandated individuals have retention, completion, and treatment outcomes comparable to or better than voluntary treatment entrants, even though they may not shift from the perception of coercion to an internalized sense of motivation. A number of approaches with DUI offenders, as one exemplar of individuals mandated to treatment, suggest that the use of brief interventions based on the principles of motivational interviewing has the potential of facilitating the change process and reducing problematic drinking and/or subsequent drinking and driving. However, these results are based on a relatively small number of studies and the effect sizes are modest. While promising, the utility of such motivational interventions, both inside and outside of the traditional DUI treatment system, warrants further investigation

SUMMARY

• An important subgroup of substance abusers meriting special attention is women, who often face significant barriers to accessing substance abuse treatment and are less likely to seek treatment.

• Women are more likely to drink in response to stress-of-life events, to have a higher prevalence of comorbid psychiatric disorders, and to be the victims of various forms of abuse.

• Women are at greater risk for health problems associated with substance use and may experience more rapid progression of alcohol-related problems then men (although this difference in progression appears to have become less pronounced in recent years).

• Issues regarding children are particularly salient for women substance abusers. These include such issues as child care responsibilities and the fear of losing custody of children.

• Women substance abusers (particularly mothers) are more subject to social stigma and are less likely to have family and/or peer support for entering treatment.

• It may be particularly beneficial to identify women problems drinkers in primary care settings and to use motivational techniques to encourage their entry into substance abuse treatment.

• Adding gender-specific approaches to traditional treatment and offering women's-only programs may be particularly beneficial for some women. However, the evidence supporting the differential effectiveness of these programs is equivocal.

• Individuals who are mandated into treatment, such as DWI offenders, comprise another group with special needs.

• Mandated DWI offenders may have less severe substance use and psychosocial problems than substance abuse patients voluntarily entering treatment. This may help explain why DWI offenders in precontemplation have been shown to have lower levels of alcohol consumption and drinking-related problems than those in the contemplation stage after treatment.

• Contrary to expectations, mandated DWI offenders have been shown to engage and remain in treatment and have treatment outcomes as good or better than noncoerced individuals.

• Mandated DWI offenders in precontemplation with less severe substance use problems may experience more negative emotional reactions to court-mandated sanctions and may be an appropriate target for brief interventions.

• DWI offenders in the contemplation stage may experience more serious problems and be at greater risk for recidivism. More intensive approaches and sanctions may be indicated for these individuals.

9

Relapse

Relapse is an old and still challenging problem in the addictive behaviors field. In the most general sense, *relapse* refers to a return to a problematic behavior. The high rates at which individuals return to substance use after stopping for any particular period of time supports the belief among many counselors and clients that, tough as it may be for a client to quit use of a substance, "staying quit" is even tougher. In this regard, Washton (1988) noted that "traditionally, relapse has been the nemesis of addiction treatment for all types of chemical dependency problems, including alcohol, heroin, and other drugs" (p. 34). Similarly, Rounsaville (1986) has argued that "relapse and relapse prevention define the major clinical problems to be faced by clinicians and researchers who do work with substance abusers" (p. 172), and Connors and Maisto (2006) more recently noted that "understanding and preventing relapse are among the greatest challenges facing those working in the field of addictions" (p. 107).

Although precise figures on the prevalence of relapse are not available, there are strong indications that relapses are anything but uncommon. In a now classic report, Hunt, Barnett, and Branch (1971) summarized relapse rates for a variety of substances. They found that individuals treated for heroin, smoking, and alcohol addiction exhibit high rates of relapse. Indeed, approximately two-thirds of these clients had relapsed within the initial 3 months following the conclusion of treatment. A similar outcome pattern was found for patients who had initiated either inpatient or outpatient treatment for alcohol dependence, although the relapse curve was not as precipitous among the outpatients studied (Lowman, Allen, Stout, & the Relapse Research Group, 1996).

A more recent review by Kirshenbaum, Olsen, and Bickel (2009) demonstrated that the relapse curve estimated by Hunt et al. consistently emerged across 20 different studies assessing outcomes among alcohol-dependent and tobacco-dependent patients.

While the data summarized within the above reports clearly highlight the prevalence of relapse events, keep in mind that *relapse* for the purposes of these reports was defined as any return to the use of the respective substances, without reference to the amount of the substance used or the duration of use. As such, persons who took one drink (in the alcohol category) and then returned to abstinence would be viewed no differently than persons who drank heavily and over an extended period of time. Clearly, use of different definitions of relapse (e.g., a single use of a drug vs. 5 days of continuous use) affects the rate of relapse indicated. The case of relapse among alcoholics serves as a useful illustration. When defining relapse as a return to pretreatment levels of drinking, Armor, Polich, and Stambul (1978) found a relapse rate of around 50% over a 12-month posttreatment follow-up period. However, when relapse has been defined as the consumption of a single drink after treatment, relapse rates as high as 90% have been reported (Orford & Edwards, 1977). Complicating this picture is the finding that drinking outcomes following treatment are highly variable. Many clients do not relapse, many who relapse do not do so immediately, and many who relapse do not remain relapsed (e.g., Annis & Ogborne, 1983; Moos et al., 1990; Polich, Armor, & Braiker, 1981; Zywiak, Kenna, & Westerberg, 2011).

While high rates of relapse following treatment are understandably discouraging, the data for months 3 through 12 are encouraging. Hunt et al. (1971), for example, found that the rates of relapse between months 3 and 12 for clients who have not relapsed by month 3 are markedly lower than the rates during the first 3 months following treatment. This indication was also evident in the Kirshenbaum et al. (2009) review, where it was found that relapse was progressively less likely to occur over time. These findings suggest the importance of preventing relapse immediately following treatment, given that the prospects for sustained abstinence are remarkably higher once an initial period of abstinence has been achieved.

In this chapter, we focus on the topics of relapse, relapse prevention, and dealing with relapses that do occur. We open with some important definitional issues, including attention to the distinction between a lapse and a relapse. We then discuss relapse in the broader context of the stages-of-change model. We highlight the potential clinical advantages of conceptualizing relapse less as a discrete event and more as a process that can be influenced. The next section keys on issues surrounding the prevention and treatment of relapses. A case example will be used to describe strategies for addressing relapse issues in the treatment setting.

DEFINITIONS AND MODELS OF RELAPSE

Despite many years of consideration of the problem of relapse, relapse still is not operationally defined in any universally accepted way. However, there has been some progress in reaching consensus on a conceptual definition of relapse. In particular, there is agreement that it is important first to distinguish between a lapse and a relapse. A *lapse* is viewed as a single episode of violation of an individual's attempt at restraint. For example, a lapse might be a person's use of heroin during the first several months following his or her treatment for heroin addiction. Relapse, however, is more abstract than the neatly defined single event of a lapse and is seen in part as a psychological construct. Relapse is the reoccurrence of some problem after a period of improvement. Importantly, there is perception of a loss of control and a marking of the failure of a behavior change effort (Brownell et al., 1986; Shiffman, 1989). A lapse does not necessarily lead to a relapse. It is essential to note, however, that, despite conceptual agreement to differentiate between lapse and relapse, the empirical literature frequently does not. Therefore, in describing or citing research we use the term "relapse" to cover both events, except where the authors distinguished between lapse and relapse.

There also has been considerable effort taken in recent years to develop models of relapse so as to help inform clinical practice and to guide future research. In this regard, Table 9.1 provides an overview of some of the more widely discussed models of relapse. The table covers only what we consider to be essential points about these models and is not meant to be a detailed review of them.

As Table 9.1 shows, the models and theories make few distinctions among different drugs as far as mechanisms of relapse are concerned. Also, the theories emphasize immediate relapse precipitants. Only the concept of "high-risk situation" could extend to more remote (from the relapse) events. Furthermore, the theories could be divided into two

TABLE 9.1. Summary of Major Models and Theories of Relapse

Model/theory	Mechanism(s) of relapse
Cognitive-behavioral (Marlatt & Gordon, 1985; Witkiewitz & Marlatt, 2004)	Interaction between "high risk" (for substance use) and the individual's self-efficacy to cope with those situations without substance use determines relapse. Expectations about the utility of drugs and alcohol in a situation also are important. Cognitive and emotional processes represented by the "abstinence violation effect" construct influence the severity and duration of relapse.
Person–situation interaction model (Litman, 1986)	Relapse is determined by an interaction among three factors: situations that the individual perceives as threatening ("high risk"), availability of an adequate repertoire of coping strategies, and the individual's perception of the appropriateness and effectiveness of available coping strategies.
Self-efficacy and outcome expectancies (Annis, 1986; Rollnick & Heather, 1982)	Initial substance use occurs from the mislabeling of negative affect and negative physical states as craving. After first substance use, expectations of control over such use decreases, along with self-efficacy. This process leads to a more severe relapse.
Opponent process (Solomon, 1980)	Through conditioning, formerly neutral internal and external stimuli become connected with various "A" and "B" states. Reexposure or reexperiencing these states may increase the individual's motivation to use drugs following a period of abstinence.
Craving and loss of control (Ludwig & Wikler, 1974)	Internal and external stimuli associated with drug withdrawal are labeled as craving. Drugs are sought as a way to relieve craving. Use of drugs then leads to a loss of control, due to inaccurate interpretation of interoceptive cues that regulate consumption.
Urges and craving (Tiffany, 1990, 1992; Wise, 1988)	Drug use and drug urges and cravings have occurred enough times to be "automatic cognitive processes." In the abstinent substance abuser, these processes can be triggered by various internal and external stimuli. Relapse may occur if an adequate "action plan" not to use drugs, a nonautomatic cognitive process, is impeded or not used. Wise adds that use of one drug may trigger urges to use another, a result of action in the brain.
Post-acute withdrawal syndrome (Gorski & Miller, 1979)	*Relapse* is defined as a "process that occurs within the patient which manifests itself in a progressive pattern of behavior that allows the symptoms of a disease or illness to become reactivated in a person that has previously arrested those symptoms" (Gorski & Miller, 1979, p. 1). The

TABLE 9.1. (*continued*)

model, developed in the context of alcohol use disorders, focuses primarily on the physiological and neurological effects of the substance on the user. When the user seeks to abstain, he or she initially goes through a period of withdrawal. This is followed by what Gorski and Miller term "post-acute withdrawal syndrome" (PAW), which primarily affects higher level cognitive functioning (e.g., abstract thinking, memory) and is linked to higher levels of emotionality and overreaction to stress. The relapse process itself follows a consistent pattern. First, the individual's attitude changes as he or she begins to question his or her well-being and ability to stay sober. The individual begins to use maladaptive coping methods, resulting in negative emotional consequences. The end result of this process is a resumption of use.

Note. Adapted from Donovan and Chaney (1985), Connors, Maisto, and Donovan (1996), and original sources.

general categories: psychological, with an emphasis on cognition (the first three theories in Table 9.1), and psychobiological (the last four theories in the table), with emphases on acquired motivation to use drugs and on urges and cravings. Within each of these classifications there is considerable overlap among theories. Except for the cognitive-behavioral and self-efficacy/outcome expectations approaches, the theories minimally if at all differentiate between a lapse and a relapse.

Across the theories, there is a consistency in what they suggest should be assessed as being relevant to relapse events. The broadest content category is stimulus conditions that are thought to be antecedents of relapse. These may be internal or external events, depending on the theory. Therefore, mood (especially negative mood), physical state, and urges and cravings are identified as important relapse antecedents. "High-risk situations" may encompass any of these antecedents as well as other psychological, social, or physical elements that may lead to substance use. Note that the mechanisms hypothesized for how different stimulus conditions come to be antecedents of relapse differ among the theories, but the implications for measurement are similar.

The psychological theories require measurement of two types of expectancies. The first is *outcome expectancies*, which refer to the individual's beliefs about the effects of a drug if it is used in a given situation. The other type of expectancy is *self-efficacy*, or the individual's estimation that he or she can successfully enact a behavior in a given situation. Finally, psychological theories require the assessment of the individual's pattern of coping in different situations that may be related to substance use.

The most discussed and clinically applied model of the relapse process has been provided by Marlatt and his colleagues. It was originally summarized by Marlatt and Gordon (1985) and subsequently updated and revised in important ways by Witkiewitz and Marlatt (2004). The basic model described by Marlatt and Gordon (1985) is shown in Figure 9.1. Marlatt hypothesized that the initiation of abstinence engenders a sense of personal control and self-efficacy, self-perceptions that become strengthened as the period of abstinence lengthens. Over this period, the substance abuser is likely to face situations that put him or her at risk for again using alcohol or drugs. Such "high-risk" situations are a central feature of the Marlatt model of relapse. The antecedents to such situations can be varied, but frequently they reflect cognitive and lifestyle factors that subsequently can place the person in a high-risk situation. When a person is placed in such a situation, the ideal response would be an effective coping behavior. When such a behavior is in the person's behavioral repertoire and is emitted, then the success experience enhances the person's self-efficacy (Bandura, 1977). This, in turn, decreases the probability of relapse in similar subsequent situations. On the other hand, if the person is unable to emit an effective coping response, then this will lead to a decreased level of self-efficacy and an increase in the attractiveness of the substance as a mechanism for dealing with the situation. This is particularly the case if the person maintains positive outcome expectancies regarding drug effects. As the attractiveness of the substance increases (in conjunction with decreased self-efficacy), it becomes more likely that the person will use the drug in that situation. If the drug is used, an abstinence violation effect (AVE) will result, involving dissonance frequently accompanied by self-attributions of guilt and low self-esteem, both of which can propel an initial use of the substance into a full-blown relapse.

On the basis of new research relevant to the components of the original relapse prevention model, Witkiewitz and Marlatt (2004) provided a revised conceptualization of the relapse process. Remaining intact as the primary basis of the Marlatt relapse model was the high-risk situation. In the new model, the following were proposed as central determinants of relapse: negative emotional states, positive emotional states, lesser levels of coping, greater outcome expectancies regarding

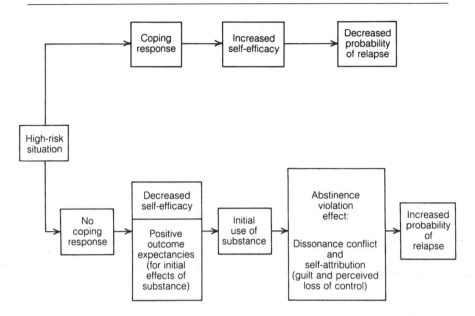

FIGURE 9.1. The Marlatt and Gordon model of the relapse process. From Marlatt (1985b, p. 38). Copyright 1985 by The Guilford Press. Reprinted by permission.

substance use, lower self-efficacy, the abstinence-violation effect, greater craving, and interpersonal relapse precipitants (Witkiewitz & Marlatt, 2007). Identified as more distal risk factors for relapse were a family history of substance abuse, a lesser extent of social support, and severity of dependence. Added and emphasized in the reconceptualized model is the timing and interrelatedness of risk factors and events. Accordingly, an individual's behavior in a given high-risk situation becomes viewed as influenced by some or many of the above-referenced determinants of relapse, which include distal risk factors (which include stable and enduring relapse vulnerabilities) and proximal risk factors (which include more immediate precipitants).

As noted above, the hallmark feature of both the original Marlatt and Gordon (1985) model and the Witkiewitz and Marlatt (2004) reconceptualized model is the high-risk situation. According to Cummings, Gordon, and Marlatt (1980), "high-risk situations are associated with a history of use of the addictive behavior as a coping response and thus represent a critical choice point for the individual" (p. 297). As such, high-risk situations often serve as precipitants to a lapse or relapse to substance use. In order to test this notion, Marlatt and Gordon (1980) performed a content analysis of situations associated with relapse. Using their schema, relapse situations were coded into two broad categories. The first represented intrapersonal–environmental determinants, which include determinants associated primarily with within-person factors and/or reactions to nonpersonal environmental events. The five subcategories of intrapersonal–environmental determinants were coping with negative emotional states, coping with negative physical–physiological states, enhancement of positive emotional states, testing personal control, or giving in to temptations or urges. The second broad category of relapse situations represented interpersonal determinants, which include factors associated with interpersonal events. The subcategories within this group were coping with interpersonal conflict, social pressure, and enhancement of positive emotional states. Table 9.2 provides a breakdown of the high-risk situations described by several groups of substance abusers. As shown, the majority of alcoholics attributed relapse to intrapersonal determinants (61% of the relapse situations). Predominant within this category were situations involving negative emotional states, such as frustration or anger. The remaining relapse situations among alcoholics (39%) included interpersonal determinants, especially interpersonal conflicts and social pressure. The relapse situations for smokers and heroin addicts differed in several ways from those reported by the alcoholics. The smokers and heroin addicts reported a lower percentage of relapses with intrapersonal determinants. This was predominantly attributable to relatively fewer endorsements of testing personal control and urges and temptations and relatively greater endorsements of positive emotional states as relapse precipitants. The smokers and heroin addicts also reported a greater frequency of interpersonal determinants, relative to the alcoholics. This difference was almost entirely attributable to the smokers and heroin addicts reporting social pressure as a relapse precipitant at a rate double that of the alcoholics. Thirty-two percent of the relapses described by smokers and 36% of those described by the heroin addicts were attributed to social pressure. The only other differences of note were between the smokers and the heroin addicts. The smokers described negative emotional states as a precipitant almost twice as often as the heroin addicts (37% vs.

TABLE 9.2. Analysis of Relapse Situations among Alcoholics, Smokers, and Heroin Addicts

Relapse situation	Frequency		
	Alcoholics	Smokers	Heroin addicts
Intrapersonal determinants			
Negative emotional states	38%	37%	19%
Negative physical states	3%	2%	9%
Positive emotional states	—	6%	10%
Testing personal control	9%	—	2%
Urges and temptations	11%	5%	5%
Total	61%	50%	45%
Interpersonal determinants			
Interpersonal conflict	18%	15%	14%
Social pressure	18%	32%	36%
Positive emotional states	3%	3%	5%
Total	39%	50%	55%

Note. Adapted from Marlatt (1985b, p. 39). Copyright 1985 by The Guilford Press. Adapted by permission.

19%), while the heroin addicts described negative physical states as a precipitant more often than the smokers (9% vs. 2%).

The pattern of findings noted above for relapse precipitants has been reported for other groups as well. Wallace (1989), for example, assessed psychological and environmental determinants of relapse among crack cocaine smokers. She found that the most frequent precursors to relapses were painful emotional states (40% of relapses), failure to enter after-care following treatment (37%), and encounters with conditioned environment stimuli (34%). In another report, Birke, Edelmann, and Davis (1990) found among illicit drug users that the most important relapse precipitants were negative affect and interpersonal conflict (but not social pressure). Finally, Lowman et al. (1996) evaluated the replicability of the Marlatt relapse precipitants taxonomy across multiple treatment sites and found them to be broadly consistent with the precipitants reported by Cummings et al. (1980). In this regard, approximately two-thirds of the precipitants to relapse events reflected negative emotional states, interpersonal conflict, or social pressure.

While the studies described above identify types of scenarios in which relapses are likely to occur, note that there are strong indications that relapses are not precipitated by a singular factor, but instead that multiple influences can operate simultaneously in leading to a relapse. This was clearly indicated by Wallace (1989). In that study, specific precipitants of relapses were identified, such as painful emotional states. However, Wallace also found that the great majority of relapses (86%) actually were multidetermined. That is, in most cases two or more categories of precipitants were acting together to set the stage for the relapse, at least among crack cocaine smokers. A similar finding has been reported by Heather, Stallard, and Tebbutt (1991) and Zywiak, Connors, Maisto, and Westerberg (1996); in each case, it was found that combinations of relapse precipitants typically operate in the context of a particular relapse event.

RELAPSE IN THE BROADER CONTEXT OF THE STAGES-OF-CHANGE MODEL

We noted earlier, in Chapter 1, that a basic feature of the stages-of-change model is that it is cyclic. A person more often will go back to an earlier stage of change after reaching a later one, generally as a result of a lapse or relapse. Such reversions (e.g., a person in action relapsing and reverting to contemplation) are generally viewed as setbacks, although the person seeking to change in most cases does not revert back to the precontemplation stage. Although individuals often relapse during the action stage, the problem of relapse is most often conceptualized and discussed in the context of the maintenance stage.

While relapse is not a stage in the stages-of-change model, it nevertheless is an important and relevant clinical issue. As noted above, clients often move back in the stage sequence as a result of a relapse. Indeed, it is not uncommon for several such reversions to occur before a durable behavioral change pattern has been established (DiClemente, 2003; Prochaska & DiClemente, 1986). In this context, relapses might well be viewed as an expected event in the overall change process. While a relapse can lead to a reversion back to the precontemplation stage, it is encouraging to note that the vast majority of regressions are to the contemplation or preparation stages (Prochaska & DiClemente, 1984).

A final point on why relapses are relevant to the stages-of-change model is that they can be viewed as the flip side of the maintenance stage. As such, a major task for the person in the maintenance stage is to avoid relapsing.

MAINTAINING ABSTINENCE AND ADDRESSING RELAPSE

For clients who have moved through the action stage and into the maintenance stage, the overarching objective is the consolidation and maintenance of gains. From a stages-of-change perspective, successful maintenance emanates from four interrelated activities (DiClemente, 2003). First is proactively countering threats to maintenance and temptations to return to substance use. Second is regularly reassessing and renewing one's commitment to the behavior changes achieved. Third is ensuring that one's decisional balance on substance use remains on the negative side for a return to substance use. Finally, the fourth activity is setting up a protective environment from substance use and establishing a lifestyle that provides satisfactions. The processes of change most centrally relevant to staying in maintenance are self-liberation, stimulus control, counterconditioning, reinforcement management, helping relationships, and social liberation.

Engagement in the four activities noted above will maximally enable clients to avoid relapsing. Nevertheless, lapses and relapses can and do occur, and it is important that clients be aware of their risk factors for relapse and be prepared to address and minimize any relapses that might occur. Accordingly, this section focuses on two treatment topics. The first is maintaining treatment gains (typically maintaining abstinence) and thus preventing relapse. The second topic is addressing relapses that do occur.

Maintaining Treatment Gains and Preventing Relapses

While a lapse or relapse is perhaps the most common outcome following substance abuse treatment, there are individuals who achieve abstinence and maintain it for extended periods. In a recent national study evaluating the response of alcoholics to different treatments, for example, 19% of the clients seen as outpatients and 35% of the clients treated in aftercare (following a more intensive inpatient or day hospital program) were abstinent throughout a 1-year follow-up period (Project MATCH Research Group, 1997a).

How is it that clients maintain durable periods of abstinence? One line of clinical research addressing this question concerns client-identified factors associated with their periods of abstinence. A pair of studies have provided some insights on these factors. In the first, McKay, Maisto, and O'Farrell (1996) interviewed male alcoholics periodically over a 30-month period following alcohol treatment that included behavioral marital therapy. At each follow-up contact, the client was asked about factors associated with any 30-day (or longer) period of continuous abstinence during the follow-up interval being assessed. Factors reflecting what were conceptualized as "active strategies" consistently emerged across each follow-up interview. In this regard, the predominant strategies were recalling the benefits of sobriety, recalling drinking problems, and remembering that sobriety is the first priority. In a second study, men and women alcoholics were similarly interviewed about factors associated with posttreatment abstinence (Connors, Maisto, & Zywiak, 1998). The methods for maintaining abstinence used most frequently (used in over 60% of the abstinent periods by both men and women) were avoiding risky people and places, recalling drinking-related problems, treatment, and self-help groups. Also used frequently by both men and women were the strategies of staying in alcohol-free environments, using treatment skills, avoiding thinking about alcohol, recalling the benefits of sobriety, and remembering sobriety as the top priority. The only difference between men and women on the endorsement of these factors as an aid in maintaining abstinence was on the method of recalling drinking problems. That strategy was used in 80% of the abstinent periods among men and in 61% of the periods among the women.

These two studies taken together suggest that clients, after treatment, use a variety of strategies in the service of maintaining abstinence. Importantly, men and women for the most part used these strategies to a comparable extent. Some specific clinical issues related to relapse, and associated clinical responses, were described earlier in Chapter 5.

Further information on the issue of maintaining abstinence has emerged from research on predictors of abstinence and other dimensions of positive posttreatment functioning. Not surprisingly, there are a considerable number of strong indications that cognitive coping skills, positive thinking, and number of available coping skills are all related to posttreatment abstinence (Connors, Longabaugh, & Miller, 1996; Litman, Eiser, Rawson, & Oppenheim, 1979; Maisto, Connors, & Zywiak, 2000; McKay et al., 1996; Moos et al., 1990). In a prospective investigation of posttreatment functioning, with a particular focus on relapse events, Miller, Westerberg, Harris, and Tonigan (1996) found that clients' coping skills were a powerful predictor of treatment outcome. More specifically, positive coping skills were associated with less subsequent drinking and avoidant coping styles predicted relapse. Similarly, Connors, Maisto, and Zywiak (1996) found that coping skills and responses generally (including available coping behaviors and perceived self-efficacy regarding the use of such behaviors) predicted a host of posttreatment outcomes (including a greater percentage of days abstinent, fewer drinking consequences, and fewer craving experiences).

These two lines of clinical research—survey assessments of factors associated with periods of abstinence and the identification of variables that are predictive of posttreatment functioning—converge in highlighting the role of active coping behaviors in maintaining abstinence and avoiding relapsing. Relatedly, treatments with the strongest evidence of efficacy prominently include those focused on developing and/or applying coping skills and altering social relationships (Miller et al., 1995).

The foregoing research also provides some guidance for helping clients set the stage for maintaining abstinence. For starters, clients should be aware of the techniques and strategies used by others to maintain abstinence, such as recalling problems associated with past drinking, participating in self-help groups, and avoiding risky people and places. Clients should identify factors associated with any of their own periods of previous abstinence, should there be such a history. The counselor and client can then focus on those strategies that appear most applicable to the client's unique needs and circumstances. It is often useful for clients to have these strategies listed on a card for their frequent review.

A key part of avoiding relapse is identifying situations in which the client is at greater risk for relapse. We presented an array of such situations earlier in this chapter. In the clinical setting, it will help to have clients identify scenarios in which they are vulnerable to substance use, either based on previous substance use patterns or anticipated situations in the immediate future. Such assessments should be conducted using open-ended questioning about high-risk situations and/or using measures specifically developed to assess domains of situations in which the client is more likely to use alcohol or drugs, such as the Situational Confidence Questionnaire (Annis, 1982b) for alcohol and the Drug-Taking Confidence Questionnaire (Annis & Martin, 1985) for other drug use (described in Chapter 3). Among outpatient alcohol abusers, for example, higher confidence to avoid drinking, assessed using the Alcohol Abstinence Self-Efficacy Scale (AASE), is associated with better treatment outcomes (Project MATCH Research Group, 1997b). Relatedly, the relationship between temptation to drink and confidence to not drink was another predictor of outcome. Clients with greater confidence relative to temptation on the AASE reported more posttreatment abstinent days and fewer drinks per drinking day. Thus, evaluating and addressing both temptations and confidence appear to be important in maximizing prospects of avoiding relapses.

Finally, a third clinical implication is to focus on the development and application of coping skills generally and especially those with relevance to high-risk situations. Interestingly, research by Miller et al. (1996) suggests that client coping skills determined the avoidance of relapse—independent of the overall amount of stress and risk to which the client was exposed. As such, treatment providers may want to incorporate into their standard practices coping skills assessment and training, should that not already be part of the treatments being offered. Among the available resources on coping skills training for substance abusers are those by Monti et al. (1989) and Kadden et al. (1992).

The foregoing interventions are intended to maximize client awareness of and sensitivity to behaviors associated with abstinence and scenarios that represent heightened risk for substance use. This endeavor has the potential for placing the client in the best position possible for productively using coping and other life-functioning skills to maintain abstinence in particular but more generally to support and engender a positive and gratifying lifestyle (see Marlatt, 1985a, for a more general discussion of lifestyle modification).

Addressing Relapses

Many clients will experience a lapse or relapse in some form. While not desirable events, these events nevertheless can be constructively used clinically in the service of reachieving abstinence for a longer period. In this regard, relapses should be framed as learning experiences, if and when they occur. Accordingly, in this section on addressing relapses we focus on preparing clients to deal with and terminate relapse episodes and reengaging the client in the change process.

Preparing Clients to Deal with and Terminate Relapses

The various high-risk scenarios in which relapse might occur for a given client were described earlier in this chapter. Ideally, client sensitivity to such situations and awareness and use of strategies to cope with these situations will preclude relapse for many. However, for those who do relapse, the ideal response on the part of the client will be to take steps immediately to minimize the extent of substance use and interrupt the relapse process.

Contingency plans for dealing with a relapse should be developed as part of treatment and before an actual relapse. Examples of behaviors a client might seek to engage in would include leaving the substance use environment, contacting one's counselor or sponsor, reinitiating self-help group attendance, and so on. Often counselors have their clients develop a written list of things to do if a relapse occurs and have them keep it in their wallets for ready access. An example of such a list is shown in Figure 9.2.

Reengaging the Client in the Change Process

Assuming the client's response to the relapse leads to a return to treatment, the counselor's tasks are similar to those faced when initiating treatment more generally. A first step would be an assessment of the client's current status in terms of substance use and immediate risk for subsequent use. Client stabilization and resolution of the relapse (if still in progress) is the most pressing clinical need. Dovetailing with this would be an assessment of the client's current stage of change. If the client was in the maintenance stage, has he or she cycled back to

---

What to do if a relapse occurs

1. Use the relapse as a learning experience.
2. See the relapse as a specific, unique event.
3. Examine the relapse openly in order to reduce the amount of guilt and/or shame you may feel (those thoughts can lead to a feeling of hopelessness and continued drinking).
4. Analyze the triggers for the relapse.
5. Examine what the expectations about drinking were at the time (What did you anticipate drinking would accomplish in that situation?).
6. Plan for dealing with the aftermath/consequences of the relapse.
7. Tell yourself that control is only a moment away.
8. Renew your commitment to abstinence.
9. Make immediate plans for recovery—don't hesitate, do it now!
10. Contact your counselor and discuss slips.

FIGURE 9.2. Reference sheet for use by clients.

contemplation—thinking about change but not acting yet? If so, interventions intended to move the client from contemplation to action would be warranted.

Regardless of the stage to which the client has cycled back, therapists should continue to use the motivational counseling techniques described earlier (in Chapter 2). In addition, attention should be placed on the reestablishment of those techniques and strategies previously used by the client to achieve and maintain abstinent periods in the past. Naturally, it may be instructive to review these techniques and strategies in light of the circumstances surrounding the relapse. Finally, supplemental treatment interventions may be necessary to address problem areas that have been exacerbated or have newly arisen as a function of the recent substance use.

CASE EXAMPLE OF A CLIENT WHO HAS RELAPSED

Angela M is now a 48-year-old woman who had achieved 21 months of sobriety, following a period of problematic drinking that extended over two decades.

Angela's background and drinking history were described earlier, in Chapter 2, in the context of a case example of a person in the maintenance stage. Briefly, Angela described a long-term problem with drinking that was characterized by a variety of negative consequences, including a pair of arrests for driving under the influence of alcohol. She also participated in treatment programs on several occasions, with some limited improvements experienced.

Angela's third course of outpatient treatment "took hold"—largely, she felt, because she was resolved to abstain completely and because she had a strong working relationship with her counselor. Her treatment sessions focused on a variety of strategies for achieving durable abstinence, developing alternatives to drinking (including stress management, avoiding situations associated with previous heavy drinking, coping with cravings and urges, and drink refusal skills), including Peter, her husband of 10 years, in portions of treatment to incorporate his support and encouragement, and developing plans to prevent relapse or at least to minimize drinking should a slip occur.

While she experienced some setbacks during the first 10 months of treatment, Angela generally rebounded quickly and, perhaps more importantly, felt she had learned valuable "sobriety lessons" from such events. Angela had incorporated a variety of change strategies that she had been using successfully, following an early period of trial and error in the application of these strategies. Now her attention was focused on what she called "cruise control," whereby she could step back from the vigilance associated with skills acquisition and application and instead let much of that behavior occur more naturally. She emphasized that cruise control still entailed paying close attention to her environment, including attention to her own thoughts and feelings. Further, Angela still spent time anticipating drinking situations and reviewed before-hand her plans to deal with such situations. She still experienced periodic thoughts and temptations regarding alcohol use, although she was pleased that she could not really classify them as cravings. Finally, it was Angela's sense that she would always need to be in a state of full awareness regarding potential challenges to her abstinence and that she would never be in a position to take her sobriety for granted.

Angela's contacts with her therapist tapered off, and she terminated treatment shortly after achieving 14 months of continuous abstinence. Seven months later she recontacted her counselor to return to treatment. Angela had relapsed and had been drinking heavily again over the preceding 2 months.

At her next session with her counselor, Angela reported that she had been doing fine during the first several months after her last treatment session. She had been doing well on her job, and her relationship with Peter continued to be positive and rewarding. The only domain in which she felt something was lacking concerned friendships. She noted that she had no close friends and relatively few acquaintances, either at work or outside work. Angela felt she had good working relationships with her coworkers but that the relationships did not extend beyond that context.

Around 4 months before returning to treatment, Angela was approached by a job "headhunter" about taking a position at a large, established company on the other side of town. She was flattered by the inquiry and decided to interview for the position. Angela afterward evaluated the advantages and disadvantages or unknowns about the new position. On the positive side, the job offered new challenges and opportunities for professional growth and advancement. It also included a significant increase in salary. The main disadvantage was leaving a relatively comfortable position where she was productive and content. Angela ultimately decided to accept the position for two reasons: the opportunities for advancement and for new social contacts. This latter advantage came to the forefront of her deliberations because she was continuing to feel the need to develop some close friendships, which were not emerging at her current job.

The job transition was a difficult one. Angela experienced almost immediately an increased level of pressure to perform, a greater workload, longer work hours, and a much more competitive environment. These combined forces resulted in a heightened general level of stress and a significant decrease in the amount of time and energy she had available for her relationship with Peter (although she reported him to be supportive of her during this difficult time). Despite these intimidations, Angela reported that she felt her work performance was satisfactory. Indeed, she found it "heady" to be working in an upscale company she felt was on the "cutting edge" of her profession. In addition, she found herself more socially involved with her coworkers than she had been at her previous place of employment. Unfortunately, although she did not immediately recognize it, most of these contacts occurred in settings where alcohol was available and used widely. For example, it was not uncommon for her coworkers to have a beer or glass of wine with lunch or dinner, and heavier drinking typically occurred at bars after work.

Angela reported that not drinking at lunch was easy. She did, however, feel more pressure internally as well as externally to drinking with her coworkers after work. The external pressures revolved around situations where someone would offer her a drink or buy a round of drinks for the group. She was, among these individuals, the only nondrinker (at that point). The internal pressures were more complicated. On the one hand, she felt she shouldn't be drinking or even thinking about it. On the other hand, she felt she was in pretty solid control of her life and that drinking in a circumscribed setting would not only be manageable but also help her fit in more with her colleagues and perhaps also better set the stage for developing the friendships she was seeking. It was on this basis that she indeed did start drinking again. Initially she drank only at the "happy hour" sessions, finding—somewhat to her surprise, she reports now—that she was able to keep it "under control." She felt she was drinking more than she should, but that it was not "really out of hand" in the eyes of the others. However, she unexpectedly found herself drinking much more when alone at home, especially when Peter was out, and it was this drinking that was causing the most tangible consequences for her. In this regard, she was becoming inconsistent in getting to work on time, she felt "fuzzy" during the first couple of hours, and she perceived a withdrawal on the part of Peter from their relationship. It was this cluster of concerns, especially the concern about the relationship with Peter, that led to Angela's decision to recontact her therapist. In addition, she was realizing gradually that her drinking in the social contexts was not leading to the development of friendships with her coworkers.

An assessment of Angela's recent drinking indicated that she was drinking with her coworkers after work around 3 days per week, typically Tuesday, Thursday, and Friday. On these occasions, she was typically consuming around three to five glasses of wine over a 2- or 3-hour period, depending on the day. At home Angela was generally consuming around three to four glasses of wine most weekday evenings, a glass or so less on evenings she was out earlier with her coworkers. She also drank on weekend days, although more sporadically; when Peter was not around, she was drinking more over the course of the day. Angela's drinking predominantly had the effect of dulling most of her senses, which was not an entirely unwelcome consequence to her.

At her return session, Angela verbalized a desire to reestablish abstinence. Over the several days before her session she had ceased drinking. Her evaluation of the pros and cons of drinking led her to this decision. The pros she had anticipated when she decided to return to drinking had not materialized—she did not fit in better with her coworkers and closer friendships did not emerge. The cons of drinking that were most striking to her at this point were the hungover feelings at work and the distancing exhibited by her husband. Further, she had not anticipated the home-bound drinking that emerged, added drinking that she felt was physically depressing her. Angela reported that she was ready to quit, and that indeed she had initiated action on this endeavor several days before. She felt the challenge before her in terms of drinking was to not relapse.

Angela's counselor devoted much of their session to a review of events since their last sessions, focusing on the time since the return to drinking. The counselor utilized a variety of the strategies described earlier in this volume in the context of motivational counseling. In the present case, Angela had determined that she wanted to continue the abstinence initiated several days earlier. They focused on the strategies utilized by Angela earlier to achieve abstinence and maintain it for over a year. For Angela, one of the strongest motivations for remaining abstinent was the recognition and continuing awareness that the resumption of drinking yielded none of the expected positives and resulted in several unanticipated negative consequences. The session keyed on here-and-now strategies, all action-oriented, for continuing the abstinence begun and for avoiding drinking and drinking-related situations during the upcoming week. In this regard, Angela determined to continue her luncheons with coworkers, where she had not been drinking, and terminate, at least for the time being, the "happy hour" excursions. This would allow continuing contact with coworkers but would be confined to a safer context. She also sought to exert more structure to her evenings, where she had gotten into the habit of drinking. Part of this structuring effort was to include planned activities, either in the house or outside, with Peter during those occasions when he was available. Finally, it was agreed at this session that subsequent sessions would focus first and foremost on maintaining abstinence and avoiding relapse, and also on developing a plan for evaluating and addressing as warranted other issues related to Angela's overall life functioning, including the development of closer friendships.

SUMMARY

- Relapse refers to a return to substance use following a period of abstinence. Lapses and relapses are common posttreatment phenomena.

- A variety of models and theories have been developed to account for the relapse process. Most emphasize immediate relapse precipitants.

- Several studies have identified a number of interpersonal and intrapersonal factors as primary determinants of relapses. However, relapses are perhaps more productively evaluated as being the result of multiple influences operating simultaneously.

- The key tasks in the maintenance stages are countering threats to abstinence, regularly reassessing and renewing one's commitment to change, ensuring that decisional balance on substance use remains in favor of abstinence, and establishing a satisfying lifestyle.

- The processes of change most centrally associated with successful maintenance are self-liberation, stimulus control, counterconditioning, reinforcement management, helping relationships, and social liberation.

- While a relapse can lead to a reversion back to the precontemplation stage of change, most regressions are to the contemplation or preparation stages.

- Studies assessing strategies used by abstinent substance abusers to maintain abstinence may provide guidance to clients seeking durable abstinence. These strategies include recalling the benefits of sobriety, recalling drinking problems, and avoiding risky people and places.

- There are strong indications that cognitive coping skills, positive thinking, and having a number of available coping skills are all related to posttreatment abstinence.

- When clients return to treatment following a relapse, the priorities are terminating the relapse episode and reengaging the client in the change process.

- While not desirable events, relapses nevertheless should be constructively used clinically in the service of reachieving abstinence for a longer period of time.

10

Applications in Opportunistic Settings

Previous chapters have addressed using the stages-of-change model in a variety of substance abuse settings. In this chapter we cover its use in venues where people are seeking treatment for issues other than substance use. These settings are often called "opportunistic" because they are places where individuals who present for a range of issues can also be identified and treated for substance use problems. These types of venues include health care settings such as primary care clinics, emergency departments, family planning clinics, trauma centers, and general hospital units. In addition, other settings, such as HIV clinics, homeless shelters, jails, prisons, and other places that serve high-risk populations often have a greater percentage of substance abusers than the general population. Interestingly, individuals with substance use problems are often more likely to seek consultations and general assistance from these types of settings than from specialist substance abuse treatment centers. In fact, the Institute of Medicine (1990) estimates that 95.5% of individuals with a diagnosable alcohol or drug disorder do not recognize that they have a problem and therefore do not seek treatment. When factoring in the additional number of individuals who do not have diagnosable substance use problems but use at risky, problematic levels, the extent of unaddressed substance use problems becomes apparent (Madras et al., 2009). Because over the course of time many of these individuals will present to a health care or other social service or community setting, these opportunistic settings are ideal places to screen and provide interventions for substance use problems.

An appealing aspect of addressing substance use in opportunistic settings is that problematic use and consequences can often be easily screened for, sometimes with just one or two questions (Seale et al., 2006; Smith et al., 2009) or with a biochemical test. Early identification and simple triaging are possible in these settings, leading to interventions that are sometimes brief and relatively informal, such as a few minutes of advice and encouragement, or longer, incorporating referral to other treatment modalities such as cognitive-behavioral or solution-focused strategies, but ideally they are tailored to the individual's stage of change. For example, while it may be counterproductive to give direct advice and discuss behavioral strategies for someone in the precontemplation stage, this approach may be more appropriate and effective for someone in the preparation stage of change. Assessment of a client's readiness to change can be easily accomplished by using simple staging rulers or algorithms or, when time permits, a more comprehensive measure such as the University of Rhode Island Change Assessment Scale (DiClemente et al., 2009). (These assessment methods were described in Chapter 3.)

In the following sections, we focus on an overview of briefer intervention modalities in opportunistic settings, followed by a discussion of specific settings in which these approaches can be utilized. Because we discuss various types of settings, at times we use the term "patient" and other times the term "client," appropriate to the setting.

BRIEF INTERVENTIONS IN OPPORTUNISTIC SETTINGS

An increasingly utilized approach for addressing substance use in opportunistic settings is termed "brief intervention" (BI). Rather than being homogeneous in nature, BIs are best thought of as a family of interventions that can vary in length, structure, and targets of intervention, and place an emphasis on personal responsibility (Heather, 1995). In general, however, BIs share a common focus on current behavior(s), utilize a collaborative dialogue, acknowledge the importance of assessing readiness to change, and allow for provision of individualized feedback.

BIs can be ideal for many opportunistic settings because they have several advantages when compared to more intensive and longer types of treatment. For example, people with less severe substance use problems, who are often seen in these opportunistic settings, may be more open to and accepting of this type of intervention, as opposed to more rigorous, traditional types of treatments. Since BIs are occurring in the context of some related concerns, these settings create "teachable moments" that take advantage of naturally occurring motivation (DiClemente, 2006). At the same time, BIs in these settings can also be useful in motivating clients with more severe problems to seek additional help (DiClemente, Schlundt, & Gemmell, 2004). Additionally, BIs are generally less expensive than more formal substance use programs, and they can also be administered by a variety of providers in a wider range of clinical settings.

Matching Brief Interventions to Client Readiness to Change

A number of studies conducted in opportunistic settings such as primary care and hospital trauma departments have found that the majority of patients who screen positive for alcohol misuse indicate some level of readiness to change; that is, they are in the contemplation stage or beyond. In addition, it appears that patients who have had more recognized consequences as a result of their alcohol use are more likely to be in the later stages of change (Apodaca & Schermer, 2003; Samet & O'Connor, 1998; Williams et al., 2006). These findings are contrary to a very commonly held stereotype that substance-abusing patients are all in precontemplation, are not interested in messages about change, or are "in denial."

Because most interventions in opportunistic settings are—out of necessity—brief, it is critical for providers to be able to select strategies that are likely to be most effective for a particular individual. When BIs specifically incorporate a motivational component to facilitate readiness to change, they are often referred to as "brief motivational interventions." These sessions typically last 10–15 minutes and have four main elements: (1) establishing rapport, (2) raising the topic and expressing concern about alcohol consumption, (3) providing feedback on the client's drinking levels and the effects of alcohol misuse, and (4) enhancing motivation to change drinking behaviors and discussing a plan of action when appropriate (D'Onofrio, 2003).

There is emerging evidence that while interventions that focus on building motivation seem effective for clients in earlier stages of readiness at baseline, this approach may not be as useful for later-staged-clients at baseline who may benefit more from receiving simple physician advice or skill-building strategies. For example, one study (Maisto et al., 2011) found that among patients presenting at primary care centers for general health issues, those in earlier stages of change prior to receiving the intervention had greater improvements in drinking outcomes at 12-month follow-up than those who were more ready prior to the intervention. This finding is consistent with some other studies conducted with treatment-seeking populations. Studies by Rohsenow et al. (2004) and Stotts, Schmitz, Rhoades, and Grabowski (2001) both found that baseline readiness to change moderated the effect of a motivational interviewing (MI) intervention such that those patients who were less ready to change prior to the intervention benefited more from MI than those who were more ready.

In integrating these stage-based findings with the stages-of-change processes, it appears that the more motivationally focused elements of an intervention likely create opportunities for evoking experiential change processes (e.g., consciousness raising, self-reevaluation) that enhance early stage movement, while later stage progression typically involves more utilization of behavioral processes (e.g., stimulus control, counterconditioning).

In sum, designing the elements of BIs to meet clients "where they are" (i.e., at their stage of change) has implications for delivering the most effective service, saving time, and judiciously dedicating limited financial resources.

Structuring Brief Interventions

When delivering interventions in opportunistic settings, the provider often starts the session by asking the client's permission to discuss the topic of substance use. In many cases, these sessions include a few brief screening questions to determine the extent of the problem behavior. These questions can be focused on drinking, drug use, smoking, or other risk behaviors. Using a conversational style (as opposed to a question-and-answer interview), the provider can then explore the patient's view of the importance of change and determine readiness. Generally, the provider offers feedback on the patient's level of use, expressing concern, and offering brief and simple advice to quit or reduce use (depending on the level of risk). The provision of advice makes sense, especially in health care settings, because some patients can modify their behaviors at the directive of their physician.

Observing how the client responds to advice can guide the provider's formulation of the next steps in the consultation, improve communication, and enhance outcomes (Zimmerman, Olsen, & Bosworth,

2000). As previously mentioned, for some clients, feedback and brief advice may be enough, while for others a more motivational approach is needed. In any case, rather than merely educating or admonishing the client, the provider *elicits* what the client already knows about the impact of the behavior on his or her health, *provides* information as needed, and *elicits*, using an open question, the client's reaction to the information (e.g., "What do you make of that?"; "What are your thoughts about that?"). The strategy for this process of information exchange is called "elicit–provide–elicit" (Rollnick et al., 2008).

Similar to a careful observation of the client's response to direct advice, the client's reactions to these types of open questions often provide additional information about his or her readiness to change and, correspondingly, serve as a guideline as to which change processes might be enhanced for a particular readiness stage. For example, if the client is in the precontemplation stage, then the intervention might include individualized feedback in order to enhance consciousness raising. If the client has been thinking about taking action (in the contemplation stage), the emphasis could be placed on resolving ambivalence by conducting a decisional balance exercise and exploring the client's perception of change benefits. If the client is preparing to take action, then the focus might be more on helping him or her develop and commit to specific change goals such as cutting down or quitting. Conversely, it may be counterproductive for a provider to advise a smoking cessation program (appropriate for those in preparation or action) for a client who is not yet considering change (i.e., in precontemplation). In the same way, a provider who does not provide adequate information about additional resources for a client who is ready to quit has also "mismatched" the intervention to the client's stage (DiClemente et al., 1992). These matching missteps can often be avoided if a provider spends a few minutes actively listening to how the client responds to opening queries. On the other hand, an observant provider will likely get a "heads up" about potential missed opportunities to structure the session to the client's stage of change when he or she notices that the client appears to become disengaged, passive, submissive, or openly resistant. Another reliable indicator of mismatching is provider frustration because the client seems "not interested . . . not really wanting to change . . . not wanting to follow advice." Importantly, this kind of frustration can be a valuable source of feedback for the provider, signaling that it is time to shift gears, listen, and reformulate the discussion.

Health Care Settings

Because of the growing evidence of the efficacy of BIs, the use of this relatively brief, problem-specific approach has become increasingly popular in the continuum of substance use care, particularly in health care settings (Moyer, Finney, Swearingen, & Vergun, 2002; Barry, 1999). In the United States, changes in reimbursement policies and a recent emphasis on managed care models have made intervening with substance abusers in opportunistic settings particularly appealing. For example, new policies allow some medical providers to be compensated for addressing substance use issues, and BIs in primary care settings are now recommended by national practice guidelines (Whitlock, Polen, Green, Orleans, & Klein, 2004). In a step toward integration of medical care and substance abuse intervention, in 2006 the American College of Surgeons (ACS) established requirements for all Level I trauma centers in the United States to provide screening for alcohol use and BIs for patients who drink at hazardous or harmful levels, regardless of the cause of the patient's injuries (American College of Surgeons, 2006). Although guidelines for levels of drinking that are considered hazardous or harmful differ by country, the World Health Organization encourages the use of BIs in opportunistic settings across the globe (Babor & Higgins-Biddle, 2001). In the United States, the guidelines provided by the National Institute on Alcohol Abuse and Alcoholism (NIAAA) are to offer interventions to anyone who drinks at risky levels (i.e., for men, more than four drinks on any day or more than 14 drinks a week; for women and those over age 65, more than three drinks on any day or more than seven drinks a week). These guidelines have increased awareness of the need to assess and address substance use in nontraditional settings, particularly those that deliver health care services.

To date, much of the research on interventions delivered in health care settings has focused on problem drinking. In a 2004 meta-analysis, Burke and colleagues found that BIs for problematic alcohol use ranked near the top in four categories: (1) total amount of research performed to investigate its efficacy, (2) the quality of that research, (3) the number of studies that showed positive outcomes, and (4) cost-effectiveness (Burke, Dunn, Atkins, & Phelps, 2004). Studies have also found that patients who received BIs prior to more formalized treatment participated more fully in treatment and drank less alcohol following that treatment than patients who did not receive a BI (Dunn, 2003). Another meta-analysis conducted by Moyer and colleagues examined 34 randomized clinical trials that compared BIs to control conditions for heavy drinkers seen in primary care settings who were not seeking treatment for substance abuse problems. In most of the studies, the BIs were delivered by physicians or other health care providers, and results demonstrated a significant reduction in alcohol consumption (Moyer et al., 2002). Consistent with these findings, other recent meta-analyses have further supported the use of BIs in health care settings for alcohol problems (Ballesteros, Duffy, Querejeta, Ariño, & González-Pinto, 2004; Kaner et al., 2009; Cuijpers, Riper, & Lemmers, 2004).

In contrast to the growing number of reports on the effectiveness of BIs with patients who have alcohol problems, investigation of BIs for patients with drug problems is more limited. This is in part because studies on illicit and prescription drug abuse are more difficult to conduct given the variability in drug(s) of choice, the degree of reported use, and issues related to the need for medication management in many settings. Although research on using BIs to increase readiness-to-change drug use is just emerging, study results to date appear promising (Estee & He, 2007; Bernstein et al., 2005). For example, a study examining the effectiveness of a single-session BI with marijuana-using patients age 16 to 20 found that participants in a BI condition, compared to an education-only condition, reported greater progression through the stages of change at 3-month follow-up and greater reductions in marijuana use (McCambridge & Strang, 2004).

Table 10.1 provides some examples that can be used in a health care setting to help facilitate client movement through the stages of change and use of the corresponding processes of change.

As noted, the predictive validity of the stages-of-change model for alcohol use is well documented in health care settings (Bertholet, Horton, & Saitz, 2009; DiClemente, Bellino, & Neavins, 1999; Heather, Hönekopp, & Smailes, 2009; Maisto et al., 2011), and progressive stage transitions are positively related to outcomes (Stein et al., 2009). Incorporating the stages-of-change model is appealing to health care providers not only because of its demonstrated efficacy, but also because it is practical and broadly applicable to a wide range of health behaviors (Peteet, Brenner, Curtiss, Ferrigno, & Kauffman, 1998; Zimmerman et al., 2000). For example, in some settings physicians and/or nurses carry pocket-sized laminated cards with scaling rulers on them. Using these cards as guides, providers can quickly assess a patient's stage for a specific behavior and plan corresponding strategies for facilitating progress to the next stage. This pocket-sized staging tool also helps the provider

TABLE 10.1. Case Examples and Provider Tasks for Facilitating Stage Movement in Health Care Settings

Stage of change	Case example	Provider tasks
Precontemplation	A 42-year-old male visits a health clinic for a sprained ankle. He drinks five drinks a night and more on the weekends. He does not have health-related consequences but his wife is concerned about the increasing number of injuries he has sustained when drinking.	• Express concern. • Raise the patient's consciousness by discussing risky drinking limits and provide feedback about how his drinking exceeds these limits. • Explore potential links between his injuries and drinking. • Ask open questions to encourage self- and environmental reevaluation (e.g., "What concerns does your wife have about your drinking?").
Contemplation	A 25-year-old male has sustained multiple injuries from an automobile accident and is admitted to a trauma center. His toxicology report indicates that he had cocaine and marijuana in his system at the time of admission. He expresses some thoughts about reviewing his current patterns of substance use.	• Discuss the pros and cons of the patient's drug use and explore ambivalence. • Reflect statements he makes about desire, ability, and reasons or need to change. • Explore ways in which his drug use conflicts with his personal goals and values. • Seek to increase his awareness of the consequences of continued drug use and the benefits of decreasing or stopping use. • Ask open questions to increase self-efficacy (e.g., "If you were to make a change in your cocaine use, how would you go about doing that?").
Preparation	A 48-year-old woman is admitted to the hospital for severe respiratory problems. She smoked one and a half packs of cigarettes a day prior to admission. She has not smoked since she entered the hospital and plans to stay quit when she is discharged. She has quit smoking in the past but relapsed after 8 months.	• Encourage self-liberation by reflecting and reinforcing statements that contain language about commitment and goal setting. • Assist the patient in developing a change plan. • Explore possible barriers and facilitators. • Provide a list of options for treatment (e.g., smoking cessation classes, quit lines, nicotine replacement therapy) and help her *(continued)*

TABLE 10.1. (*continued*)

Stage of change	Case example	Provider tasks
		plan how to obtain the treatment that is best for her.
		• Ask open questions and elicit her ideas about controlling the stimuli in her environment, and planning alternative behaviors (e.g., "How might you go about avoiding situations in which you are tempted to smoke? What helped you the most during your last quit attempt?").
Action	A 30-year-old male is being treated in the emergency department for a hand injury that required stitches. He is in recovery for alcohol and has been sober for 35 days. He attends AA meetings at least three times a week.	• Reinforce the patient's accomplishments and discuss any barriers he might anticipate. (This might include exploring the potential effect of his taking pain medication if it is prescribed.) • Assess relapse prevention skills and shore up skills to maintain sobriety as needed. Encourage him to identify potential helping relationships (including AA members). • Identify additional resources as needed.

appreciate the notion that change is an incremental process, accept and respect the client's current stage, avoid "getting too far ahead" of the client and provoke resistance, and apply the most appropriate counseling strategy for each stage of change.

An example of a pocket-sized card developed for use in a health care setting is presented in Figure 10.1. After determining level of drinking risk based on the patient's gender and age, the provider assesses readiness to change (i.e., to drink below risky levels) by showing the patient the ruler card and soliciting his or her response. Subsequently, the provider may refer to the card for examples of open questions to facilitate a conversation about change.

In the following case example, a health care provider has assessed a patient's stage and determined that the patient is in the contemplation stage. The goal in this exchange is to explore ambivalence, tip the decisional balance in favor of change, and elicit ideas about any next steps.

Please mark the point on the ruler that best describes how ready you are *at the present time* to drink below risk levels:

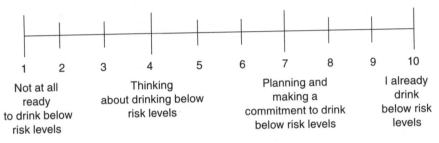

| 1 | 2 | 3 | 4 | 5 | 6 | 7 | 8 | 9 | 10 |

Not at all ready to drink below risk levels

Thinking about drinking below risk levels

Planning and making a commitment to drink below risk levels

I already drink below risk levels

Example scaling questions, depending on the patient's response:

Tell me why you picked a __ and not a __?" [Always start with the higher number.]

What would it take for you to move from a ____ to a ____? [Start with lower number.]

You've picked quite a high number. What are your plans, if any, for making this change?

Let's suppose you were a 10 sometime in the future. How do you think your life might be different?

Ask for elaboration. (LISTEN!)

FIGURE 10.1. Sample card for assessing readiness to change drinking to below risk levels.

Sam R is a 30-year-old single male who made an appointment with his family physician because of a sore throat and upper respiratory infection. Sam has a part-time job as a security guard in a local mall, and he is also attending a community college. In response to a general screening questionnaire, he reported that he occasionally drinks more than 10 beers a day. After Sam's lab work had been completed, he and his health care provider reviewed some screening information he had provided and assessed his readiness to change. As they discussed his general health, Sam said that he really looks forward to a Friday night out with some of his buddies—he likes to blow off steam and have a good time. At the same time, he said with a laugh that he didn't enjoy the hangover the next morning, especially since he sometimes has had to call in sick at work because he felt so lousy. In the review of the screening results, Sam's conversation revealed some potential concerns and an awareness of how his binging episodes were beginning to impact his life. These kinds of emerging issues are the hallmark of the contemplation stage as the ambivalence about the benefits of the behavior versus the costs or consequences of it are experienced as somewhat unsettling or divergent with larger goals, personal values, or self-concept. In order to explore and enhance these issues and provide opportunities for creating a discrepancy between Sam's alcohol use pattern and his overall goals and values, after offering a reflection, his physician asked Sam about the pros and cons of his drinking.

> "So, you enjoy hanging out with your friends and having some beers—helps you decompress a bit after a long week. What are some of the other good things about drinking for you?"

Sam said that he really liked the taste of beer and that it loosened him up a bit, made him less shy. Following a brief summary, his physician asked about any possible "cons."

> "It tastes good and you are more outgoing, more sociable when you are drinking. What might be some not-so-good things about drinking for you?"

In response to this query, Sam said that he felt terrible the next day, and that he was a little worried that calling in sick might get him fired. When the physician asked what else might concern him, Sam said that while he had always thought he could hold his liquor, after he had had an entire case of beer one Saturday he realized that he wasn't exactly superman—that even his friends had gotten concerned when they had a hard time waking him up. At this point the provider, in a neutral, empathic fashion, utilized a double-sided reflection and then asked if he could offer some information.

> "Part of you really likes the way beer makes you feel—more outgoing, less shy, and part of you doesn't like the hangover problems the next day, especially maybe risking your job. Would it be okay if I shared some information that other patients have found helpful? One thing we've learned is that risky drinking—which, as we've discussed, is more than five drinks in a single day for men—can put people at risk for a number of difficulties, such as trouble with the law, accidents, or even alcohol poisoning. Of course, I don't know how any of this might fit for you. What are your thoughts about this?"

Acute Care Settings

Two other opportunistic settings that have placed particular emphasis on substance use interventions are trauma centers and emergency departments because, in part, substance use is associated with all modes of injury requiring treatment. For example, it is estimated that up to 50% or more of patients test positive for alcohol at the time of admission (Gentilello et al., 1999; Soderstrom et al., 2007). Having sustained a major injury also creates a window of opportunity for medical professionals to assess for substance use and deliver brief interventions that may change the course of many lives (DiClemente, 2005a).

Although unaddressed alcohol problems in trauma patients can result in recurrent injury requiring readmission to a trauma center and/or death, studies indicate that BIs in emergency or trauma settings reduce alcohol consumption, subsequent injuries, and other alcohol-related problems (Gentilello et al., 1999; Longabaugh et al., 2001; Mello et al., 2005; Schermer, Moyers, Miller, & Bloomfield, 2006; Soderstrom et al., 2007). For example, in a seminal study, Gentilello and colleagues (1999) found that trauma center adult patients who received a BI, compared to a control group, decreased alcohol consumption significantly at 12 months. In addition, this work demonstrated a 47% reduction in injuries requiring either emergency or trauma center admission at 1-year follow-up and a 48% reduction in injuries requiring hospital admission at 3-year follow-up. Schermer and colleagues determined that a motivational BI addressing alcohol use significantly reduced the risk of DUI arrest at 3-year follow-up such that for every nine interventions conducted, there was a reduction of one DUI arrest (Schermer et al., 2006). In a cost analysis, Gentilello and colleagues found that for every dollar spent there was $3.81 saved in direct injury-related medical costs (Gentilello et al., 2005). These findings indicate that if BIs could be offered to every eligible injured person in U.S. emergency or trauma centers, the resulting annual savings from health care costs alone would be approximately $1.82 billion. Needless to say, given the clear individual and social benefits of this cost-effective approach, studies such as these have gained the interest not only of the medical community, but of policymakers as well.

As the stages-of-change model continues to contribute significantly to the development of BIs for acute care settings, a number of researchers and clinicians have written about the importance of matching intervention strategies in these types of venues to patients' stages of change.

For example, Dunn, Hungerford, Field, and McCann (2005) found that patients admitted to a trauma center are much more likely to be in the later stages of change than they are to be in precontemplation, and that interventions should be tailored accordingly. In their study of 346 patients receiving BIs in a Level I trauma center, only 24% were in precontemplation, and 72% were in either contemplation or preparation. These findings are similar to those of another study that also explored readiness to change alcohol use in patients hospitalized in a Level 1 trauma center. In that study, Apodaca and Schermer (2003) found that of 50 patients with an alcohol-related injury, 84% were in the contemplation or action stages of change for reducing or quitting their alcohol use, and only 16% were in precontemplation. This reflects the motivational opportunity provided by the teachable moment, however, and may be fleeting if not enhanced by a BI.

Studies of adolescents in trauma settings are consistent with those of adults, as there appears to be little support for the notion that most substance users—whether adolescents or adults—lack any motivation to change. For example, Barnett et al. (2002) found that 51% of 254 injured adolescents sampled in an emergency department in an urban hospital were in the preparation or action stages of change. In a study of 120 young adults (age 15–24) admitted to a Level 1 center with major trauma and positive alcohol/toxicology screens, Yonas et al. (2005) found that 87% of those using alcohol and 85% of those using other drugs were either in the contemplation or action stages of change.

Given these findings, there is an emerging interest in exploring the efficacy of BIs for adolescents in acute care settings. Currently, there are only six outcome studies in the literature, and, so far, the results are mixed. In reviewing evidence on BIs for risky alcohol use among adolescent patients in trauma or emergency departments, Yuma-Guerrero et al. (2012) found that of the studies comparing BIs to usual care, only half demonstrated a significant intervention effect. Five of the six studies, however, showed reduction in substance use and/or negative alcohol-related consequences regardless of the study condition. These findings suggest that although BI for adolescents in acute care settings may be efficacious, further exploration is needed.

The following example concerns a patient in an acute care setting who is in the preparation stage of change. This patient, who had been diagnosed as alcohol-dependent in the past, was admitted to a trauma center after an automobile accident. At the time of admission, his blood alcohol level was 0.19, which is over twice the legal limit in his state.

Martin S is a 63-year-old divorced man who has been hospitalized several times over the past few years because of health issues including depression, stomach problems, and hypertension. After test results during his last physical exam revealed early stage liver disease, Martin began to consider that he might have to make some hard changes in his life but he had not yet taken action. This is the first time he has been injured as a result of his drinking and he considers his automobile accident to be a "wake-up call." Although Martin acknowledges that he has had alcohol-related illnesses in the past, it is only now that he feels ready to change. He acknowledges that he would really miss alcohol, as he has relied on it for many years to help him forget his problems and just get by. He says that although he had tried several times to cut down, the shakes and terrible anxiety got to him—he just couldn't handle it. Although Martin has made some initial inquires about local resources and expresses a vague interest in getting an AA sponsor, he says that he just wishes that he could quit cold turkey on his own.

As is often typical for someone in the preparation stage, Martin is really considering the need to change his alcohol use as he has begun to see that problems associated with his drinking far outweigh the advantages he once associated with it. One thing he lacks at this point, however, is an articulated plan of action that is appropriate for individuals who are likely alcohol-dependent. Thus, although he appreciates the seriousness of his situation and has taken some preliminary steps toward change, strategies that strengthen motivation, build self-efficacy, and specify incremental behaviors will help him move past the preparation threshold into action. One approach that helps accomplish this task is the collaborative development of a change plan. Such a plan can incorporate the primary change talk elements that capture the most important reasons the patient has for making the change, specify things to do to begin the change, identify how other people can be of help, anticipate and design strategies to deal with relapse triggers and temptations, and describe what success will look like. Chapter 5 contains an illustration of a change plan worksheet. In Martin's case, he and the provider might have a dialogue similar to the following to prepare for completing the change plan and helping Martin move into the action stage of change.

PROVIDER: We've talked about your accident and you've had some feedback about your blood alcohol level when they brought you into the hospital. You've given this some serious thought and you worry about the connection between your injury and your drinking, and also about the consequences of alcohol on your future health. You seem ready to make some significant changes in your drinking. For some people, developing what we call a change plan can be helpful. Is it okay with you if we go through this process together?

MARTIN: Sure. I think I'm ready, but I know there will be some times when it's really hard for me to stay away from drinking.

PROVIDER: Some people find it helpful to think about times in the past when they've made behavior changes. For example, you mentioned that you've quit drinking before. While we complete your change plan, I'll be interested in learning about the steps you've taken in the past to accomplish your goals, as well as any obstacles you might face and how you might handle them. So if you like, we can go through the worksheet together and discuss the areas that stand out for you.

Social Service and Community Settings

Interventions in community service settings may not be quite as time-limited as those in primary or acute care medical settings, but they are often successfully delivered in relatively brief formats. In the section below, we discuss settings in which clinicians used the stages and/or processes of change to develop and deliver substance abuse interventions or to determine the need for future services.

Settings for Women at Risk of Alcohol-Exposed Pregnancies

Women who drink during pregnancy expose their babies to a set of conditions called "fetal alcohol spectrum disorder" (FASD) that can encompass a range of problems from attention and behavioral problems to birth defects, mental retardation, and neurodevelopmental disorders. Although many women know that they should not drink while they are pregnant, nearly half of pregnancies in the United States are unplanned, and many women with a planned or unplanned pregnancy do not realize they are pregnant until they are well into the first trimester. As a result, many pregnant women who are drinking at risk levels may be unintentionally exposing their developing fetus to alcohol. Because the early weeks of pregnancy are a critical period of fetal susceptibility to alcohol, alcohol-related effects on the fetus often happen before a woman knows she is pregnant (Floyd, Decoufle, & Hungerford, 1999).

To reduce alcohol-exposed pregnancies (AEP), interventions should be conducted in settings that serve women of childbearing age who drink at risky levels and have sex without effective contraception. Examples of these types of settings are not only substance abuse treatment centers, but also jails, prisons, reproductive health clinics, and college campuses. A series of studies, called "Project CHOICES," that were designed to reach women in a number of these high-risk settings occurred in three phases: identifying opportunistic settings with high-risk populations (Project CHOICES Research Group, 2002); testing the feasibility and impact of the intervention (Project CHOICES Intervention Research Group, 2003); and testing the efficacy of the intervention in a randomized trial in 12 different opportunistic settings such as primary care, urban jails, and hospital-based obstetric/gynecology practice (Floyd et al., 2007; Velasquez et al., 2010). The intervention consisted of up to four counseling sessions based on the stages of change that incorporated motivational interviewing, relapse prevention strategies, and provision of information on preventing FASD, as well as the offer of a session with a family planning provider for individualized birth control education and optional gynecologic and birth control services. Results indicated that women in the intervention group were twice as likely to be at reduced risk for an alcohol-exposed pregnancy at 12-month follow-up compared to the group that received information only (Floyd et al., 2007). A two-session version of CHOICES has also been tested in a randomized study on a college campus with positive outcomes (Ceperich & Ingersoll, 2011). The results of the Project CHOICES efficacy study have been widely disseminated, and the intervention is now used in several federal initiatives and community settings both in the United States and abroad (e.g., STD and HIV clinics, primary care community clinics, and criminal justice settings). A current study in hospitals and community health clinics is testing the efficacy of a briefer, two-session version of the CHOICES intervention with the addition of screening and referral of smokers to an evidence-based smoking cessation program.[1]

Settings for Men at Risk of HIV

Settings that provide services for individuals with HIV also provide opportunities to deliver substance use interventions. HIV-positive

---

[1]The four-session Project CHOICES intervention training curriculum, counselors manual, and participant workbook are available for free through the CDC website (*www.cdc.gov/ncbddd/fasd/freematerials.html*).

persons often report high levels of alcohol and other drug use, both of which are associated with sexual risk taking (Colfax et al., 2004; Irwin, Morgenstern, Parsons, Wainberg, & Labouvie, 2006; Vanable et al., 2004). In addition to the concerns about the role that substance use may play in the sexual risk practices of this population, it also has implications for overall health and immune functioning (Lucas, Gebo, Chaisson, & Moore, 2002; Meyerhoff, 2001; Nath et al., 2002). For example, heavy alcohol users are less likely to respond positively to HIV medication regimens (Ena, Amador, Benito, Fenoll, & Pasquau, 2003; Palepu, Horton, Tibbetts, Meli, & Samet, 2004), and HIV medication adherence is negatively affected by heavy drinking (Cook et al., 2001; Halkitas, Parsons, Wolitski, & Remien, 2003). Thus, there is a critical need to design and implement effective interventions to reduce alcohol use among those living with HIV.

Positive Choices is an example of a stages-of-change-based intervention that was developed for men at risk of HIV. The purpose of this study was to evaluate the efficacy of a stage-based behavioral intervention in a randomized clinical trial designed to prevent HIV among alcohol-abusing men who have sex with men (Velasquez et al., 2009). The participants were recruited in gay, bisexual, and/or HIV/AIDS settings (e.g., AIDS service organizations, mainstream venues such as bars and cafes in predominantly gay neighborhoods). The intervention used both individual counseling and education/support peer groups, and it emphasized the stages and processes of change. Participants in the control condition received materials about HIV prevention and a resource referral list. (The intervention is described in more detail in Chapter 6 and by Velasquez et al., 2009). The major findings were that, relative to the control group, the intervention group significantly reduced number of drinks per drinking day, number of heavy drinking days, and number of days on which both heavy drinking and unprotected sex occurred.

Settings for the Homeless

Homeless shelters and other organizations that serve the homeless also offer opportunities to intervene with substance abusers. More than half a million people in the United States are considered "homeless" at any given time, and an estimated 100 million people are homeless worldwide (Office of the United Nations High Commission on Human Rights, 2005). Thirty to forty percent of homeless individuals are estimated to have alcohol disorders (Burt, 2001; Hartwell, 2003), and more than 15% have other substance use disorders (McCarty, Argeriou, Huebner, & Lubran, 1991). Compounding the problems associated with substance use, as many as 50% of the homeless population have some form of mental illness, with 70–80% having had a mental illness diagnosis at some point in their lifetime (Scott, 1993). As is abundantly clear, substance use has a major impact on the physical health and safety of the homeless as it increases the probability of high-risk life-endangering behaviors, severe trauma, and serious health problems such as liver disease, nutritional deficiencies, hypertension, chronic obstructive pulmonary disease, gastrointestinal disorders, and arterial disease (Harris, Mowbray, & Solarz, 1994).

In contrast to other opportunistic settings we have discussed, organizations that serve the homeless are likely to serve individuals who are in the earlier stages of change. This is not surprising in light of the numerous and complex problems that the homeless face. Individuals in precontemplation in this population may be demoralized and discouraged (DiClemente & Hughes, 1990) rather than actively denying that they have a problem. Additionally, because of the serious problems and challenging circumstances with which the homeless deal, they are harder to engage in treatment and often do not attend self-help groups or other substance abuse services that might be available in the community (Schutt & Garrett, 1992).

These general difficulties point to the need for developing innovative substance abuse interventions in opportunistic settings that literally meet the individuals where they are, both in terms of physical locations and in their stage of change. Unfortunately, many settings for the homeless deny services to those who are actively using alcohol or drugs. As a result, clients are often required to submit to random toxicology screens to assure that they are "clean" in order to qualify for services. When substance abuse services are available, they are typically action-oriented, require abstinence, and are focused only on relapse prevention. In some cases, the primary service for homeless clients is a referral to 12-step community programs, which they generally fail to attend (Schutt & Garrett, 1992).

Much work is needed to study the diverse challenges of the homeless and to develop integrative services to address their issues, many of which are related to the need for increased motivation for positive, sustained change. In terms of substance use, rather than "referring out," requiring abstinence, or offering a "one-size-fits-all" type of service, programs might incorporate the stages and processes of change in terms of the specific needs of specific individuals in multiple domains of their lives. Several researchers have called for this type of programming in venues serving the homeless.

In an early study assessing the needs of the homeless, DeLeon, Sacks, Staines, and McKendrick (1999) explored motivation, readiness, and suitability for treatment among homeless substance abusers in community settings. The researchers concluded that programs needed to be tailored to client readiness to change and the circumstances of this population. In another study, Velasquez, Crouch, von Sternberg, and Grosdanis (2000) assessed substance use, psychological distress, and stage-of-change treatment needs of 100 homeless individuals participating in a large urban day shelter program. Eighty percent reported using alcohol in the past 6 months, 65% were drinking at risky levels, and 60% had used illicit drugs. While the majority of participants reported that they drank and/or used drugs "too much," most indicated that they were not ready to change. Fifty-four percent of those who had drunk alcohol in the past 6 months were classified into the precontemplation stage (no intention of quitting in the next 6 months) and 40% were in the contemplation stage (currently using but intending to quit within the next 6 months). Only 4% of the drinkers were in the action stage for quitting their drinking (have not consumed alcohol for 30 days and intend to "stay off forever"). In terms of other drugs, 30% of the participants who had used drugs in the past 6 months were in the precontemplation stage, 60% were in the contemplation stage, and 10% were in the action stage.

Study findings for adolescent homeless substance abusers are similar to those for adults. In one of the few randomized trials conducted with homeless youth, the STARRS study (Baer, Peterson, & Wells, 2004) tested the efficacy of a brief motivational intervention for homeless substance abusers in youth-serving agencies. The intervention, based on the stages of change, matched services to the clients' stage for reducing or quitting alcohol use and drugs. At baseline assessment, most were in precontemplation for abstaining from drugs or alcohol (74% and 81%, respectively). In contrast, however, when the youth were asked informally about their interest in *reducing* alcohol or substance use, far fewer were in the precontemplation stage (47% for alcohol, 52% for drugs), and many more were in the contemplation or preparation stages (43%

for alcohol, 43% for drugs). An interesting finding from this study is that homeless youth reported being much more open to harm reduction goals than abstinence goals. In terms of outcomes, there was a significant intervention effect for illicit drug use (with the exception of marijuana), but not for alcohol.

SUMMARY

• The majority of individuals with a diagnosable alcohol or drug use disorder do not recognize that they have a problem and therefore do not seek treatment in traditional substance abuse settings.

• Stage-based brief interventions delivered in opportunistic settings have several advantages when compared to more intensive and longer types of treatment. They take advantage of teachable moments, identify problematic use earlier, and offer motivational enhancement at an opportune moment.

• Assessment of a patient's readiness to change can be easily accomplished in opportunistic settings using readiness rulers. Interventions can be tailored accordingly.

• Interventions that focus on building motivation appear to be effective and useful for clients in earlier stages of readiness but later-stage clients may benefit more from receiving advice or skill-building strategies.

• Complex cases require staging of multiple intervention targets and selection of the prime intervention target to avoid overwhelming the client.

11

Final Thoughts and Future Directions

Since its introduction, the transtheoretical stages-of-change model has sought to understand and elucidate client motivation to change problem behaviors. Our goal in writing this book, and in revising the first edition, has been to provide readers with up-to-date research and clinical information about using the stages-of-change model and the corresponding processes of change with substance abusers. In the previous chapters we have presented the most current thinking on the stages and processes of change and described a number of research studies in which these constructs have been related to client progress and outcomes. We have also offered a number of questions that remain to be explored.

As Miller and Rose (2009) note, the stages-of-change model revolutionized addiction treatment and more generally how professionals think about facilitating change. This model popularized a recognition that many substance abusers, even those entering treatment systems, are not yet committed to change and that interventions should therefore be adjusted to the individual's current level of readiness. Rather than being a specific clinical method to enhance personal motivation for change, the transtheoretical model is intended to provide a comprehensive conceptual framework of how and why changes occur. Within this framework, interventions can be matched to specific client characteristics.

In order for good models and theories to develop, it is necessary to question them, modify them as necessary and allow the science to guide decision making. As Whitelaw et al. (2000) and Hodgins (2005) note, perhaps the greatest need for rigorous examination and critique is when an idea becomes "accepted" as has the stages-of-change model. Given the widespread popularity and utilization of the stages-of-change model, it appears to have gained this accepted status. In this volume, we have looked critically at the various components of the model and discussed what parts seem to be most functional and what parts may need further development. As we continue to explore how to understand and influence change—both in treatment settings and in everyday life—we have seen an increasing interest in other variables in the stages-of-change model, particularly the experiential and behavioral processes of change.

So, as we often ask our clients, "Where does that leave us?" In this final chapter, we offer answers to some essential questions. One question we've heard is "Are the stages, as they are currently identified, the 'right ones'?" Albert Bandura (1997) writes that stages are nonpermeable and distinct as when a caterpillar turns into a butterfly—once the change is made, there is no going back. In contrast, the stages of change are actually more about tasks that, when accomplished, promote change. Thus, the model's stages are thought of as dynamic constructs that have overlapping edges, as opposed to an "either/or" design (DiClemente, 2005c). We do know that the process of change is not linear—it is messier than that. Some people move forward, some move backward. Relapse and recycling is happening all the time.

We believe the more compelling and useful questions are about how elements of the model can be used to create an authentically client-centered intervention, provide practical clinical utility, articulate the roles of the client and therapist, and improve our understanding of the nature of the change process. These issues will be addressed in this chapter. Additionally, this chapter discusses questions regarding the contributions and critiques of the model and provide some thoughts about future directions.

A related focus of this chapter is how to help clients as they prepare for change. Clinically, one important question is determining the points during treatment at which we should switch or vary our intervention approaches. For example, when working with a substance-abusing client who begins treatment low in readiness to change, when should we move from an approach such as motivational interviewing to more of a cognitive-behavioral or relapse-prevention focus as the client becomes more ready for change? How do we most efficiently assess readiness in order to fine-tune our sessions? In Chapter 6, we provided a table that suggested specific intervention strategies that can be utilized depending on the client's stage of change. In this chapter, we focus on the importance of tailoring treatment to each client's particular process of change and on the important differences between treatment planning and helping clients as they develop plans for lasting behavior change.

AUTHENTIC CLIENT-CENTERED TREATMENT

A central tenet underlying the stages and processes of change is that the client owns and manages the change process. Indeed, the insights behind the stages-of-change model came from individuals describing how they traveled the often frustrating path toward successful change. That path included false starts, progression and regression, becoming stuck, small successes, significant failures, multiple attempts, and successive approximations that often led to successful change. Although treatments interact with this path, they are necessarily ancillary to the client's own change process since it is the client who has to make and sustain the behavior change. This is the real meaning of client-centered therapy.

The idea that behavior change is complex and involves a path or process is not new. Therapists and counselors from many different theoretical orientations have described complex mechanisms to promote change (see Prochaska & Norcross, 1999). These ideas include making the unconscious conscious (Freud), removing conditions of worth (Rogers), employing various schedules of reinforcement (Skinner), exposure and emotional release (Wolpe, Perls), changing cognitions (Beck, Ellis), and shifting family systems (Minuchin), among others. Most of these theories describe defenses and barriers that make change difficult as well as critical moments or incidents that foster change and involve insight, behavior, or emotions. Some of them target broader problems (meaning, self-actualization, the Oedipus complex) and others concentrate on behavior-specific problems (fear of flying, panic attacks). All of them, however, acknowledge the difficulty of achieving long-term successful change. Many of these theories inform our current substance abuse treatments.

Researchers testing these treatments, however, have focused mostly on what the therapist does and what the treatment prescribes and not as much on the critical element of the client's own process of change. As we have discussed in earlier chapters, the stages of change and the experiential and behavioral processes provide ways of identifying where an individual client is in the process of changing a behavior and using that knowledge in "real time" to guide the selection of intervention goals and strategies.

Over the past 30 years, clinical trial research studies have compared treatments derived from very different theories to find which ones were superior to others. This "horse race" research design has not found a single specific treatment for substance abuse that consistently outperforms all the others. In fact, most psychosocial treatments finish in a dead heat against one another (Luborsky, Singer, & Luborsky, 1975). Recent trials in substance abuse treatment have demonstrated similar results. For example, the Collaborative Cocaine Treatment Study showed little difference among the different treatment conditions (Crits-Christoph et al., 1999). Project MATCH, a large alcohol-focused treatment matching trial comparing three treatment approaches that differed significantly in intensity and in philosophy, also found few differences in client outcomes with clients in all three conditions significantly reducing their alcohol use (Project MATCH Research Group, 1997a, 1997b, 1998a). Even the large multisite National Institute of Mental Health (NIMH) depression trial comparing medication with two types of psychotherapy (interpersonal and cognitive) found that there were few differences in long-term outcomes with these very different types of treatments (Elkin et al., 1989). The COMBINE Study, a trial that evaluated the efficacy of medication, behavioral therapies, and their combinations for treatment of alcohol dependence, did find support for some combinations of medication and psychosocial treatments. In this study, participants in all of the treatment conditions made gains; however, participants who received combinations of one or both psychosocial treatments along with naltrexone reduced their drinking more than did those in a placebo control condition (Anton et al., 2006).

Although in most studies no one specific psychotherapeutic approach appears to be more effective than another, there is a growing consensus among researchers that common elements or a common path of change may underlie all psychosocial treatments (Norcross & Goldfried, 1992). Some researchers have identified commonalities in the treatment relationship, therapist variables, or client demographic variables as the source of the common outcomes (Beutler & Clarkin, 1990; Norcross & Wampold, 2011). It seems equally plausible, however, that the common element across treatments is how the treatments interact with the individual's process of change that we have highlighted in this book. Moreover, the importance of client motivation, ambivalence, and commitment is supported by the more recent focus on approaches such as motivational interviewing, which highlights various tasks identified by the stages of change (DiClemente & Velasquez, 2002; Miller & Rollnick, 1991).

The stages-of-change model offers neither a theory of personality nor an extensive exposition of the biopsychosocial factors that contribute to the development of the problem. The focus of the model is on identifying important components that are common to the change process, whether that change occurs with or without the aid of formal treatment (Prochaska & DiClemente, 1983, 1984; DiClemente & Prochaska, 1998). This perspective emerged from early attempts to look across systems of psychotherapy to find common processes of change (Prochaska, 1979), and it has become more explicit and client-focused in the exploration of addictive behaviors (DiClemente & Prochaska, 1982, 1985; DiClemente et al., 1991; Prochaska & DiClemente, 1982, 1984; Prochaska et al., 1992).

The development of the stages-of-change model has been influenced by many discoveries in both psychotherapy and addiction research. During the 1970s, there was growing interest in how attitudes and decision making influenced behavior change (Janis & Mann, 1977). Behavior therapy and behavior modification increased awareness that identifying and concentrating on specific behaviors could increase the effectiveness of our treatments (Craighead, Craighead, & Ilardi, 1995). These trends led to the growth in the influence of the social learning perspective and the development of cognitive-behavioral therapy (Bandura, 1986; Meichenbaum, 1995). In addition, there was growing recognition of the problem of relapse in addictive behaviors (Brownell et al., 1986). Once treatment researchers began including long-term follow-up of treated clients, they realized that maintenance of behavior change did not automatically follow short-term success (Marlatt & Gordon, 1985; Brownell et al., 1986). In the area of smoking cessation and alcoholism treatment, in particular, there was growing awareness that knowledge, education, and social support were necessary but not sufficient to produce behavior change (Glynn, Boyd, & Gruman, 1990). Relapse was recognized as a persistent and rather intractable problem (Lichtenstein, 1971). As the complexity and multiple aspects of change became clearer, some researchers began to delineate distinguishable steps or tasks that were involved in creating sustained change of addictive behaviors (Horn, 1976; DiClemente & Prochaska, 1982).

The increasing eclecticism among therapists and the increasing number of discoveries related to the process of change laid the foundation for the development of the stages-of-change model. The model offered an understandable and clinically useful perspective on the process of change. These stages divided up the process of change into segments that highlighted the critical issues of resistance to change, decision making, anticipation, action, relapse, and maintenance for specific behavioral problems. This wide-angle view of the process of change was the initial insight that caught the attention of therapists and counselors and gave them a terminology to describe their experiences with clients in treatment. Treatment professionals from New England to New Zealand and from Scotland to South Africa began to use the terminology and to recognize clients as being in precontemplation or contemplation for change, rather than expecting all of them to be either ready for action or "in denial." That this process of change appeared to be cyclical and not linear was another concept that resonated with the experiences of addiction counselors and therapists. The concept of stages of change and the notion that clients recycle through these stages highlighted not only where the client was in regard to the change process at a particular point in time but also where the client had been in terms of his or her change history. The ability of the stages to capture descriptively what many therapists had experienced in practice accounted for the initial success and spread of the stages-of-change construct (Joseph, Breslin, & Skinner, 1999).

What has been most interesting in the research findings about stages of change is that stage status is reliably related to change mechanisms or coping activities that have been labeled processes of change and to a variety of markers of motivation, decision making, and self-efficacy. Evidence from a number of studies indicates that in the preaction stages the cognitive and experiential processes of change are differentially important. Certain processes, like consciousness raising and self-reevaluation, increase in the earlier stages of change and then sometimes decrease during action and maintenance, while behavioral processes are more important in the later action stages of change (Prochaska et al., 1991; Perz et al., 1996; Velicer, DiClemente, Rossi, & Prochaska, 1990; Chapter 2, this volume). This is especially true when cessation of a target behavior is the goal (Carbonari & DiClemente, 2000; DiClemente, 2003; DiClemente & Prochaska, 1985). If stage of change were not related to coping activities and other markers of change like decisional balance and self-efficacy, stages would simply represent descriptive labels offering little or no direction for treatment. It is the interaction of the stages and the processes of change across multiple problem behaviors that offers critical support for the integrative and comprehensive nature of this model in which the client is the central figure in decision making, action, and resolution.

CLINICAL UTILITY OF THE STAGES AND PROCESSES OF CHANGE

As noted above, the most significant contribution of the stages-of-change model to clinical practice is the identification and specification of different tasks and challenges that face the client and the therapist at different points in the process of changing addictive behaviors (Miller & Rollnick, 1991; DiClemente, 1991, 2003, 2005c; DiClemente & Prochaska, 1998; Prochaska & DiClemente, 1984). In this section we highlight several key contributions of the stages-of-change model to the treatment of substance abuse. The clinical utility of this model derives from the clarification of the role of the client and therapist in the process of change, recognition of critical stage-specific tasks, distinguishing between treatment and change, and identification of the cyclical and spiral nature of the process of change.

The Role of the Client

It is the client who owns and manages the process of change. Even the more recent success of approaches such as contingency management, that have increased attendance at treatment or the production of drug-free urines, supports this reality (Higgins, Silverman, & Heil, 2007; Petry, 2000). Clients often respond to incentives even when they are alcohol- or drug-dependent. Moreover, research supports the existence of a common process of intentional human behavior change that seems to be essentially the same whether individuals change a problem behavior with or without formal treatment (DiClemente, 2006; DiClemente & Prochaska, 1982, 1998). Studies that have examined self-change as well as those that have concentrated on treatment seekers have uncovered many similarities in the reported mechanisms and experiences of this process of change (Sobell, Cunningham, Sobell, & Toneatto, 1993; Klingemann, 1991; Tucker et al., 1995; DiClemente & Prochaska, 1985; DiClemente, Carbonari, Zweben, et al., 2001). Thus, the reality is that the client is in charge of the change process and that this process of change begins well before he or she enters treatment and does not end with the completion of treatment (DiClemente & Prochaska, 1998; DiClemente, 1999a, 2003; Penberthy et al., 2007).

The perspective of the stages of change highlights the multiple tasks encountered on the road to recovery from addiction. This focus on tasks to be accomplished allows clients and therapists to evaluate those current critical steps that the client needs to take for progression in the change process. These stage tasks require effort and energy on the part of the client. Moreover, adequacy of completion of each of the tasks can vary significantly between clients. Factors such as the strength of the client's interest and concern, the degree to which the client is determined to change, the depth of the commitment, and how well a change plan is formulated will have an important influence on successful instigation and maintenance of a behavior change. When multiple substances are being used, clients can be at different places in the process of change for each substance, thus requiring different tasks depending on the degree of readiness for changing each substance. Integrated treatment and change plans that take these considerations into account have the highest degree of likelihood for success.

Many individuals have difficulty making and sustaining the change that leads to recovery. For many years these difficulties were attributed to the problem of denial, addiction, craving, or to the strength of the cues in the environment. Although problem dimensions and environment are important, recovery seems to have more to do with negotiating successfully the change process than with dimensions of the substance abuse problems. In fact, in Project MATCH severity of alcohol dependence, often viewed as a negative indicator of success, was a predictor of success and not failure (Project MATCH Research Group, 1997b, 1998a). There are many reasons why some clients are not successful in their attempts to change. Some clients appear not to know what to do. Others seem to have insufficient motivation and are focused on other life problems. Still others appear to be trying too hard with inadequate assistance or ineffective strategies. Although the process is a complicated one, it is the client who must ultimately become sufficiently motivated, make the decisions, create a viable plan, and get committed and follow through on that plan in order for the substance abuse behavior to change.

The Role of the Therapist

Research consistently shows that one of the biggest contributing factors to client success in substance abuse treatment is the therapist who provides the treatment (Norcross & Wampold, 2011). The therapist role has been described as similar to that of a coach or a midwife to this unfolding process of change (DiClemente, 1991). The client is seen as having responsibility for completing tasks that enable movement from one stage to another and for using appropriate processes of change that foster that movement to enter into recovery. Although the ultimate responsibility for change lies with the client, the therapist does have the ethical and clinical responsibility to meet clients where they are in the change process and to support that process. Therapists should first "do no harm" to the client or to the change process, and should offer support and strategies to assist clients to complete stage tasks as competently and completely as possible. Thus, when a client turns to a therapist or counselor for help, the client is asking for help not simply with a problem but with his or her change process. Therapist strategies must be tailored to client process-of-change challenges. However, an important note of caution is needed here: while clients are responsible for their own change, this responsibility for the process of change should not be equated to the moral model view of substance abuse that blames clients for the problem and orders them to clean up their act and change (Donovan & Marlatt, 1988).

Although the client is in charge of the change process, the therapist is not simply an idle bystander or an authoritarian/parental figure. Treatments and therapists are not inert, inactive elements in the process of change. A therapist cannot make a client change, but he or she can support or interfere with the process of change (Project MATCH Research Group, 1998b; DiClemente, 1999a). Although therapists are responsible for instigating and supporting the process of change, they are not responsible for implementing the required tasks and activities needed for a client to move through the process (Tucker et al., 1995). That is, treatments and therapists are catalysts that can create the atmosphere for change, highlight and evoke intrinsic motivation, and contribute important elements to the client's behavior change processes, but the therapist does not *make* the change happen. The stages-of-change model provides a perspective on the process of change that offers a roadmap to the therapist. This roadmap indicates what to do to assist the client to move forward through the stages and through the recycling in order to achieve successful, sustained recovery from the substance abuse problem. It also offers guidance on working with the client to facilitate use of particular experiential and behavioral change processes depending on the client's stage of change.

Treatment Plans and Change Plans in Client-Centered Therapy

It is often suggested that matching treatments to particular client characteristics may improve substance abuse treatment outcomes. In our opinion, the ideal treatment matching would be to have the therapist and the client consciously collaborating on the same goals and tasks that are required at each stage in the change process. If the counselor or therapist is offering action options when the client is in precontemplation, treatment will be experienced as imposing change and will most often fail to obtain sustained change. It is the client's process of change that must be accurately tracked. Hence, knowing the location of the client in the process of change and using that knowledge to guide the selection of intervention goals and strategies are both important. It should be kept in mind that change happens both inside and outside of the therapy session, so therapists should track the client's motivation and change process activity frequently and adjust their treatment strategies accordingly (see Chapter 5).

Just as there are different roles for client and therapist, there is a critical distinction to be made between a *treatment plan* and a *change plan*. The treatment plan details what the therapist or counselor will do or offer to the client. The change plan is what the client is going to do to make the behavior change. The change plan is always more important than the treatment plan and the treatment plan should always be in the service of the change plan. Just because a client comes to treatment does not mean that he or she is committed to or engaged in changing substance use behaviors. However, if the treatment plan and change plan are in synchrony, there should be better engagement and outcomes. This seems to be the underlying rationale for including a motivational dimension in most treatments and the realization that preaction as well as action treatment strategies are needed in any comprehensive treatment program (DiClemente, Garay, & Gemmell, 2011; Martino, Carroll, Nich, & Rounsaville, 2006; Mueser, Noordsy, Drake, & Fox, 2003).

The Cyclical and Spiral Nature of Change

The stages-of-change model's characterization of the flow of the process of change as cyclical or spiral in nature, and ultimate success as reflecting successive approximations, also has proved helpful to clinicians. Addictions are complicated habits involving biological, psychological, and environmental components. As clients become addicted, they learn how to access, use, and hide their drugs of choice. They modify their lives to accommodate the substance abuse. Thus, there is an important learning component to the creation of these habits. There is also a learning component to the modification of these habits (DiClemente, 1999a, 2003; Donovan & Marlatt, 1988; Rotgers, Keller, & Morgenstern, 1996; Tucker et al., 1995; Werch & DiClemente, 1994). Substance abusers must learn how problematic their drug or alcohol problems are, what the pros and cons are for change, how firm a commitment to make, what strategies to use, and how to change their lives to eliminate those problem behaviors. These things are not ordinarily learned in a single day or in a single successful attempt to change. False starts, regression, and relapse are all part of the learning process (DiClemente, Holmgren & Rounsaville, 2010). Recycling through the stages appears to be a normal part of the process of recovery. However, the cycling should not be endless. Rapid and unproductive cycling through the stages indicates a serious problem in the process of change (Carbonari et al., 1999; DiClemente & Prochaska, 1998; DiClemente & Scott, 1997). Recycling, at its most productive, represents a learning process of successive approximations wherein the individual and the therapist learn what will and will not work for that individual to change successfully. Thus, the process is described as a spiral one in which the client moves through the stages repeatedly until he or she reaches sustained change. This notion apparently has brought comfort and direction to many clients and therapists, enabling them to reconceptualize the work of breaking away from addictions in a more realistic and helpful manner.

EVALUATING CURRENT STATUS AND CRITIQUES OF THE STAGES-OF-CHANGE MODEL

The widespread use of the stages and processes of change in the treatment of addictive behaviors has not been uniformly well received. Some clinicians and researchers have expressed concerns about the model and its utility (Bandura, 1997; Davidson, 1992; Farkas et al., 1996; Herzog, 2008; Pierce, Farkas, Zhu, Berry, & Kaplan, 1996; Sutton, 1996; West, 2005). In this section, we highlight some of these concerns and discuss them. The stages-of-change model has been proposed as one that isolates critical dimensions of the intentional behavior change process. In addition to its clinical utility and popularity with many addiction counselors and researchers, in order for it to be relevant the model should also prove useful for tracking and predicting change. Research findings should support the contentions of the model or at least be relatively consistent with the constructs outlined by the model. While research can never prove a theory, it can weaken or disprove various aspects of a theory if the findings consistently contradict the basic assumptions of the model. It is critically important, however, that when we are evaluating a model or a theory we must first make sure that assumptions, definitions, and constructs are well described and understood.

Stages or a Continuous Process?

Are there really stages of change, or is the process of change better viewed as a continuous one? Difficulties in classifying people into the specific stages (Joseph et al., 1999) and the criticism that stage models are not helpful for viewing process activities (Bandura, 1997) have produced challenges to the validity of the stage perspective. Critics question whether it is more useful to view the process of change as similar to a single stream that flows around curves and barriers, as a chaotic, nonlinear random series of events, or as a series of stages that are distinct, sequential, and interconnected. The critiques of the stages of change appear to be based on the view that the process of change must either be a multidimensional continuous one, a nonlinear random one, or one that has distinct stages. If only one of these competing views of the process of change must be chosen, research and anecdotes indicates that a multidimensional view that allows for progression and regression, learning, failure and trying, and the subtle and not-so-subtle influence of random events seems most appealing. However, according to the developers of the stages-of-change model, these different conceptualizations do not have to be at odds (Prochaska & DiClemente, 1998; DiClemente, 2005c). Depending on how one defines stages, the permeability of the boundaries between stages, whether there is a strict assumption of linearity, and how broad a perspective is taken, the process of human behavior change can be viewed as a continuous but not inevitable process with important discrete steps influenced by multiple internal and external determinants that occur over time in a rather disorderly fashion. For example, continuity and a stepwise function are not necessarily incompatible. A staircase is really a continuous straight line from one floor to another. However, without the steps it would be difficult to negotiate the passage. A lifespan view of recovery from alcoholism (Vaillant, 1995) can identify a course of change over time that for some clients looks like a steady stream of activity leading to successful problem resolution and recovery. In fact, the famous Jellinek U-shaped curve depicted the process of becoming addicted and recovering as a smooth curvilinear function, indicating that the individual descended into addiction, hit bottom, and then moved upward into recovery (DiClemente & Scott, 1997). However, the process does not appear to be continuous, linear, or curvilinear for many (DiClemente, 2006) and lifespan views for many look more like a series of hills and valleys or the path of a pinball bouncing around multiple consequences and obstacles.

That same lifespan view of addiction and recovery indicates that most individuals have followed problematic paths over many years and made multiple attempts to change before being successful (Vaillant, 1995). Longitudinal research indicates that individuals get stuck at certain points in this process of change and invest more time and energy in *not* changing or thinking about change than in activities that would promote change. For some, the goal of recovery is elusive even with multiple attempts to change and the road ends in death before a more complete recovery. Taking actions that result in relapse or maintenance represent important distinct steps in successful recovery. For most, however, the process of change is filled with periods of movement as well as long periods of time spent maintaining the status quo of the habit. As we tie together the different events in a life of addiction and recovery, there seems to be both ebb and flow in the process of change precipitated by teachable moments and important, distinct tasks that mark the process. Continuous, chaotic, and discrete-stage perspectives on the process of change are not necessarily contradictory. In fact, they can be complementary (Prochaska & DiClemente, 1998; DiClemente, 2005a). "Continuous" does not mean that there are not tasks that need to be accomplished. "Chaotic" and "nonlinear" do not mean that there is no order but simply that we cannot always see connections in the randomness of events.

The stages are a way of segmenting the process of change into useful but rather fluid states (DiClemente & Prochaska, 1998). Individuals can move forward and backward through the stages, and they can do so quickly. A 15- to 20-minute motivation-enhancing conversation often can generate the interest and concern needed to help someone who is in precontemplation for a particular change to move to contemplation. A thoughtful discussion of a change plan can help a client move from preparation to action. As well as moving forward, a client can sometimes shift backward in stage in the course of a session. For example, a client might move from preparation back to contemplation for a short time when the client and therapist recognize that some earlier stage tasks must be accomplished before moving on. An example of this would be the need to enhance the client's process of self-reevaluation through a thoughtful discussion of what life might be like after making the change. This fluidity is normal and an insightful therapist can use it as an opportunity to elicit the client's fears or concerns about change as well as reinforcing talk about change and commitment.

The critical defining feature of a stage seems to be whether there are important distinguishable tasks that need to be accomplished to achieve movement toward successful behavior change. However, these tasks, though related, do not have the identical markers or characteristics from one stage to the next, as would be observed in developmental stage theories that mark the growth of an organism. Growth indicators like increases in height or the transition from caterpillar to butterfly have only a single direction and never proceed in opposite directions. Butterflies never become caterpillars, and people become taller until reaching full development. These developmental stages are unidirectional, discrete, self-contained states that are discontinuous. Rather than being purely developmental in nature, the stages of change represent a series of tasks that need to be accomplished to some degree so the individual can move from one stage to the next stage. These tasks involve dimensions (motivation, decision making, efficacy, and coping activities) that have been identified in many different models of change. The tasks are somewhat independent but connected and have an ongoing influence on the change process, can be accomplished quickly or slowly, and can be done more or less completely. From this perspective, the quality and completeness of the execution of the stage-specific tasks would impact success in the subsequent stages, recycling, and long-term success.

These stages of change, therefore, seem to be unlike developmental, discontinuous steps and more like the stage dimensions of personality development proposed by Erikson (1963). Erikson viewed the psychological growth and maturation of an individual as a series of bipolar tasks (trust vs. mistrust) that build on one another, become salient at certain points in the development of the individual, and can be more or less resolved as the individual moves through life. If unresolved, these tasks create problems for future development and success. If stages of change are envisioned more like Eriksonian stages, then the debate over a continuous versus a discrete stage process seems less important and the debate about whether the stages are linear or nonlinear becomes less of an issue.

The research to date appears to support a process of change for substance abusers that can be described as a series of steps or phases that require different strategies and address different issues. Processes of change, decision-making self-evaluations, and relevant efficacy evaluations vary significantly by stage of change (DiClemente & Prochaska, 1998; DiClemente, Prochaska, & Gibertini, 1985; DiClemente et al., 1991; Smith et al., 1995; Prochaska et al., 1991, 1992; Prochaska, Velicer, et al., 1994; Velasquez et al., 1999). There is also evidence that shifting process activity from more experiential processes to more behavioral ones as someone moves from contemplation and preparation to action is the more effective way to achieve successful smoking cessation (Perz et al., 1996). Movement through the process of change does not appear to be a case of doing more of the same thing, as would be expected in a purely continuous model, but instead a case of doing the right thing at the right time. The research examining a success profile at the end of treatment that related to successful modification of drinking in the posttreatment period seems to indicate that there are some process markers that are reliably related to success so that recovery would not be best represented as chaotic and nonlinear (Carbonari & DiClemente, 2000). This provides the very exciting possibility of therapists assessing key client variables during the course of treatment (such as the stages of change, temptation, self-efficacy, and the pros and cons of change) and adjusting treatment accordingly to help the client achieve the profile with the highest likelihood of success.

The developers of the model have proposed that the research evidence of significant differences among individuals in the different stages of change on decisional balance, self-efficacy, and processes of change offer support for the importance of the discrete stage perspective. The interrelationship between the stages and these other critical dimensions of change are at the heart of the larger model of the intentional change process. The fact that these differences between stages have been found with changes across different types of behaviors (exercise adoption, modification of alcohol problems, smoking cessation, condom use) seems to offer significant support for that contention. It is interesting that when examining relationships across time and stages for subgroups of individuals, the graphic representations of process activity, efficacy, and decisional considerations by stages appear continuous and represent either a linear or curvilinear shape across the different stages (Prochaska et al., 1991). Pros and cons for change do seem to rise or fall across the stages in a curvilinear fashion (Prochaska, Velicer, et al., 1994). Self-efficacy appears to rise as individuals move from precontemplation through the stages to maintenance (DiClemente et al., 1985). Some processes appear to rise in early stages and then decline in occurrence during action and maintenance (Prochaska et al., 1991). However, when one looks at the multiple patterns of change over time that include all of the lapse, relapse and recycling events and episodes, the shapes are clearly not linear. Instead, over a 2-year period, over 40 different patterns of change were found (Prochaska et al., 1991).

Relapse as an Event

It is also interesting to note how the proponents of the model have handled the issue of relapse. Initially relapse was viewed as a potential stage of change (Prochaska & DiClemente, 1982). However, as data on the processes of change used by relapsers became clearer, relapse appeared to be better categorized as a distinct event or process rather than a stage of change (DiClemente & Prochaska, 1998). In fact, all relapsers can be categorized in terms of their current stage of change. Thus, it makes more sense to envision and classify individuals who recently relapsed as recycling through the earlier stages of precontemplation, contemplation, and preparation rather than being in a separate stage (Prochaska & DiClemente, 1984; DiClemente & Prochaska, 1998; DiClemente, 2003). There do appear to be important distinctions among the events that occur on the road to recovery before and after a lapse or relapse that have implications for moving through the stages of change. For example, a lapse can be an important indicator that the plan developed in preparation and enacted in the action stages has one or more flaws and needs to be revised if action is to be continued. An unsuccessful attempt to quit the substance, labeled "a relapse," can indicate that the individual is better prepared to make another attempt that may be more successful. Some definitions of the preparation stage include a recent quit attempt (DiClemente et al., 1991), since smokers who had made a prior quit attempt were more prepared and likely to make another more successful one. Once again, this seems to indicate that stages are based on particular tasks that have continuity but often result in a circuitous route to recovery from substance abuse and dependence to sobriety and abstinence.

Evolution of the Stages of Change

As with any good model, the thinking on stages of change has evolved as research has revealed areas for development. As such, there have been different stages proposed in earlier and later versions of the model. An early version presented only the precontemplation, contemplation, action, and maintenance stages, with the preparation stage added later (DiClemente et al., 1991). Some authors reporting on an early version of the model identify a stage that was labeled "determination" (Miller & Rollnick, 1991). The proponents of the model claim that measuring the determination (early version) or preparation (later version) stage has been challenging, and therefore some versions of the model have included only four stages since these were the only ones that could be reliably measured (Prochaska & DiClemente, 1984). More current versions of the model have included a preparation stage (DiClemente, 2003; DiClemente & Prochaska, 1998).

The issue of assessment of stages is a particularly complicated one, and we will examine it in detail later. However, it does seem to be reasonable that assessment and theory building be integrated. If a construct cannot be measured, it cannot be evaluated. One can hypothesize the existence of many different constructs, as the history of clinical psychology will attest. However, many of these constructs have not been able to be tested because they have not been operationalized (defined in a measurable way). The attempt to make assumptions and to revise the model based on empirical data seems to be a strength rather than a weakness. Although changing names and constructs does sometimes pose problems for those wanting to apply the model, this attention to research and dedication to modifying constructs as more is learned about the process of change is probably what have made the stages-of-change model so relevant to real-life substance abuse treatment. In the end, the test will be whether these stages can be identified, measured, and used in ways that are helpful to clinicians and supported by research.

Prediction of Outcomes

Another concern is whether the stages are related to outcomes, as expected by the model. Although the data are not conclusive, a growing body of literature appears to support the relationship of stage indicators to important clinical outcomes. In many studies, stage status or readiness measured using a stage-based assessment have been related to participation in program activities like reading self-help materials (DiClemente et al., 1991), attendance at treatment sessions (Smith et al., 1995), and outcomes of interventions (DiClemente et al., 1991; Project MATCH Research Group, 1997a).

Changes in stage from one time point to another (Carbonari et al., 1999) and increasing and decreasing levels of process of change activities by stage (Prochaska et al., 1991) also support the relationship of stage status with progress and the process of recovery. Stages and the related concept of readiness to change have been predictive of the amount and extent of change. In several studies, stage-related status predicted attempts to change and successful outcomes (Carbonari & DiClemente, 2000; DiClemente et al., 1991; Tsoh, 1995; Project MATCH Research Group, 1997a, 1997b, 1998a). Clinical trials testing interventions based on the stages and processes of change have also found that clients' increased use of the processes is predictive of improved outcomes in drinking among HIV-positive men (Velasquez, 2006; Velasquez et al., 2009), reduction of drinking in women at risk for fetal alcohol spectrum disorder (Floyd et al., 2007; Mullen, Velasquez, von Sternberg, Cummins, & Green, 2005), and reductions in cocaine use in group treatment participants (Velasquez, von Sternberg, & Stephens, 2011).

In Project MATCH, a microanalysis of the influence of client readiness to change assessed as individuals entered outpatient treatment indicated that readiness predicted client evaluations of the quality of the therapeutic relationship, level of coping activities both during and at the end of treatment, and drinking quantity and frequency during posttreatment (DiClemente, Carbonari, Zweben, et al., 2001; Connors et al., 2000). Further, there was partial support for a treatment-matching effect between baseline motivation and the Project MATCH motivational enhancement treatment (Witkiewitz, Hartzler, & Donovan, 2010). Although there is intriguing support for the role of motivation and stages in the prediction of outcomes for substance abuse treatments, more research is needed. In addition, studies are needed that examine the interaction of stage status with a variety of other variables so that the combined and unique predictive ability of all these variables can be better understood. There is evidence that currently supports the predictive validity of the stages among substance abusers. These studies have been conducted in settings ranging from college campuses to substance abuse treatment programs to health care settings (DiClemente, Schumann, Greene, & Earley, 2011; DiClemente et al., 1999; Fromme & Corbin, 2004; Heather et al., 2009; Maisto et al., 2011; Stein et al., 2009). However, the evidence is not conclusive at the present time. Complex modeling is needed since process variables are interrelated, interactive, and shift over time.

Labels—or Aids to Intervention?

When considering the stages of change, it is important to remember that they represent client states and not traits. The difference, of course, is that a *trait* is a relatively permanent individual characteristic whereas a *state* is temporary and subject to change. The critique that stages are simply labels would be justified if providers treated them as traits instead of states and, for example, identified some clients as "precontemplators" in order to deny services instead of seeing them as "individuals in precontemplation" capable of moving forward. Providers should use these stages as a way to conceptualize what is going on for the client in that particular stage and how to help him or her move to the next step. If stages were used simply as labels to stigmatize people (e.g., as hopeless precontemplators), they would be at best useless, at worst harmful. This would be similar to viewing everyone who is not ready for action as being in denial. However, on the whole, utilization of the stages has spurred many clinicians to develop alternative strategies for welcoming substance abusers who are in precontemplation into treatment and addressing their specific needs. Miller and Rollnick (1991), originally inspired by the dilemma of early-stage clients, have outlined motivational interviewing procedures to address individuals in precontemplation and contemplation. Clinicians and researchers have come together to outline strategies and procedures to move individuals through each of the stages of change (Miller, 1999; Rollnick et al., 1999; Shaffer, 1992; Velasquez et al., 2001). Programs have been developed to reach out proactively to those in precontemplation and to engage them in the process of change with good success (DiClemente, 2003; DiClemente & Prochaska, 1998; Heather et al., 2009; Soderstrom et al., 2006; Velicer et al., 1993). In general, the stage construct does appear to have utility beyond mere categorization of individuals and has generated innovative approaches to treatment of substance abusers.

Measuring the Stages

Although intuitively easy to understand, measurement of stages of change poses a particular problem for the practitioner and the researcher. How to assess the stage status of individuals with different substance abuse problems and in different types of programs has created significant frustration with the construct of stages (Carey et al., 1999; Joseph et al., 1999). Multiple measures have been used, including categorical algorithms, ladders or rulers, grids, and multiple item, multiple subscale questionnaires like the URICA (McConnaughy et al., 1989), the SOCRATES (Miller & Tonigan, 1996), and readiness-to-change scales (Carbonari, DiClemente, & Zweben, 1994; DiClemente & Prochaska, 1998; Heather et al., 1993). The good news is that many different measures have been able to divide the population of changers into subgroups that make sense and are most often consistent with the characteristics based on the idea of stages (Carney & Kivlahan, 1995; DiClemente et al., 1991; Isenhart, 1994; Willoughby & Edens, 1996). However, the not-so-good news is that there is no single measure of stage status for all behaviors. It is also significant that the different measures do not always cross-classify individuals into the same stage of change (Belding et al., 1996; Carey et al., 1999; Joseph et al., 1999; Rothfleisch, 1997) because of the reactivity of self-reporting in various types of settings. However, the importance of readiness to change is supported in many different studies (DeLeon et al., 1994; DiClemente, 1999b; Simpson & Joe, 1993; Project MATCH Research Group, 1997a).

Although it is not unusual to have multiple measures for a construct, as is evident for depression, anxiety, spirituality, and drinking, specific problems with assessing stage status appear to be related to four issues. First, the target goal of the behavior change often is poorly specified. Second, measures have been poorly constructed and inadequately evaluated. Third, measures must rely on self-report and the accuracy and honesty of the individual reporting his or her behavior and attitudes. Fourth, stage status is difficult to assess since it represents a mobile state and not a static trait. Here we address each of these issues in turn.

Specification of Target Behaviors

Evaluating stages for any behavior change necessitates identification of a clear behavioral target (e.g., cocaine use or drinking behavior, abstinence or reduction), making a clear distinction between those individuals in action stages and those who are not yet engaged and are in preaction stages. Then it is important to identify attitudes or intentions of those in preaction toward changing that behavior in the future (next 6 months or next month). For those in action it is critical to specify accepted indicators of actual behavior change and length of time the change has been sustained (DiClemente & Prochaska, 1998; DiClemente, Schlundt, & Gemmell, 2004). Addressing all of these dimensions of behavior change is not a simple matter, particularly when the target behavior is complex and multifaceted or when there are multiple potential goals with regard to the target behavior. For example, reducing drinking and abstaining from drinking represent two different potential goals for an alcohol abuser. Stage status related to these two distinct goals could be very different for a given individual. Some polysubstance-abusing clients are prepared to take action with regard to one drug but not another, so a generic stage status related to use of illegal drugs would likely miss client readiness with one or the other drug. Specificity of behavior and of the change goal is critical for accurate assessment of stage. Identifying what constitutes action and what maintenance would look like are also critical. Would action be defined as never having a binge episode of more than five drinks on an occasion? Is maintenance never having even a taste of alcohol?

Multiple Measures of Stage

The multiple measures of stage status are a mixed blessing. The fact that different measures can be used successfully supports both the notion that the process of change can be segmented and the existence of some underlying construct, like stages of change. These assessments create ways to identify whether the individual is in earlier or later segments of the process of change. Some measures attempt to create stage subgroups; others are satisfied with simply identifying individuals who are more or less ready to change. However, using either continuous measures or stage-based classifications, individuals earlier in the process differ from individuals in later stages on measures of change-process activity, decisional considerations, and self-efficacy in expected ways (DiClemente, 2005c;

DiClemente, Schlundt, & Gemmell, 2004). Although measuring these stages in different behaviors has proved challenging, various measures seem to have identified individuals at different points in the process of change with many addictive and health behaviors. The important thing to remember is that one needs to make sure that the assessment strategy fits the specific target behavior and the type of setting. Just translating stage assessments used for smoking cessation and applying them indiscriminately to a court-ordered population of cocaine users will yield inaccurate and misleading assessment of stage status or readiness.

Reliance on Self-Report

Research on the stages requires accurate assessment of where clients are in the process of change. That assessment is almost completely reliant on the self-report of the individual substance abuser. Some biochemical assessments can verify the self-report of abstinence from certain substances. Samples of blood, breath, saliva, urine, and even hair can be used to see whether an individual has used a particular substance within the immediate past day, week or, at best, few weeks. These tests yield only an assessment of abstinence and typically cannot examine reduction in use, binge episodes, and other irregular patterns of use. So, even for the evaluation of action and maintenance stage status, the therapist must necessarily rely on the self-report of the substance abuser. And it is clear that reliable reporting of attitudes and behavior is even more critical to the assessment of earlier stages.

Although social pressure, situational demands, and self-deception can influence self-reports of substance abusers, there is no reason to abandon self-report. The client's perspective is the most important one in the treatment process. The key objective is to create an environment in which the client can report honestly and to ask questions that allow the client to characterize his or her attitudes and behaviors in ways that are comfortable. Asking a client who comes to treatment as a condition of parole whether he or she wants to stop using cocaine on the first day in the clinic is problematic. This would be particularly true if the client believed that saying yes was essential to entry into treatment. However, cigarette smoking evokes less concern, and most of the time asking a series of questions about current smoking and readiness to quit smoking yields a pretty good assessment of a smoker's stage of change (DiClemente & Prochaska, 1998). However, there have been numerous problems with using a similar set of questions during intake to a drug abuse program (Rothfleisch, 1997; Belding et al., 1996). A less direct approach may be needed with other substance abuse behaviors. As described in the assessment chapter, the SOCRATES and versions of the URICA have been rather successful in assessing readiness to change and stage-related groups but can be tricky to use (DiClemente & Hughes, 1990; DiClemente, Schlundt, & Gemell, 2004; Carney & Kivlahan, 1995; Willoughby & Edens, 1996). In both of these assessments, clients are asked a series of questions representing a number of attitudes and views that they can endorse by using a range of responses and not simply yes or no. When given the opportunity to endorse a little or a lot, clients give a more accurate view of where they are in the process of change. However, additional research on how to evaluate stage status in different settings and with different substance abuse problems is needed.

The Nature of the Stages

Some of the difficulty in assessing stage status is due to the nature of the stages of change. Stages represent the current state of the individual with respect to changing a single behavior. Stage status can persist for a long time or could change in a very short time. An individual who is in precontemplation about quitting smoking today could be in preparation or action tomorrow after learning about the death of his best friend from lung cancer. Assessing this moving target and then using that single intake assessment to predict change outcomes is problematic. It is all the more impressive that the stage variables have been very potent predictors in many studies despite all the problems described above. A measure should operationalize a construct in a satisfactory manner. However, no measure is ever a complete measure of a construct. For example, there are multiple behavior-specific measures of the construct of self-efficacy. Each measure is only an approximation of the efficacy construct applied to a particular behavior and behavioral goal. Similarly, multiple assessments of stages must be viewed as unique efforts at approximating the stage status of an individual.

Multiple Problems and a Common Process

An early concern about the model was that it was applied mostly to smoking cessation. The concern was whether it could be used with other behaviors and if it could be applied to behavior changes needed in psychiatric disorders. However, after years of application to a range of behaviors, it seems that one of the advantages for those who are using the stages-of-change model in treatment is that the process of change outlined in the model is assumed to be the same for substance abuse problems as well as other life problems when behavior change is involved. The model has been applied to changing many different behaviors, including positive health behaviors like exercise and cancer screening as well as problems such as medication compliance, anxiety and depression, and obesity (Beitman et al., 1994; Bowen & Trotter, 1995; DiClemente, Ferentz, & Velasquez, 2004; DiClemente, Nidecker, & Bellack, 2008; Grimley, Riley, Bellis, & Prochaska, 1993; Marcus, Rossi, Selby, Niaura, & Abrams, 1992; McConnaughy et al., 1989). Stages and processes of change have been evaluated in a variety of these behaviors. The process appears to be similar across the various behaviors and among subgroups of clients. Clinicians who use the model can think about the various problems that the substance-abusing client has on entry to treatment in a similar way (DiClemente et al., 1992). Some clients are very ready to deal with one problem while being in early stages with regard to another problem. The ability to view the multiple problems of a client, be they various drugs of abuse or problems in other areas of life, in terms of a single change process appears to be an important advantage for the clinician (DiClemente, 2003).

Treatment of substance abuse has often been viewed as very different from treatment of mental health, relationships, adjustment, and physical health problems. In that way, substance abuse treatment has been isolated and "carved out" of traditional health care considerations. Although some critics view the breadth of application of the stages-of-change model to multiple problem areas to be a negative, substance abuse treatment providers can use this breadth of scope to assist them in dealing with the many other problems of the substance abuser. Moreover, the commonality of this process of change across different types of behaviors argues for substance abuse treatment to be included in the broad continuum of care that should be provided to individuals in the community rather than being an isolated treatment service (DiClemente, 1999a; McLellan, Arndt, Metzger, Woody, & O'Brien, 1993).

Adequacy of the Stages-of-Change Model

A final critique of the stages of change model is that it focuses on individual change dimensions and has a limited perspective. Some critics argue that there exist other more comprehensive and explanatory theories, like Bandura's social cognitive theory (1986) that can explain change. The implication is that the stages-of-change model omits important dimensions and is not comprehensive. There is a significant difference between a model and a theory. The architects of the stages-of-change model have focused the model on the process of intentional behavior change and claim that the model has a narrower focus than the more global theories of human functioning (DiClemente & Prochaska, 1998; Joseph et al., 1999). Nonetheless, the stages do cover a considerable amount of ground, since the process of intentional behavior change is central in the life of the individual, with major implications for human growth and development.

The stages of change have been applied to multiple types of behavior changes, from sunscreen use to cocaine addiction. There are few models that can be applied to such a variety of behaviors with such similar and consistent results. However, the application of the model to these multiple behaviors is sometimes conducted without proper attention being paid to important differences among these behaviors. For example, there are distinct patterns of change depending on whether one is initiating a new behavior, stopping a problematic behavior, or otherwise modifying a current pattern of behavior. This lack of precision fuels some of the criticism about the model reaching beyond its scope or appropriate applicability. It may also be true that some proponents appear to make claims for the model that encourage critics to compare the model to a more general theory of human functioning. The model should be judged in the context of the rather narrow focus of intentional behavior change (rather than all human functioning). In this context, the broad applicability to behavior change despite the clear differences among these behaviors (exercise, drinking, smoking, condom use) supports the construct validity of the stages and processes of change. Attempts to use this as a broad theory of human functioning or to compare it to such a theory, however, are misguided.

FUTURE DIRECTIONS

Although a substantial number of studies have applied the stages-of-change model to substance abuse problems, there is still much to learn about the stages and how the model can most productively be used in clinical practice. Some domains of particular importance include the following.

Promoting Stage Progression

In this volume we have identified issues, strategies, and interventions that are relevant to individuals in the various stages of change. However, clinicians and researchers must continue to examine how to support movement through the stages more effectively and efficiently and to identify which techniques or strategies would be most successful with clients in these stages. In particular, we need to know how to get individuals moving who are stuck in the precontemplation and contemplation stages of change, understand the critical parameters of planning needed in the preparation stage, and evaluate the most effective ways to promote recycling. There is a role for more basic research as well. Understanding how self-regulation skills impact the completing of stage tasks, whether individuals can quickly move through stages seeming to move forward without consciously or deliberately completing the tasks, and whether there are some critical tasks that if done well can produce successful change are interesting and important questions. We also need more information on the point in the change process at which clinicians should shift strategies and which approaches are most effective at which stages of change. Specifics about how the process of change works with different groups of individuals in recovery, such as those who only go to Alcoholics Anonymous (Snow, Prochaska, & Rossi, 1994; DiClemente, 1993), those who are dually diagnosed (Bellack & DiClemente, 1999; DiClemente et al., 2008; Heesch, Velasquez, & von Sternberg, 2005; Velasquez et al., 1999), and those who change as a result of brief interventions (DiClemente, 2006) are also needed. Another important challenge concerns the training of individuals to deliver interventions that effectively engage appropriate processes of change across the entire spectrum of intentional change.

Substance abusers as well as other types of changers take a long time to move through these stages of change once they have a well-established pattern of drug or alcohol dependence. Over a 6-month period without intervention, the majority of smokers in the earlier stages of change will remain in precontemplation or contemplation (Carbonari et al., 1999). Previous research has identified large numbers of individuals in contemplation who remain in contemplation for long periods of time and has labeled these individuals "chronic contemplators" (Prochaska et al., 1991). Encouraging movement out of these initial stages is not easy for "virgin quitters" as they move through the stages making a first attempt to stop drinking or drugging. Once individuals have been through the cycle and failed, it can be even harder to get them to move through again. Treatment should help individuals to accomplish stage tasks and move more efficiently or more effectively through the process. However, it is important to remember that the process of change occurs in the natural environment and not simply during treatment or intervention (DiClemente, 1999a, 2005c, 2006). Most individuals who come into treatment, therefore, are not naive "change virgins" who have never tried to modify or stop their problematic substance use. Many have been through the cycle of change on their own several times before asking for help (DiClemente & Scott, 1997). Sometimes they expect treatment to make change happen with little effort on their part. At other times they need to be convinced that it would be worthwhile to leave precontemplation or contemplation again to make another attempt to solve the drug abuse problem.

Several strategies have been identified that can be used as motivational enhancement strategies (DiClemente, Garay, & Gemmell, 2011; Miller & Rollnick, 1991; Miller, 1999). However, continued thought and effort should be dedicated to researching and designing ways of specifically encouraging individuals to move out of precontemplation and contemplation. As the legal system becomes more aggressive in mandating drug and alcohol offenders to treatment, the need to develop strategies that engage the client in an intentional process of change during mandated interventions or an imposed suspension of the drug abuse behavior become more important. There is room for creativity and ingenuity on the part of the clinician and researcher alike to design and evaluate new interventions to help these early-stage individuals break the logjam and move forward in the process of change.

One of the important parts of preparing individuals for action is promoting and increasing commitment to action. The descriptions of the preparation stage detail both developing a change plan and increasing commitment as the two critical tasks to be accomplished during that stage. Clinicians are given little training in how to enhance commitment to follow through on an action plan. Albert Ellis and colleagues have written about defeating procrastination (Ellis & Dryden, 1987), which seems to be part of the problem. However, techniques and strategies that address commitment enhancement are in only limited use in substance abuse counseling programs. Goal setting, choice, and going public have all been identified as potential commitment enhancement tools (Miller, 1999; Miller & Rose, 2009). These and other similar techniques need to be evaluated in the context of preparation stage activity in order to see which are the most important. How to increase commitment effectively represents a significant challenge for the field.

Relapse and Recycling

Another important issue in the treatment of substance abuse involves the reality of relapse and how relapse impacts movement through the stages of change. The stages model has identified a recycling process in which relapse becomes an event that creates a cyclical movement back through the stages of change. However, how this occurs, what the critical dimensions of the recycling events are, and what interventions yield the most efficient recycling have not yet been established. Relapse appears to be a critical event in the process of recovery that influences how long recovery will take for any given individual. It is an important learning experience that can encourage, discourage, or derail positive movement through the change process. Although there has been extensive research on relapse and relapse prevention (Marlatt, 1996; Marlatt & Donovan, 2005; Marlatt & Gordon, 1985), knowledge about the event, its precipitants, and, most importantly, its role in the overall view of recovery remains lacking. Efficacy and temptation have been key dimensions related to successful long-term outcomes in the process profiles derived at the end of the Project MATCH treatments (Carbonari & DiClemente, 2000). More recent research indicates that relapse vulnerability can be measured by examining the relationships between levels of temptation to drink and levels of confidence to abstain. Holmgren and DiClemente (2012) found that, defined in this manner, relapse vulnerability predicted time to first drink, number of drinks on the first drinking day, and number of drinking days in the first week of drinking after abstinence. Clinicians and researchers need to take a broader view of the process of recovery when dealing with clients or designing studies. Where the client has been in the process of change prior to entering treatment and how successfully he or she has completed tasks seems as important as the specific goals of the client.

Assessing Stage Status and Task Completion

Relapse is not the only area where additional research is needed to assist clinicians in applying the stages and processes of change. Other critical areas that need clarification and better understanding include measurement of the stages-of-change tasks, the relationship of stage transitions to long-term outcomes, and how different treatments interact with the process of change. Although there sometimes are difficulties in formally conducting research assessments, clinicians seem to have less of a problem identifying stage status when they can talk with an individual client openly and honestly and when they can access thoughts and feelings as well as watch the client's behavior over time. What seem to be needed are multiple indicators that would enable the clinician and researcher to pinpoint the stage status of an individual across several dimensions. In the book *Health Behavior Change,* Rollnick and colleagues (1999) discussed the importance of the change and the confidence to make the change as important and rather independent dimensions that can influence readiness to change. Decisional balance considerations or the relations between the pros and cons of change would be another possible indicator. Appropriate change-process activity could also become a marker of stage status once we have some norms for individuals seeking treatment. In any case, there is a need for significant additional research in assessing the stages and related constructs so that clinicians can better classify individuals along the steps in the process of change.

Even more importantly, clinicians need to understand and find ways to evaluate the comprehensiveness or quality of a client's completion of stage tasks. This leads to several important questions. How important is the completion of stage-specific tasks to the overall achievement of successful maintenance? Is it better to have individuals make some half-hearted attempts to change or to have them wait and make only serious ones? How does external pressure to enter treatment affect the movement from one stage to the next for individuals in precontemplation versus contemplation? Is there an ideal amount of time that needs to be spent in a stage, or is it completely variable? Do individuals who are stuck in a particular stage for a long period of time fare better or worse in achieving their ultimate goal? Should they just be encouraged to jump-start the process? Some of the most informative data we have about these issues comes from following smokers over long periods of time. However, it is not clear if the patterns and process for smoking cessation are exactly the same as the ones for other substances, such as heroin, cocaine, or alcohol. There has not been enough research to make all the comparisons needed, and there is still much to learn about the process of recovery for smoking cessation as well as other drugs of abuse. Longitudinal research with large numbers of individuals is needed to answer these questions. Capturing this process in the natural environment is not an easy task. It is not easy to accumulate the numbers of individuals needed to have the power to be able to predict outcomes for each stage of change. With so many individuals being stuck in stages for long periods of time, it is difficult to capture enough changers at any one time to make certain predictions with very large numbers of research participants willing to participate over many years. Nevertheless, the need for such research to resolve some basic questions about the process of change for substance abusers is obvious.

Understanding this process of change is of paramount importance. However, it probably cannot be studied without examining the relationship between the process and the various treatments to which substance abusers are exposed. How treatment interacts with the process of change is another important avenue for continued research. At present, the evidence indicates that different types of treatments influence the process of change in similar ways (Prochaska, DiClemente, Velicer, & Rossi, 1993; DiClemente, Carbonari, Zweben, et al., 2001). In Project MATCH, the three different treatments (cognitive-behavioral, motivational enhancement, and 12-step facilitation) resulted in very similar client process activity and equivalent levels of abstinence self-efficacy. Miller and Rollnick (1991) indicate that motivational interviewing is particularly important for individuals in early stages of change. However, research evidence for these claims needs to be gathered. A question remaining is whether we can find treatments that differentially impact processes of change so as to match clinical interventions to specific stages.

Finally, there are some interesting phenomena that can be explored using the stages-of-change perspective. Research on smoking cessation with pregnant women indicates that these women may temporarily stop during pregnancy rather than quit smoking permanently (Stotts, DiClemente, Carbonari, & Mullen, 1996). Even after extensive periods of abstinence during pregnancy, women relapse at very high rates immediately postpartum. They seem to be suspending the behavior rather than changing it, and their attitudes toward postpartum smoking appear to be critical in predicting the return to smoking (Stotts, DiClemente, Carbonari, & Mullen, 2000). These findings lead to a broader discussion of imposed and extrinsically motivated change compared to intrinsic and chosen change (DiClemente, 1999b, 2003). With the increasing use of court-mandated treatment and efforts to provide treatment in prison settings, the issues of extrinsic and intrinsic motivations for change and how they interact with the process of change need an extensive examination and additional research.

A similar issue arises when discussing harm reduction strategies. Do harm reduction strategies interfere with successful movement through the process of change outlined in this volume? Do they enhance it? Harm reduction and recovery from substance abuse problems do not have to be at odds since the same concerns that encourage individuals to take some harm reduction steps could also serve to tip the decisional balance toward action for a more complete change. For clients who use at-risk levels but are not dependent, it might be that reduction of use, rather than total abstinence, is a more realistic target behavior. However, whether each of the specific harm reduction strategies does or does not function as a facilitator of change, or at least does not prove to be a barrier to complete recovery, requires extensive research into how harm reduction affects the process of change.

Change-Generating and Change-Regulating Mechanisms

A final issue that must be addressed as we continue to develop a better understanding of the process of change is specifying the role of self-regulation in this process (DiClemente, 2007). There is an important role for self-control in the change process. Almost all treatments include self-observations, self-management, and self-reflection. All of these activities depend on a more generic self-regulation process and the self-control "muscle" (Muraven & Baumeister, 2000). Understanding how these more generic, change-regulating mechanisms relate to the more specific, change-generating mechanisms of stage tasks, decision making, efficacy, and coping processes of change may be a new frontier for research and practice.

CONCLUSION

This volume offers clinicians a view of treatment that is informed by the stages-of-change model. The recommendations are based on our view of the current literature and the clinical applications of this model. Since researchers and practitioners continue to apply this model to different populations and problems and to refine the constructs, clinical application continues to be a work in progress. Additional knowledge and insights will undoubtedly emerge as this work progresses. We hope we have provided the clinician some new strategies and views with which to assist those struggling with substance abuse problems to move forward on the road to recovery.

SUMMARY

• The stages-of-change model focuses on the identification of important components in the process of intentional behavior change. The stages highlight the critical issues of denial, decision making, anticipation, action, relapse, and maintenance for specific behavioral problems.

• A significant contribution of the model is the identification of different tasks and challenges faced by the client and the therapist at different points in the process of changing addictive behaviors.

• Clinicians should identify where a client is in the process of change and use that knowledge to guide the selection of intervention goals and strengths.

• It is important to avoid overly simplistic views of motivation for treatment or for change. It is likely that approaches to facilitating change processes need to differ, depending on the client.

• It should be kept in mind that the use of the experiential and behavioral processes and other change variables happens both inside and outside of the treatment session.

• It is necessary to track motivation and change-process use frequently and adjust treatment strategies accordingly.

• There is debate in the literature on some aspects of the stages-of-change model. One particular issue of note is whether the process of change is most productively viewed as involving stages of change or as a continuous process. It is argued here that the process of change for substance abusers involves a series of stages or phases that require different strategies and address different issues.

• While much has been written about the application of the stages-of-change model to substance abuse problems, there is more to be learned about the stages and how the model can be most productively used in clinical practice. Additional knowledge and insights will undoubtedly emerge as researchers and practitioners continue to apply the model to different populations and problems.

References

Addiction Research Foundation. (1993). *Directory of client outcome measures for addictions treatment programs.* Toronto: Author.

Agency for Health Care Policy and Research. (1996). *Clinical practice guideline for smoking cessation.* AHCPR Guideline Number 18. Washington, DC: Author.

Agrawal, A., & Lynskey, M. T. (2006). The genetic epidemiology of cannabis use, abuse and dependence. *Addiction, 101,* 801–812.

Agrawal, A., & Lynskey, M. T. (2008). Are there genetic influences on addiction?: Evidence from family, adoption and twin studies. *Addiction, 103,* 1069–1081.

Ahijevych, K., & Wewers, M. E. (1992). Processes of change across five stages of smoking cessation. *Addictive Behaviors, 17,* 17–25.

Allan, C. A., & Cooke, D. J. (1985). Stressful life events and alcohol misuse in women: A critical review. *Journal of Studies on Alcohol, 46,* 147–152.

Allen, J. C., & Columbus, M. (Eds.). (1995). *Assessing alcohol problems.* Rockville, MD: National Institute on Alcohol Abuse and Alcoholism.

Allen, J. P., & Litten, R. Z. (1992). Techniques to enhance compliance with disulfiram. *Alcoholism: Clinical and Experimental Research, 16,* 1035–1041.

Allen, J. P., Sillanaukee, P., Strid, N., & Litten, R. Z. (2003). Biomarkers of heavy drinking. In J. P. Allen & V. Wilson (Eds.), *Assessing alcohol problems: A guide for clinicians and researchers* (2nd ed., pp. 37–53). Bethesda, MD: National Institute on Alcohol Abuse and Alcoholism.

Allen, J. P., & Wilson, V. (Eds.). (2003). *Assessing alcohol problems: A guide for clinicians and researchers* (2nd ed.). Bethesda, MD: National Institute on Alcohol Abuse and Alcoholism.

Alvanzo, A. A., Storr, C. L., La Flair, L., Green, K. M., Wagner, F. A., & Crum, R. M. (2011). Race/ethnicity and sex differences in progression from drinking initiation to the development of alcohol dependence. *Drug and Alcohol Dependence, 118,* 375–382.

American College of Surgeons. (2006). *Resources for optimal care of the injured patient 2006.* Chicago: Author.

American Psychiatric Association. (1994). *Diagnostic and statistical manual of mental disorders* (4th ed.). Washington, DC: Author.

Amrhein, P. C., Miller, W. R., Yahne, C. E., Palmer, M., & Fulcher, L. (2003). Client commitment language during motivational interviewing predicts drug use outcomes. *Journal of Consulting and Clinical Psychology, 71,* 862–878.

Anderson, C. M., & Stewart, S. (1983). *Mastering resistance: A practical guide to family therapy.* New York: Guilford Press.

Anderson, D. J. (1981). *The psychopathology of denial.* Minneapolis: Hazelden.

Annis, H. M. (1982a). *Inventory of Drinking Situations.* Toronto: Addiction Research Foundation.

Annis, H. M. (1982b). *Situational Confidence Questionnaire.* Toronto: Addiction Research Foundation.

Annis, H. M. (1986). A relapse prevention model for treatment of alcoholics. In W. R. Miller & N. Heather (Eds.), *Treating addictive behaviors* (pp. 407–433). New York: Plenum Press.

Annis, H. M. (1987). *Situational Confidence Questionnaire (SCQ-39).* Toronto: Addiction Research Foundation.

Annis, H. M., & Graham, J. M. (1988). *Situational Confidence Questionnaire (SCQ-39) user's guide.* Toronto: Addiction Research Foundation.

Annis, H. M., & Graham, J. M. (1995). Profile types on the Inventory of Drinking Situations: Implications for relapse prevention counseling. *Psychology of Addictive Behaviors, 9,* 176–182.

Annis, H. M., Graham, J. M., & Davis, C. S. (1987). *Inventory of Drinking Situations (IDS) user's guide.* Toronto: Addiction Research Foundation.

Annis, H. M., & Martin, G. (1985). *Drug-Taking Confidence Questionnaire.* Toronto: Addiction Research Foundation.

Annis, H. M., & Martin, G. (1993a). *The Inventory of Drug-Taking Situations.* Toronto: Addiction Research Foundation.

Annis, H. M., & Martin, G. (1993b). *The Drug-Taking Confidence Questionnaire.* Toronto: Addiction Research Foundation.

Annis, H. M., & Ogborne, A. C. (1983). *The temporal stability of alcoholism treatment outcome results.* Unpublished manuscript, Addiction Research Foundation, Toronto.

Annis, H. M., Schober, R., & Kelly, E. (1996). Matching addiction outpatient counseling to client readiness for change: The role of structured relapse prevention counseling. *Experimental and Clinical Psychopharmacology, 4,* 37–45.

Annis, H. M., Turner, N. E., & Sklar, S. M. (1997). *Inventory of Drug-Taking Situations: User's guide.* Toronto: Addiction Research Foundation.

Anton, R. F., Lieber, C., Tabakoff, C., & CDTect Study Group. (2002). Carbohydrate deficient transferrin (CDT) and gamma glutamyltransferase for the detection and monitoring of alcoholics. *Alcoholism: Clinical and Experimental Research, 26,* 1215–1222.

Anton, R. F., Litten, R. Z., & Allen, J. P. (1995). Biological assessment of alcohol consumption. In J. P. Allen & M. Columbus (Eds.), *Assessing alcohol problems* (pp. 31–40). Rockville, MD: National Institute on Alcohol Abuse and Alcoholism.

Anton, R. F., O'Malley, S. S., Ciraulo, D. A., Cisler, R. A., Couper, D., Donovan, D. M., et al. (2006). Combined pharmacotherapies and behavioral interventions for alcohol dependence: The COMBINE Study: A randomized controlled trial. *Journal of the American Medical Association, 295,* 2003–2017.

Apodaca, T. R., & Schermer, C. R. (2003). Readiness to change alcohol use after trauma. *Journal of Trauma, Injury, Infection, and Critical Care, 54,* 990–994.

Armor, D., Polich, J., & Stambul, H. (1978). *Alcoholism and treatment.* New York: Wiley.

Ashley, O. S., Marsden, M. E., & Brady, T. M. (2003). Effectiveness of substance abuse treatment programming for women: A review. *American Journal of Drug and Alcohol Abuse, 29,* 19–53.

Azrin, N. H. (1976). Improvements in the community-reinforcement approach to alcoholism. *Behaviour Research and Therapy, 14,* 339–348.

Babor, T. F. (1993). Alcohol and drug use history, patterns, and problems. In B. J. Rounsaville,

F. M. Tims, A. M. Horton, & B. J. Sowder (Eds.), *Diagnostic source book on drug abuse research and treatment* (pp. 19–34). Bethesda, MD: National Institute on Drug Abuse.

Babor, T. F., & Higgins-Biddle, J. C. (2000). Alcohol screening and brief intervention: Dissemination strategies for medical practice and public health. *Addiction, 95*, 677–686.

Babor, T. F., & Higgins-Biddle, J. C. (2001). *Brief intervention for hazardous and harmful drinking: A manual for use in primary care.* Geneva, Switzerland: World Health Organization.

Babor, T. F., McRee, B. G., Kassebaum, P. A., Grimaldi, P. L., Ahmed, K., & Bray, J. (2007). Screening, brief intervention, and referral to treatment (SBIRT): Toward a public health approach to the management of substance abuse. *Substance Abuse, 28*, 7–30.

Backinger, C. L., Thorton-Bullock, A., Miner, C., Orleans, C. T., Siener, K., DiClemente, C. C., et al. (2010). Building consumer demand for tobacco-cessation products and services. *American Journal of Preventive Medicine, 38*, S307–S311.

Baer, J. S., Peterson, P. L., & Wells, E. A. (2004). Rationale and design of a brief substance use intervention for homeless adolescents. *Addiction Research and Theory, 12*, 317–334.

Bailey, K. A., Baker, A. L., Webster, R. A., & Lewin, T. J. (2004). Pilot randomized controlled trial of a brief alcohol intervention group for adolescents. *Drug and Alcohol Review, 23*, 157–166.

Balgopal, P. R., & Hull, R. F. (1973). Keeping secrets: Group resistance for patients and therapists. *Psychotherapy: Theory, Research, and Practice, 10*, 334–336.

Ballesteros, J., Duffy, J. C., Querejeta, I., Ariño, J., & González-Pinto, A. (2004). Efficacy of brief interventions for hazardous drinkers in primary care: Systematic review and meta-analyses. *Alcoholism: Clinical and Experimental Research, 28*, 608–618.

Bandura, A. (1977). Self-efficacy: Toward a unifying theory of behavioral change. *Psychological Review, 84*, 191–215.

Bandura, A. (1986). *Social foundations of thought and action: A social cognitive theory.* Englewood Cliffs, NJ: Prentice-Hall.

Bandura, A. (1997). The anatomy of stages of change [Editorial]. *American Journal of Health Promotion, 12*, 8–10.

Barber, J. G., & Gilbertson, R. (1997). Unilateral interventions for women living with heavy drinkers. *Social Work, 42*, 69–78.

Barnett, N. P., Lebeau-Craven, R., O'Leary, T. A., Colby, S. M., Woolard, R., Rohsenow, D. J., et al. (2002). Predictors of motivation to change after medical treatment for drinking-related events in adolescents. *Psychology of Addictive Behaviors, 16*, 106–112.

Barrie, K. (1991). Motivational counseling in groups. In R. Davidson, S. Rollnick, & I. MacEwan (Eds.), *Counseling problem drinkers* (pp. 115–131). London: Tavistock/Routledge.

Barry, K. L. (1999). *Brief interventions and brief therapies for substance abuse* (Treatment Improvement Protocol Series, No. 34, DHHS Publication No. [SMA] 99–3353). Rockville, MD: U.S. Department of Health and Human Services.

Basu, D., Ball, S. A., Feinn, R., Gelernter, J., & Kranzler, H. R. (2004). Typologies of drug dependence: Comparative validity of a multivariate and four univariate models. *Drug and Alcohol Dependence, 73*, 289–300.

Baumberg, B. (2006). The global economic burden of alcohol: A review. *Drug and Alcohol Review, 25*, 537–551.

Beckman, L. J. (1984). Treatment needs of women alcoholics. *Alcoholism Treatment Quarterly, 1*, 101–114.

Beckman, L. J. (1994). Treatment needs of women with alcohol problems. *Alcohol Health and Research World, 18*, 206–211.

Beckman, L. J., & Amaro, H. (1986). Personal and social difficulties faced by women and men entering alcoholism treatment. *Journal of Studies on Alcohol, 47,* 135–145.

Beitman, B. D., Beck, N. C., Deuser, W., Carter, C., Davidson, J., & Maddock, R. (1994). Patient stages of change predicts outcome in a panic disorder medication trial. *Anxiety, 1,* 64–69.

Belding, M., Iguchi, M., & Lamb, R. J. (1996). Stages of change in methadone maintenance: Assessing the convergent validity of two measures. *Psychology of Addictive Behaviors, 10,* 157–166.

Belding, M. A., Iguchi, M. Y., & Lamb, R. J. (1997). Stages and processes of change as predictors of drug use among methadone maintenance patients. *Experimental and Clinical Psychopharmacology, 5,* 65–73.

Bellack, A. S., & DiClemente, C. C. (1999). Treating substance abuse among patients with schizophrenia. *Psychiatric Services, 50,* 75–80.

Benishek, L. A., Kirby, K. C., & Dugosh, K. L. (2011). Prevalence and frequency of problems of concerned family members with a substance-using loved one. *American Journal of Drug and Alcohol Abuse, 37,* 82–88.

Berg, I. K., & Miller, S. D. (1992). *Working with the problem drinker: A solution-focused approach.* New York: Norton.

Bernstein, J., Bernstein, E., Tassiopoulos, K., Heeren, T., Levenson, S., & Hingson, R. (2005). Brief motivational intervention at a clinic visit reduces cocaine and heroin use. *Drug and Alcohol Dependence, 77,* 49–59.

Bertholet, N., Horton, N. J., & Saitz, R. (2009). Improvements in readiness to change and drinking in primary care patients with unhealthy alcohol use: A prospective study. *BMC Public Health, 9,* 101.

Beutler, L. E., & Clarkin, J. F. (1990). *Systematic treatment selection.* New York: Brunner/Mazel.

Bien, T., Miller, W., & Boroughs, J. (1993). Motivational interviewing with alcohol outpatients. *Behavioral and Cognitive Psychotherapy, 21,* 347–356.

Biener, L., & Abrams, D. B. (1991). The Contemplation Ladder: Validation of a measure of readiness to consider smoking cessation. *Health Psychology, 10,* 360–365.

Bierut, L. J., Dinwiddie, S. H., Begleiter, H., Crowe, R. R., Hesselbrock, V., Nurnberger, J. I., Jr., et al. (1998). Familial transmission of substance dependence: Alcohol, marijuana, cocaine, and habitual smoking. *Archives of General Psychiatry, 55,* 982–988.

Birke, S. A., Edelmann, R. J., & Davis, P. E. (1990). An analysis of the abstinence violation effect in a sample of illicit drug users. *British Journal of Addiction, 85,* 1299–1307.

Bischof, G., Rumpf, H. J., Hapke, U., Meyer, C., & John, U. (2001). Factors influencing remission from alcohol dependence without formal help in a representative population sample. *Addiction, 96,* 1327–1336.

Bland, R. C., Newman, S. C., & Orn, H. (1997). Help-seeking for psychiatric disorders. *Canadian Journal of Psychiatry, 42,* 935–942.

Blume, A. W., Morera, O. F., & Garcia de la Cruz, B. (2005). Assessment of addictive behaviors in ethnic-minority populations. In D. M. Donovan & G. A. Marlatt (Eds.), *Assessment of addictive behaviors* (2nd ed., pp. 49–70). New York: Guilford Press.

Blume, A. W., Resor, M. R., & Kantin, A. V. (2009). Addiction treatment disparities among ethnic and sexual minority populations. In P. M. Miller (Ed.), *Evidence-based addiction treatment* (pp. 313–325). San Diego: Elsevier.

Bolton, J. M., Robinson, J., & Sareen, J. (2009). Self-medication of mood disorders with alcohol and drugs in the National Epidemiologic Survey on Alcohol and Related Conditions. *Journal of Affective Disorders, 115,* 367–375.

Booth, P. G., Dale, B., & Ansari, J. (1984). Problem drinkers' goal choice and treatment outcome: A preliminary study. *Addictive Behaviors, 9,* 357–364.

Bowen, A., & Trotter, R. (1995). HIV risk in intravenous drug users and crack cocaine smokers: Predicting stage of change for condom use. *Journal of Consulting and Clinical Psychology, 63*, 238–248.

Bradley, K. A., Boyd-Wickizer, J., Powell, S. H., & Burman, M. L. (1998). Alcohol screening questionnaires in women: A critical review. *Journal of the American Medical Association, 280*, 166–171.

Bradley, K. A., Bush, K. R., Epler, A. J., Dobie, D. J., Davis, T. M., Sporleder, J. L., et al. (2003). Two brief alcohol-screening tests from the Alcohol Use Disorders Identification Test (AUDIT): Validation in a female Veterans Affairs patient population. *Archives of Internal Medicine, 163*, 821–829.

Bradley, K. A., DeBenedetti, A. F., Volk, R. J., Williams, E. C., Frank, D., & Kivlahan, D. R. (2007). AUDIT- C as a brief screen for alcohol misuse in primary care. *Alcoholism: Clinical and Experimental Research, 31*, 1208–1217.

Brady, K. T., & Randall, C. L. (1999). Gender differences in substance use disorders. *Psychiatric Clinics of North America, 22*, 241–252.

Brady, K. T., Verduin, M. L., & Tolliver, B. K. (2007). Treatment of patients comorbid for addiction and other psychiatric disorders. *Current Psychiatry Reports, 9*, 374–380.

Breslin, F. C., Sobell, L. C., Sobell, M. B., & Agrawal, S. (2000). A comparison of a brief and long version of the Situational Confidence Questionnaire. *Behaviour Research and Therapy, 38*, 1211–1220.

Brook, D. W. (2008). Group therapy. In M. Galanter & H. D. Kleber (Eds.), *The American Psychiatric Publishing textbook of substance abuse treatment* (4th ed., pp. 413–427). Arlington, VA: American Psychiatric Publishing.

Brown, R. L., Leonard, T., Saunders, L. A., & Papasouliotis, O. (2001). A two-item conjoint screen for alcohol and other drug problems. *Journal of the American Board of Family Practice, 14*, 95–106.

Brown, T. G., Dongier, M., Ouimet, M. C., Tremblay, J., Chanut, F., Legault, L., et al. (2010). Brief motivational interviewing for DWI recidivists who abuse alcohol and are not participating in DWI intervention: A randomized controlled trial. *Alcoholism: Clinical and Experimental Research, 34*, 292–301.

Brownell, K. D., Marlatt, G. A., Lichtenstein, E., & Wilson, G. T. (1986). Understanding and preventing relapse. *American Psychologist, 41*, 765–782.

Bucholz, K. K., Homan, S. M., & Helzer, J. E. (1992). When do alcoholics first discuss drinking problems? *Journal of Studies on Alcohol, 53*, 582–589.

Burke, A. C., & Gregoire, T. K. (2007). Substance abuse treatment outcomes for coerced and noncoerced clients. *Health and Social Work, 32*, 7–15.

Burke, B. L., Arkowitz, H., & Menchola, M. (2003). The efficacy of motivational interviewing: A meta-analysis of controlled clinical trials. *Journal of Consulting and Clinical Psychology, 71*, 843–861.

Burke, B. L., Dunn, C. W., Atkins, D. C., & Phelps, J. S. (2004). The emerging evidence base for motivational interviewing: A meta-analytical and qualitative inquiry. *Journal of Cognitive Psychotherapy, 18*, 309–322.

Burling, T. A., Reilly, P. M., Molzen, J. O., & Ziff, D. C. (1989). Self-efficacy and relapse among inpatient drug and alcohol abusers: A predictor of outcome. *Journal of Studies on Alcohol, 6*, 354–360.

Burns, E., Gray, R., & Smith, L. A. (2010). Brief screening questionnaires to identify problem drinking during pregnancy: A systematic review. *Addiction, 105*, 601–614.

Burt, M. (2001). *What will it take to end homelessness?* Washington, DC: Urban Institute.

Bush, K., Kivlahan, D. R., McDonell, M. B., Fihn, S. D., & Bradley, K. A. (1998). The AUDIT alcohol consumption questions (AUDIT- C). *Archives of Internal Medicine, 158*, 1789–1795.

Caldeira, K. M., Kasperski, S. J., Sharma, E., Vincent, K. B., O'Grady, K. E., Wish, E. D., et al. (2009). College students rarely seek help despite serious substance use problems. *Journal of Substance Abuse Treatment, 37,* 368–378.

Campbell, C. I., Alexander, J. A., & Lemak, C. H. (2009). Organizational determinants of outpatient substance abuse treatment duration in women. *Journal of Substance Abuse Treatment, 37,* 64–72.

Carbonari, J. C., & DiClemente, C. C. (2000). Using transtheoretical model profiles to differentiate levels of alcohol abstinence success. *Journal of Consulting and Clinical Psychology, 68,* 810–817.

Carbonari, J. P., DiClemente, C. C., Addy, R., & Pollack, K. (1996). *Alternate short forms of the Readiness to Change Scale.* Paper presented at the Fourth International Congress on Behavioral Medicine, Washington, DC.

Carbonari, J. P., DiClemente, C. C., & Sewell, K. B. (1999). Stage transitions and the transtheoretical "stages of change" model of smoking cessation. *Swiss Journal of Psychology, 58,* 134–144.

Carbonari, J., DiClemente, C., & Zweben, A. (1994, November). A readiness to change scale: Its development, validation and usefulness. In C. C. DiClemente (Chair), *Assessing critical dimensions for alcoholism treatment.* Symposium presented at the annual meeting of the Association for Advancement of Behavior Therapy, San Diego.

Carey, K. B., Purnine, D. M., Maisto, S. A., & Carey, M. P. (1999). Assessing readiness to change substance abuse: A critical review of instruments. *Clinical Psychology: Science and Practice, 6,* 245–266.

Carise, D., Gurel, O., McLellan, A. T., Dugosh, K., & Kendig, C. (2005). Getting patients the services they need using a computer-assisted system for patient assessment and referral—CASPAR. *Drug and Alcohol Dependence, 80,* 177–189.

Carney, M. M., & Kivlahan, D. R. (1995). Motivational subtypes among veterans seeking substance abuse treatment: Profiles based on stages of change. *Psychology of Addictive Behaviors, 9,* 135–142.

Carroll, K. M. (1996a). Integrating psychotherapy and pharmacotherapy in substance abuse treatment. In F. Rotgers, D. S. Keller, & J. Morgenstern (Eds.), *Treating substance abuse: Theory and technique* (pp. 286–318). New York: Guilford Press.

Carroll, K. M. (1996b). Relapse prevention as a psychosocial treatment: A review of controlled clinical trials. *Experimental and Clinical Psychopharmacology, 4,* 46–54.

Carroll, K. M. (1999). Behavioral and cognitive behavioral treatments. In B. S. McCrady & E. E. Epstein (Eds.), *Addiction: A comprehensive guidebook* (pp. 250–267). New York: Oxford University Press.

Carroll, K. M., & Onken, L. S. (2005). Behavioral therapies for drug abuse. *American Journal of Psychiatry, 162,* 1452–1460.

Carter, R. E., Haynes, L. F., Back, S. E., Herrin, A. E., Brady, K. T., Leimberger, J. D., et al. (2008). Improving the transition from residential to outpatient addiction treatment: Gender differences in response to supportive telephone calls. *American Journal of Drug and Alcohol Abuse, 34,* 47–59.

Cartwright, A. (1987). Group work with substance abusers: Basic issues and future research. *British Journal of Addiction, 82,* 951–953.

Casswell, S., You, R. Q., & Huckle, T. (2011). Alcohol's harm to others: Reduced well-being and health status for those with heavy drinkers in their lives. *Addiction, 106,* 1087–1094.

Catanzaro, S. J., & Laurent, J. (2004). Perceived family support, negative mood regulation expectancies, coping, and adolescent alcohol use: Evidence of mediation and moderation effects. *Addictive Behaviors, 29,* 1779–1797.

Cavaiola, A. A. (1984). Resistance issues in the treatment of the DWI offender. *Alcoholism Treatment Quarterly, 1*, 87–100.

Center for Substance Abuse Treatment. (2009a). *Substance abuse treatment: Group therapy* (Treatment Improvement Protocol Series, No. 41, DHHS Publication No. [SMA] 09–3991). Washington, DC: U.S. Government Printing Office.

Center for Substance Abuse Treatment. (2009b). *Substance abuse treatment: Addressing the specific needs of women* (Treatment Improvement Protocol Series No. 51, DHHS Publication No. [SMA] 09–4426). Rockville, MD: Substance Abuse and Mental Health Services Administration.

Ceperich, S. D., & Ingersoll, K. S. (2011). Motivational interviewing and feedback intervention to reduce alcohol-exposed pregnancy risk among college binge drinkers: Determinants and patterns of response. *Journal of Behavioral Medicine, 34*, 381–395.

Cermak, T. L. (1989). Al-Anon and recovery. In M. Galanter (Ed.), *Recent developments in alcoholism* (Vol. 7, pp. 91–104). New York: Plenum Press.

Chafetz, M. E. (1970). Practical and theoretical considerations in the psychotherapy of alcoholism. In M. E. Chafetz, H. T. Blane, & M. J. Hill (Eds.), *Frontiers of alcoholism* (pp. 6–15). New York: Science House.

Chang, G., Behr, H., Goetz, M. A., Hiley, A., & Bigby, J. (1997). Women and alcohol abuse in primary care. Identification and intervention. *American Journal on Addictions, 6*, 183–192.

Chang, G., Fisher, N. D., Hornstein, M. D., Jones, J. A., & Orav, E. J. (2010). Identification of risk drinking women: T-ACE screening tool or the medical record. *Journal of Women's Health, 19*, 1933–1939.

Chang, I., & Lapham, S. C. (1996). Validity of self-reported criminal offences and traffic violations in screening of driving-while-intoxicated offenders. *Alcohol and Alcoholism, 31*, 583–590.

Chessick, R. D. (1974). *Technique and practice of intensive psychotherapy*. New York: Jason Aronson.

Cialdini, R. B. (1988). *Influence: Science and practice* (2nd ed.). Glenview, IL: Scott Foresman.

Claus, R. E., Orwin, R. G., Kissin, W., Krupski, A., Campbell, K., & Stark, K. (2007). Does gender-specific substance abuse treatment for women promote continuity of care? *Journal of Substance Abuse Treatment, 32*, 27–39.

Colfax, G., Vittinghoff, E., Husnik, M. J., McKirnan, D., Buchbinder, S., Koblin, B., et al. (2004). Substance use and sexual risk: A participant- and episode-level analysis among a cohort of men who have sex with men. *American Journal of Epidemiology, 159*, 1002–1012.

Connors, G. J. (1995). Screening for alcohol problems. In J. A. Allen & M. Columbus (Eds.), *Assessing alcohol problems* (pp. 17–29). Rockville, MD: National Institute on Alcohol Abuse and Alcoholism.

Connors, G. J., Carroll, K. M., DiClemente, C. C., Longabaugh, R., & Donovan, D. M. (1997). The therapeutic alliance and its relationship to alcoholism treatment participation and outcome. *Journal of Consulting and Clinical Psychology, 65*, 588–598.

Connors, G. J., DiClemente, C. C., Dermen, K. H., Kadden, R., Carroll, K. M., & Frone, M. R. (2000). Predicting the therapeutic alliance in alcoholism treatment. *Journal of Studies on Alcohol, 61*, 139–149.

Connors, G. J., Longabaugh, R., & Miller, W. R. (1996). Looking forward and back to relapse: Implications for research and practice. *Addiction, 91*(Suppl.), 191–196.

Connors, G. J., & Maisto, S. A. (2006). Relapse in the addictive behaviors. *Clinical Psychology Review, 26*, 107–108.

Connors, G. J., Maisto, S. A., & Donovan, D. M. (1996). Conceptualizations of relapse: A summary of psychological and psychobiological models. *Addiction, 91*(Suppl.), 5–13.

Connors, G. J., Maisto, S. A., & Zywiak, W. H. (1996). Understanding relapse in the broader context of posttreatment functioning. *Addiction, 91*(Suppl.), 173–189.

Connors, G. J., Maisto, S. A., & Zywiak, W. H. (1998). Male and female alcoholics' attributions regarding the onset and termination of relapses and the maintenance of abstinence. *Journal of Substance Abuse, 10,* 27–42.

Connors, G. J., & Volk, R. J. (2003). Screening for alcohol problems among adults. In J. P. Allen & V. Wilson (Eds.), *Assessing alcohol problems: A guide for clinicians and researchers* (2nd ed., pp. 21–35). Bethesda, MD: National Institute on Alcohol Abuse and Alcoholism.

Cook, C. A. L., Booth, B. M., Blow, F. C., Gogineni, A., & Bunn, J. Y. (1992). Alcoholism treatment, severity of alcohol-related medical complications, and health services utilization. *Journal of Mental Health Administration, 19,* 31–40.

Cook, R. L., Sereika, S. M., Hunt, S. C., Woodward, W. C., Erlen, J. A., & Conigliaro, J. (2001). Problem drinking and medication adherence among persons with HIV infection. *Journal of General Internal Medicine, 16,* 83–88.

Copeland, J., & Hall, W. (1992). A comparison of women seeking drug and alcohol treatment in a specialist women's and two traditional mixed-sex treatment services. *British Journal of Addictions, 87,* 1293–1302.

Copeland, J., Hall, W., Didcott, P., & Biggs, V. (1993). A comparison of a specialist women's alcohol and other drug treatment service with two traditional mixed-sex services: Client characteristics and treatment outcome. *Drug and Alcohol Dependence, 32,* 81–92.

Copello, A., & Orford, J. (2002). Addiction and the family: Is it time for services to take notice of the evidence? *Addiction, 97,* 1361–1363.

Copello, A., Templeton, L., Orford, J., Velleman, R., Patel, A., Moore, L., et al. (2009). The relative efficacy of two levels of a primary care intervention for family members affected by the addiction problem of a close relative: A randomized trial. *Addiction, 104,* 49–58.

Copello, A. G., Templeton, L., & Velleman, R. (2006). Family interventions for drug and alcohol misuse: Is there a best practice? *Current Opinion in Psychiatry, 19,* 271–276.

Copello, A., Velleman, R. D., & Templeton, L. J. (2005). Family interventions in the treatment of alcohol and drug problems. *Drug and Alcohol Review, 24,* 369–385.

Costantini, M. F., Wermuth, L., Sorensen, J. L., & Lyons, J. S. (1992). Family functioning as a predictor of progress in substance abuse treatment. *Journal of Substance Abuse, 9,* 331–335.

Craig, R. J. (2005). Assessing contemporary substance abusers with the MMPI MacAndrews Alcoholism Scale: A review. *Substance Use and Misuse, 40,* 427–450.

Craighead, W. E., Craighead, L. W., & Ilardi, S. S. (1995). Behavior therapies in historical perspective. In B. Bongar & L. E. Beutler (Eds.), *Comprehensive textbook of psychotherapy* (pp. 64–83). New York: Oxford University Press.

Cranford, J. A., Floyd, F. J., Schulenberg, J. E., & Zucker, R. A. (2011). Husbands' and wives' alcohol use disorders and marital interactions as longitudinal predictors of marital adjustment. *Journal of Abnormal Psychology, 120,* 210–222.

Crits-Christoph, P., Siqueland, L., Blaine, J., Frank, A., Luborsky, L., Onken, L. S., et al. (1999). Psychosocial treatments for cocaine dependence: National Institute on Drug Abuse Collaborative Cocaine Treatment Study. *Archives of General Psychiatry, 57,* 493–502.

Cuijpers, P., Riper, H., & Lemmers, L. (2004). The effects of mortality on brief interventions for problem drinking: A meta-analysis. *Addiction, 99,* 839–845.

Cummings, A. M., Gallop, R. J., & Greenfield, S. F. (2010). Self-efficacy and substance use outcomes for women in single-gender versus mixed-gender group treatment. *Journal of Groups in Addiction and Recovery, 5,* 4–16.

Cummings, C., Gordon, J. R., & Marlatt, G. A. (1980). Relapse: Prevention and prediction. In W. R. Miller (Ed.), *The addictive behaviors* (pp. 291–321). New York: Pergamon Press.

Cunningham, J. A., Sobell, L. C., Sobell, M. B., Agrawal, S., & Toneatto, T. (1993). Barriers to treatment: Why alcohol and drug abusers delay or never seek treatment. *Addictive Behaviors, 18,* 347–353.

Cunningham, J. A., Sobell, L. C., Sobell, M. B., & Gaskin, J. (1994). Alcohol and drug abusers' reasons for seeking treatment. *Addictive Behaviors, 19,* 691–696.

Cunningham, J. A., Sobell, M. B., Sobell, L. C., Gavin, D. R., & Annis, H. (1995). Heavy drinking and negative affective situations in a general population and treatment sample: Alternative explanations. *Psychology of Addictive Behaviors, 9,* 123–127.

Cyr, M. G., & McGarry, K. A. (2002). Alcohol use disorders in women: Screening methods and approaches to treatment. *Postgraduate Medicine, 112,* 39–40, 43–47.

Cyr, M. G., & Wartman, S. A. (1988). The effectiveness of routine screening questions in the detection of alcoholism. *Journal of the American Medical Association, 259,* 51–54.

D'Amico, E. J., Osilla, K. C., & Hunter, S. B. (2010). Developing a group motivational interviewing intervention for adolescents at–risk for developing an alcohol or drug use disorder. *Alcoholism Treatment Quarterly, 28,* 417–436.

Daniels, J. W. (1998). *Coping with the health threat of smoking: An analysis of the precontemplation stage of smoking cessation.* Unpublished doctoral dissertation, University of Maryland, Baltimore County.

Davidson, R. (1992). Prochaska & DiClemente's model of change: A case study? *British Journal of Addictions, 87,* 821–822.

De Alba, I., Samet, J. H., & Saitz, R. (2004). Burden of medical illness in drug- and alcohol-dependent persons without primary care. *American Journal on Addictions, 13,* 33–45.

De Leon, G., Melnick, G., Kressel, D., & Jainchill, N. (1994). Circumstances, motivation, readiness and suitability (The CMRS Scales): Predicting retention in therapeutic community treatment. *American Journal of Drug and Alcohol Abuse, 20,* 101–106.

De Leon, G., Sacks, S., Staines, G., & McKendrick, K. (1999). Modified therapeutic community for homeless mentally ill chemical abusers: Emerging subtypes. *American Journal of Drug and Alcohol Abuse, 25,* 495–515.

Dick, D. M., & Bierut, L. J. (2006). The genetics of alcohol dependence. *Current Psychiatry Reports, 8,* 151–157.

DiClemente, C. C. (1991). Motivational interviewing and the stages of change. In W. R. Miller & S. Rollnick (Eds.), *Motivational interviewing: Preparing people to change addictive behavior* (pp. 191–202). New York: Guilford Press.

DiClemente, C. C. (1993). Alcoholics Anonymous and the structure of change. In B. S. McCrady & W. R. Miller (Eds.), *Research on Alcoholics Anonymous: Opportunities and alternatives* (pp. 79–97). New Brunswick, NJ: Rutgers Center of Alcohol Studies.

DiClemente, C. C. (1999a). Prevention and harm reduction for chemical dependency: A process perspective. *Clinical Psychology Review, 19,* 473–486.

DiClemente, C. C. (1999b). Motivation for change: Implications for substance abuse. *Psychological Science, 10,* 209–213.

DiClemente, C. C. (2003). *Addiction and change: How addictions develop and addicted people recover.* New York: Guilford Press.

DiClemente, C. C. (2005a). The challenge of change. *Journal of Trauma: Injury, Infection, and Critical Care, 59,* S3–S4.

DiClemente, C. C. (2005b). Conceptual models and applied research: The ongoing contribution of the transtheoretical model. *Journal of Addictions Nursing, 16,* 5–12.

DiClemente, C. C. (2005c). A premature obituary for the transtheoretical model: A response to West (2005). *Addiction, 100*, 1046–1048.

DiClemente, C. C. (2006). Natural change and the troublesome use of substances. In W. R. Miller & K. M. Carroll (Eds.), *Rethinking substance abuse: What the science shows and what we should do about it* (pp. 81–96). New York: Guilford Press.

DiClemente, C. C. (2007). Mechanisms, determinants and process of change in the modification of drinking behavior. *Alcoholism: Clinical and Experimental Research, 31*(Suppl. 3), 13S–20S.

DiClemente, C. C., Bellino, L. E., & Neavins, T. M. (1999). Motivation for change and alcoholism treatment. *Alcohol Research and Health, 23*, 86–92.

DiClemente, C. C., Carbonari, J. P., Daniels, J., Donovan, D. M., Bellino, L. E., & Neavins, T. M. (2001). Self-efficacy as a matching hypothesis: Causal chain analysis. In R. Longabaugh & P. W. Wirth (Eds.), *Project MATCH: A priori matching hypotheses, results, and mediating mechanisms* (National Institute on Alcohol Abuse and Alcoholism Project MATCH Monograph Series, Vol. 8, pp. 251–269). Rockville, MD: National Institute on Alcohol Abuse and Alcoholism.

DiClemente, C. C., Carbonari, J. P., Montgomery, R. P. G., & Hughes, S. O. (1994). The Alcohol Abstinence Self-Efficacy Scale. *Journal of Studies on Alcohol, 55*, 141–148.

DiClemente, C. C., Carbonari, J. P., & Velasquez, M. M. (1992). Alcoholism treatment mismatching from a process of change perspective. In R. R. Watson (Ed.), *Treatment of drug and alcohol abuse* (pp. 115–142). Totowa, NJ: Humana Press.

DiClemente, C. C., Carbonari, J., Zweben, A., Morrel, T., & Lee., R. E. (2001). Motivational hypothesis causal chain analysis. In R. Longabaugh & P. W. Wirtz (Eds.), *Project MATCH: A priori matching hypotheses, results, and mediating mechanisms* (National Institute on Alcohol Abuse and Alcoholism Project MATCH Monograph Series, Vol. 8, pp. 218–234). Rockville, MD: National Institute on Alcohol Abuse and Alcoholism.

DiClemente, C. C., Delahanty, J. C., & Fiedler, R. M. (2010). The journey to the end of smoking. *American Journal of Preventive Medicine, 38*, S418–S428.

DiClemente, C. C., Doyle, S. R., & Donovan, D. (2009). Predicting treatment seekers readiness to change their drinking behavior in the COMBINE study. *Alcoholism: Clinical and Experimental Research, 33*, 879–892.

DiClemente, C. C., Ferentz, K., & Velasquez, M. M. (2004). Health behavior change and the problem of "noncompliance." In L. J. Haas (Ed.), *Handbook of primary care psychology* (pp. 157–172). New York: Oxford University Press.

DiClemente, C. C., Garay, M., & Gemmell, L. (2011). Motivation enhancement in the treatment of substance abuse. In M. Galanter & H. D. Kleber (Eds.), *American Psychiatric Publishing textbook of substance abuse* (5th ed., pp. 125–152). Washington, DC: American Psychiatric Publishing.

DiClemente, C. C., Holmgren, M. A., & Rounsaville, D. (2010). Relapse prevention and recycling in addiction. In B. A. Johnson (Ed.), *Addiction medicine: Science and practice* (pp. 765–782). New York: Springer.

DiClemente, C. C., & Hughes, S. O. (1990). Stages of change profiles in outpatient alcoholism treatment. *Journal of Substance Abuse, 2*, 217–235.

DiClemente, C. C., Nidecker, M., & Bellack, A. S. (2008). Motivation and the stages of change among individuals with severe mental illness and substance abuse disorders. *Journal of Substance Abuse Treatment, 34*, 25–35.

DiClemente, C. C., & Prochaska, J. O. (1982). Self-change and therapy change of smoking behavior: A comparison of processes of change in cessation and maintenance. *Addictive Behaviors, 7*, 133–142.

DiClemente, C. C., & Prochaska, J. O. (1985). Processes and stages of change: Coping and competence in smoking behavior change. In S. Shiffman & T. A. Wills (Eds.), *Coping and substance abuse* (pp. 319–342). New York: Academic Press.

DiClemente, C. C., & Prochaska, J. O. (1998). Toward a comprehensive, transtheoretical model of change: Stages of change and addictive behaviors. In W. R. Miller & N. Heather (Eds.), *Treating addictive behaviors* (2nd ed., pp. 3–24). New York: Plenum Press.

DiClemente, C. C., Prochaska, J. O., Fairhurst, S. K., Velicer, W. F., Velasquez, M. M., & Rossi, J. S. (1991). The process of smoking cessation: An analysis of precontemplation, contemplation, and preparation stages of change. *Journal of Consulting and Clinical Psychology, 59,* 295–304.

DiClemente, C. C., Prochaska, J. O., & Gibertini, M. (1985). Self-efficacy and the stages of self-change of smoking. *Cognitive Therapy and Research, 9,* 181–200.

DiClemente, C. C., Schlundt, D., & Gemmell, L. (2004). Readiness and stages of change in addiction treatments. *American Journal on Addictions, 13,* 103–119.

DiClemente, C. C., Schumann, K., Greene, P. A., & Earley, M. D. (2011). A transtheoretical model perspective on change: Process-focused intervention in mental health-substance use. In D. B. Cooper (Ed.), *Intervention in mental health-substance use* (pp. 69–87). London: Radcliffe.

DiClemente, C. C., & Scott, C. W. (1997). Stages of change: Interactions with treatment compliance and involvement. In L. S. Onken, J. D. Blaine, & J. J. Boren (Eds.), *Beyond the therapeutic alliance: Keeping the drug-dependent individual in treatment* (National Institute on Drug Abuse Research Monograph No. 165, pp. 131–156). Rockville, MD: National Institute on Drug Abuse.

DiClemente, C. C., & Velasquez, M. (2002). Motivational interviewing and the stages of change. In W. R. Miller & S. Rollnick, *Motivational interviewing: Preparing people for change* (2nd ed., pp. 201–216). New York: Guilford Press.

Dill, P. L., & Wells-Parker, E. (2006). Court-mandated treatment for convicted drinking drivers. *Alcohol Research and Health, 29,* 41–48.

D'Onofrio, G. (2003). Treatment for alcohol and other drug problems: Closing the gap. *Annals of Emergency Medicine, 41,* 814–817.

Donovan, D. M. (1998). Continuing care: Promoting the maintenance of change. In W. R. Miller & N. Heather (Eds.), *Treating addictive behaviors* (2nd ed., pp. 317–336). New York: Plenum Press.

Donovan, D. M. (1999). Assessment strategies and measures in addictive behaviors. In B. S. McCrady & E. E. Epstein (Eds.), *Addiction: A comprehensive guidebook* (pp. 187–215). New York: Oxford University Press.

Donovan, D. M. (2003). Assessment to aid in the treatment planning process. In J. P. Allen & V. Wilson (Eds.), *Assessing alcohol problems: A guide for clinicians and researchers* (2nd ed., pp. 125–188). Bethesda, MD: National Institute on Alcohol Abuse and Alcoholism.

Donovan, D. M. (in press). Assessment strategies and measures in addictive behaviors. In B. S. McCrady & E. E. Epstein (Eds.), *Addiction: A comprehensive guidebook* (2nd ed.). New York: Oxford University Press.

Donovan, D. M., & Chaney, E. F. (1985). Alcoholic relapse prevention and intervention: Models and methods. In G. A. Marlatt & J. R. Gordon (Eds.), *Relapse prevention* (pp. 351–416). New York: Guilford Press.

Donovan, D. M., & Marlatt, G. A. (Eds.). (1988). *Assessment of addictive behaviors.* New York: Guilford Press.

Donovan, D. M., & Marlatt, G. A. (Eds.). (2005). *Assessment of addictive behaviors* (2nd ed.). New York: Guilford Press.

Dunn, C. (2003). Brief motivational interviewing interventions targeting substance abuse in the acute care medical setting. *Seminars in Clinical Neuropsychiatry, 8,* 188–196.

Dunn, C., Hungerford, D. W., Field, C., & McCann, B. (2005). The stages of change: When are trauma patients truly ready to change? *Journal of Trauma: Injury, Infection, and Critical Care, 59,* S27–S32.

DuPont, R. L., & McGovern, J. P. (1996). Co-dependence. In *The Hatherleigh guide to issues in modern therapy* (pp. 69–91). New York: Hatherleigh Press.

DuPont, R. L., & Selavka, C. M. (2008). Testing to identify recent drug use. In M. Galanter & H. D. Kleber (Eds.), *Textbook of substance abuse treatment* (4th ed., pp. 655–664). Washington, DC: American Psychiatric Publishing.

Ehrman, R. N., & Robins, S. J. (1994). Reliability and validity of 6 month timeline reports of cocaine and heroin use in a methadone population. *Journal of Consulting and Clinical Psychology, 6,* 843–850.

Elder, R. W., Voas, R., Beirness, D., Shults, R. A., Sleet, D. A., Nichols, J. L., et al. (2011). Effectiveness of ignition interlocks for preventing alcohol-impaired driving and alcohol-related crashes: A Community Guide systematic review. *American Journal of Preventive Medicine, 40,* 362–376.

Elkin, I., Shea, M. T., Watkins, J. T., Imber, S. D., Sotsky, S. M., Collins, J. F., et al. (1989). National Institute of Mental Health Treatment of Depression Collaborative Research Program: General effectiveness of treatments. *Archives of General Psychiatry, 46,* 971–982.

Ellis, A. (1983a). Rational-emotive therapy (RET) approaches to overcoming resistance: I. Common forms of resistance. *British Journal of Cognitive Psychotherapy, 1,* 28–38.

Ellis, A. (1983b). Rational-emotive therapy (RET) approaches to overcoming resistance: II. How RET disputes clients' irrational, resistance-creating beliefs. *British Journal of Cognitive Psychotherapy, 1,* 1–16.

Ellis, A. (1984). Rational-emotive therapy (RET) approaches to overcoming resistance: III. Using emotive and behavioral techniques of overcoming resistance. *British Journal of Cognitive Psychotherapy, 2,* 11–26.

Ellis, A. (1985). Approaches to overcoming resistance: IV. Handling special kinds of clients. *British Journal of Cognitive Psychotherapy, 1,* 26–42.

Ellis, A., & Dryden, W. (1987). *The practice of rational-emotive therapy.* New York: Springer.

Ellis, A., McInerney, J. F., & DiGiuseppe, R. (1988). *Rational-emotive therapy with alcoholics and substance abusers.* Elmsford, NY: Pergamon Press.

Ellis, D. A., Zucker, R. A., & Fitzgerald, H. E. (1997). The role of family influences in development and risk. *Alcohol Health and Research World, 21,* 218–226.

Ena, J., Amador, C., Benito, C., Fenoll, V., & Pasquau, F. (2003). Risk and determinants of developing severe liver toxicity during therapy with nevirapine- and efavirenz-containing regimens in HIV-infected patients. *International Journal of STD and AIDS, 14,* 776–781.

Epler, A., Kivlahan, D. R., Bush, K. R., Dobie, D. J., & Bradley, K. A. (2005). A brief readiness to change drinking algorithm: Concurrent validity in female VA primary care patients. *Addictive Behaviors, 30,* 389–395.

Epstein, E. E., & McCrady, B. S. (1998). Behavioral couples treatment of alcohol and drug use disorders: Current status and innovations. *Clinical Psychology Review, 18,* 689–711.

Erikson, E. H. (1963). *Childhood and society* (rev. ed.). New York: Norton.

Estee, S., & He, L. (2007). *Use of alcohol and other drugs declined among emergency department patients who received brief interventions for substance use disorders through WASBIRT* (Analysis RaD, Contract No. 4.60.WA.2007.1). Olympia, WA: Washington State Department of Social and Health Services.

Faber, E., & Keating-O'Connor, B. (1991). Planned family intervention: Johnson Institute method. *Journal of Chemical Dependency Treatment, 4,* 61–71.

Farkas, A. J., Pierce, J. P., Zhu, S. H., Rosbrook, B., Gilpin, E. A., Berry, C., et al. (1996).

Addiction versus stages of change models in predicting smoking cessation. *Addiction,* *91,* 1271–1280.

Fell, J. C., Tippetts, A. S., & Ciccel, J. D. (2011). An evaluation of three driving-under-the-influence courts in Georgia. *Annals of Advances of Automotive Medicine, 55,* 301–312.

Fenichel, O. (1945). *The psychoanalytic theory of neurosis.* New York: Norton.

Fernandez, A. C., Begley, E. A., & Marlatt, G. A. (2006). Family and peer interventions for adults: Past approaches and future directions. *Psychology of Addictive Behaviors, 20,* 207–213.

Finney, J. W., Moos, R. H., & Timko, C. (1999). The course of treated and untreated substance use disorders: Remission, resolution, relapse, and mortality. In B. S. McCrady & E. E. Epstein (Eds.), *Addiction: A comprehensive guidebook* (pp. 30–49). New York: Oxford University Press.

Floyd, R. L., Decoufle, P., & Hungerford, D. W. (1999). Alcohol use prior to pregnancy recognition. *American Journal of Preventive Medicine, 17,* 101–107.

Floyd, R. L., Sobell, M., Velasquez, M. M., Ingersoll, K., Nettleman, M., Sobell, L., et al. (2007). Preventing alcohol-exposed pregnancies: A randomized controlled trial. *American Journal of Preventive Medicine, 32,* 1–10.

Freyer, J., Coder, B., Bischof, G., Baumeister, S. E., Rumpf, H. J., John, U., et al. (2007). Intention to utilize formal help in a sample with alcohol problems: A prospective study. *Drug and Alcohol Dependence, 87,* 210–216.

Freyer, J., Tonigan, J. S., Keller, S., John, U., Rumpf, H. J., & Hapke, U. (2004). Readiness to change versus readiness to seek help for alcohol problems: The development of the Treatment Readiness Tool (TReaT). *Journal of Studies on Alcohol, 65,* 801–809.

Freyer, J., Tonigan, J. S., Keller, S., Rumpf, H. J., John, U., & Hapke, U. (2005). Readiness for change and readiness for help-seeking: A composite assessment of client motivation. *Alcohol and Alcoholism, 40,* 540–544.

Freyer-Adam, J., Coder, B., Ottersbach, C., Tonigan, J. S., Rumpf, H.-J., Ulrich, J., et al. (2009). The performance of two motivation measures and outcome after alcohol detoxification. *Alcohol and Alcoholism, 44,* 77–83.

Fromme, K., & Corbin, W. (2004). Prevention of heavy drinking and associated negative consequences among mandated and voluntary college students. *Journal of Consulting and Clinical Psychology, 72,* 1038–1049.

Gainsbury, S., & Blaszczynski, A. (2010). A systematic review of Internet-based therapy for the treatment of addictions. *Clinical Psychology Review, 31,* 490–498.

Galanter, M., Castaneda, R., & Franco, H. (1991). Group therapy and self-help groups. In R. J. Frances & S. I. Miller (Eds.), *Clinical textbook of addictive disorders* (pp. 431–451). New York: Guilford Press.

Galanter, M., & Kleber, H.D. (Eds.). (2008). *Textbook of substance abuse treatment* (4th ed.). Washington, DC: American Psychiatric Publishing.

Garrett, J., Landau, J., Shea, R., Stanton, M. D., Baciewicz, G., & Brinkman-Sull, D. (1998). The ARISE intervention: Using family and network links to engage addicted persons in treatment. *Journal of Substance Abuse Treatment, 15,* 333–343.

Garrett, J., Landau-Stanton, J., Stanton, M. D., Stellato-Kabat, J., & Stellato-Kabat, D. (1997). ARISE: A method for engaging reluctant alcohol- and drug-dependent individuals in treatment. *Journal of Substance Abuse Treatment, 14,* 235–248.

Garrett, J., Stanton, M. D., Landau, J., Baciewicz, G., Brinkman-Sull, D., & Shea, R. (1999). The "concerned other" call: Using family links and networks to overcome resistance to addiction treatment. *Substance Use and Misuse, 34,* 363–382.

Gastfriend, D. R., Donovan, D. M., Lefebvre, R., & Murray, K. T. (2005). Developing a baseline assessment battery: Balancing patient time burden with essential clinical and research monitoring. *Journal of Studies on Alcohol, 66*(Suppl. 15), 94–103.

Gavin, D. R., Sobell, L. C., & Sobell, M. B. (1998). Evaluation of the Readiness to Change Questionnaire with problem drinkers in treatment. *Journal of Substance Abuse, 10,* 53–58.

Gayman, M. D., Cuddeback, G. S., & Morrissey, J. P. (2011). Help-seeking behaviors in a community sample of young adults with substance use disorders. *Journal of Behavioral Health Services and Research, 38,* 464–477.

Gentilello, L. M., Duggan, P., Drummond, D., Tonnesen, A., Degner, E. E., Fischer, R. P., et al. (1988). Major injury as a unique opportunity to initiate treatment in the alcoholic. *American Journal of Surgery, 156,* 558–561.

Gentilello, L. M., Ebel, B. E., Wickizer, T. M., Salkever, D. S., & Rivara, F. P. (2005). Alcohol interventions for trauma patients treated in emergency departments and hospitals: A cost benefit analysis. *Annals of Surgery, 241,* 541–550.

Gentilello, L. M., Rivara, F. P., Donovan, D. D., Jurkovich, G. J., Daranciang, E., Dunn, C. W., et al. (1999). Alcohol interventions in a trauma center as a means of reducing the risk of injury recurrence. *Annals of Surgery, 230,* 473–483.

Gibbs, L. E. (1983). Validity and reliability of the Michigan Alcoholism Screening Test: A review. *Drug and Alcohol Dependence, 12,* 279–285.

Gil-Rivas, V., Fiorentine, R., & Anglin, M. D. (1996). Sexual abuse, physical abuse, and posttraumatic stress disorder among women participating in outpatient drug abuse treatment. *Journal of Psychoactive Drugs, 28,* 95–102.

Gil-Rivas, V., Fiorentine, R., Anglin, M. D., & Taylor, E. (1997). Sexual and physical abuse: Do they compromise drug treatment outcomes? *Journal of Substance Abuse Treatment, 14,* 351–358.

Gillet, C., Paille, F., Wahl, D., Aubin, H. J., Pirollet, P., & Prime, T. (1991). Outcome of treatment in alcoholic women. *Drug and Alcohol Dependence, 29,* 189–194.

Glynn, T. J., Boyd, G. M., & Gruman, J. C. (1990). Essential elements of self-help/minimal intervention strategies for smoking cessation. *Health Education Quarterly, 17,* 329–345.

Golden, W. L. (1983). Resistance in cognitive-behavior therapy. *British Journal of Cognitive Psychotherapy, 1,* 33–42.

Gomberg, E. S. (2003). Treatment for alcohol-related problems: Special populations: Research opportunities. *Recent Developments in Alcoholism, 16,* 313–333.

Goodwin, D. W., & Warnock, J. K. (1991). Alcoholism: A family disease. In R. J. Frances & S. I. Miller (Eds.), *Clinical textbook of addictive disorders* (pp. 485–500). New York: Guilford Press.

Gordon, S. M. (2007). Barriers to treatment for women. *Counselor: The Magazine for Addiction Professionals, 8,* 22–28.

Gorski, T. T., & Miller, M. (1979). *Counseling for relapse prevention.* Hazel Creste, IL: Alcoholism Systems Associates.

Graham, J. R. (1999). *MMPI-2: Assessing personality and psychopathology* (3rd ed.). New York: Oxford University Press.

Graham, K., Annis, H. M., Brett, P. J., & Venesoen, P. (1996). A controlled field trial of group versus individual cognitive-behavioural training for relapse prevention. *Addiction, 91,* 1127–1140.

Green, C. A. (2006). Gender and use of substance abuse treatment services. *Alcohol Research and Health, 29,* 55–62.

Green, C. A., Polen, M. R., Dickinson, D. M., Lynch, F. L., & Bennett, M. D. (2002). Gender differences in predictors of initiation, retention, and completion in an HMO-based substance abuse treatment program. *Journal of Substance Abuse Treatment, 23,* 285–295.

Greenfield, L., Burgdorf, K., Chen, X., Porowski, A., Roberts, T., & Herrell, J. (2004).

Effectiveness of long-term residential substance abuse treatment for women: Findings from three national studies. *American Journal of Drug and Alcohol Abuse, 30,* 537–550.

Greenfield, S. F., Back, S. E., Lawson, K., & Brady, K. T. (2010). Substance abuse in women. *Psychiatric Clinics of North America, 33,* 339–355.

Greenfield, S. F., Brooks, A. J., Gordon, S. M., Green, C. A., Kropp, F., McHugh, R. K., et al. (2007a). Substance abuse treatment entry, retention, and outcome in women: A review of the literature. *Drug and Alcohol Dependence, 86,* 1–21.

Greenfield, S. F., & Grella, C. E. (2009). What is "women-focused" treatment for substance use disorders? *Psychiatric Services, 60,* 880–882.

Greenfield, S. F., Potter, J. S., Lincoln, M. F., Popuch, R. E., Kuper, L., & Gallop, R. J. (2008). High psychiatric symptom severity is a moderator of substance abuse treatment outcomes among women in single vs. mixed gender group treatment. *American Journal of Drug and Alcohol Abuse, 34,* 594–602.

Greenfield, S. F., Trucco, E. M., McHugh, R. K., Lincoln, M., & Gallop, R. J. (2007b). The Women's Recovery Group Study: A Stage I trial of women-focused group therapy for substance use disorders versus mixed-gender group drug counseling. *Drug and Alcohol Dependence, 90,* 39–47.

Greenson, R. R. (1967). *The technique and practice of psychoanalysis* (Vol. 1). New York: International Universities Press.

Greenstein, D. K., Franklin, M. E., & McGuffin, P. (1999). Measuring motivation to change: An examination of the University of Rhode Island Change Assessment Questionnaire (URICA) in an adolescent sample. *Psychotherapy: Theory, Research, Practice, Training, 36,* 47–55.

Grella, C. E. (2008). From generic to gender-responsive treatment: Changes in social policies, treatment services, and outcomes of women in substance abuse treatment. *Journal of Psychoactive Drugs, 40*(Suppl. 5), 327–343.

Grella, C. E., & Greenwell, L. (2004). Substance abuse treatment for women: Changes in the settings where women received treatment and types of services provided, 1987–1998. *Journal of Behavioral Health Services and Research, 31,* 367–383.

Grimley, D. M., Riley, G. E., Bellis, J. M., & Prochaska, J. O. (1993). Assessing the stages of change and decision-making for contraceptive use for the prevention of pregnancy, sexually transmitted diseases, and acquired immunodeficiency syndrome. *Health Education Quarterly, 20,* 455–470.

Gruber, K. J., & Taylor, M. F. (2006). A family perspective for substance abuse: Implications from the literature. *Journal of Social Work Practice in the Addictions, 9,* 1–29.

Gurman, A. S. (1984). Transference and resistance in marital therapy. *American Journal of Family Therapy, 12,* 70–73.

Hagan, T. A., Finnegan, L. P., & Nelson-Zlupko, L. (1994). Impediments to comprehensive treatment models for substance dependent women: Treatment and research questions. *Journal of Psychoactive Drugs, 26,* 163–171.

Halkitis, P. N., Parsons, J. T., Wolitski, R. J., & Remien, R. H. (2003). Characteristics of HIV antiretroviral treatments, access and adherence in an ethnically diverse sample of men who have sex with men. *AIDS Care, 15,* 89–102.

Harris, S. N., Mowbray, C. T., & Solarz, A. (1994). Physical health, mental health, and substance abuse problems of shelter users. *Health and Social Work, 19,* 37–45.

Hartera, S. L. (2000). Psychosocial adjustment of adult children of alcoholics: A review of the recent empirical literature. *Clinical Psychology Review, 20,* 311–337.

Hartwell, S. (2003). Deviance over the life course: The case of homeless substance abusers. *Substance Use and Misuse, 38,* 475–502.

Harwood, H. (2000). *Updating estimates of the economic costs of alcohol abuse in the*

United States: Estimates, update methods, and data. Rockville, MD: National Institute on Alcohol Abuse and Alcoholism.

Hasin, D. S. (1991). Diagnostic interviews for assessment: Background, reliability, validity. *Alcohol Health and Research World, 15,* 293–302.

Hasin, D. S. (1994). Treatment/self-help for alcohol-related problems: Relationship to social pressure and alcohol dependence. *Journal of Studies on Alcohol, 55,* 660–666.

Hawkins, C. A. (1997). Disruption of family rituals as a mediator of the relationship between parental drinking and adult adjustment in offspring. *Addictive Behaviors, 22,* 219–231.

Heath, A. W., & Stanton, M. D. (1998). Family-based treatment: Stages and outcomes. In *Clinical textbook of addictive disorders* (2nd ed., pp. 496–520). New York: Guilford Press.

Heather, N. (1995). Interpreting the evidence on brief interventions for excessive drinkers: The need for caution. *Alcohol and Alcoholism, 30,* 287–296.

Heather, N., & Hönekopp, J. (2008). A revised edition of the Readiness to Change Questionnaire [Treatment Version]. *Addiction Research and Theory, 16,* 421–433.

Heather, N., Hönekopp, J., Smailes, D., & UKATT Research Team. (2009). Progressive stage transition does mean getting better: A further test of the transtheoretical model in recovery from alcohol problems. *Addiction, 104,* 949–958.

Heather, N., Luce, A., Peck, D., Dunbar, B., & James, I. (1999). Development of a treatment version of the Readiness to Change Questionnaire. *Addiction Research, 7,* 63–83.

Heather, N., Rollnick, S., & Bell, A. (1993). Predictive validity of the Readiness to Change Questionnaire. *Addiction, 88,* 1667–1677.

Heather, N., Stallard, A., & Tebbutt, J. (1991). Importance of substance cues in relapse among heroin users: Comparison of two methods of investigation. *Addictive Behaviors, 16,* 41–49.

Hecksher, D., & Hesse, M. (2009). Women and substance use disorders. *Mens Sana Monographs, 7,* 50–62.

Heesch, K. C., Velasquez, M. M., & von Sternberg, K. (2005). Readiness for mental health treatment and for changing alcohol use in patients with comorbid psychiatric and alcohol disorders: Are they congruent?. *Addictive Behaviors, 30,* 531–643.

Heffner, J. L., Blom, T. J., & Anthenelli, R. M. (2011). Gender differences in trauma history and symptoms as predictors of relapse to alcohol and drug use. *American Journal of Addiction, 20,* 307–311.

Herkov, M. (2010). About group therapy. *Psych Central.* Retrieved November 12, 2011, from *psychcentral.com/lib/2006/about-group-therapy.*

Hernandez-Avila, C. A., Rounsaville, B. J., & Kranzler, H. R. (2004). Opioid-, cannabis- and alcohol-dependent women show more rapid progression to substance abuse treatment. *Drug and Alcohol Dependence, 74,* 265–272.

Herzog, T. A. (2008). Analyzing the transtheoretical model using the framework of Weinstein, Rothman, and Sutton (1998): The example of smoking cessation. *Health Psychology, 27,* 548–556.

Hesselbrock, V. M., & Hesselbrock, M. N. (2006). Are there empirically supported and clinically useful subtypes of alcohol dependence? *Addiction, 101*(Suppl. 1), 97–103.

Higgins, S. T. (1999). Potential contributions of the community reinforcement approach and contingency management to broadening the base of substance abuse treatment. In J. A. Tucker, D. M. Donovan, & G. A. Marlatt (Eds.), *Changing addictive behavior: Bridging clinical and public health strategies* (pp. 283–306). New York: Guilford Press.

Higgins, S. T., Budney, A. J., Bickel, W. K., Hughes, J. R., Forerq, F., & Badger, G. (1993). Achieving cocaine abstinence with a behavioral approach. *American Journal of Psychiatry, 150,* 763–769.

Higgins, S. T., Silverman, K., & Heil, S. H. (2007). *Contingency management in substance abuse treatment*. New York: Guilford Press.

Higgins, S. T., Tidey, J. W., & Stitzer, M. L. (1998). Community reinforcement and contingency management interventions. In A. W. Graham, T. K. Schultz, & B. B. Wilford (Eds.), *Principles of addiction medicine* (pp. 675–690). Chevy Chase, MD: American Society of Addiction Medicine.

Hingson, R., Mangione, T., Meyers, A., & Scotch, N. (1982). Seeking help for drinking problems. *Journal of Studies on Alcohol, 43*, 273–288.

Hingson, R., & Winter, M. (2003). Epidemiology and consequences of drinking and driving. *Alcohol Research and Health, 27*, 63–78.

Hinkin, C. H., & Kahn, M. (1995). Psychological symptomatology in spouses and adult children of alcoholics: An examination of the hypothesized personality characteristics of codependency. *International Journal of the Addictions, 30*, 843–861.

Hodgins, D. C. (2005). Weighing the pros and cons of changing change models: A comment on West (2005). *Addiction, 100*, 1042.

Hogue, A., Dauber, S., & Morgenstern, J. (2010). Validation of a contemplation ladder in an adult substance use disorder sample. *Psychology of Addictive Behaviors, 24*, 137–144.

Holder, H. D. (1998). The cost offsets of alcoholism treatment. In M. Galanter (Ed.), *Recent developments in alcoholism* (Vol. 14, pp. 361–374). New York: Plenum Press.

Holder, H. D., Lennox, R. D., & Blose, J. O. (1992). The economic benefits of alcoholism treatment: A summary of twenty years of research. *Journal of Employee Assistance Research, 1*, 63–82.

Holmgren, M. A., & DiClemente, C. C. (2012). *Relapse vulnerability predicting post-treatment severity of relapse in Project MATCH*. Unpublished data, University of Maryland, Baltimore County.

Hook, M. K. (2011). Alcohol addiction and families. In D. Capuzzi & M. D. Stauffer. *Foundations of addiction counseling* (pp. 278–300). Upper Saddle River, NJ: Prentice-Hall.

Horn, D. A. (1976). A model for the study of personal choice health behavior. *International Journal of Health Education, 19*, 89–98.

Horn, J. L., Wanberg, K. W., & Foster, F. M. (1987). *Guide to the Alcohol Use Inventory (AUI)*. Minneapolis: National Computer Systems.

Hser, Y. I., Evans, E., Huang, D., & Messina, N. (2011). Long-term outcomes among drug-dependent mothers treated in women-only versus mixed-gender programs. *Journal of Substance Abuse Treatment, 41*, 115–123.

Hser, Y. I., & Niv, N. (2006). Pregnant women in women-only and mixed-gender substance abuse treatment programs: A comparison of client characteristics and program services. *Journal of Behavioral Health Services and Research, 33*, 431–442.

Huang, S., Trapido, E., Fleming, L., Arheart, K., Crandall, L., French, M., et al. (2011). The long-term effects of childhood maltreatment experiences on subsequent illicit drug use and drug-related problems in young adulthood. *Addictive Behaviors, 36*, 95–102.

Humeniuk, R. E., Ali, R. A., Babor, T. F., Farrell, M., Formigoni, M. L., Jittiwutikarn, J., et al. (2008). Validation of the Alcohol, Smoking and Substance Involvement Screening Test (ASSIST). *Addiction, 103*, 1039–1047.

Humphreys, K., & Moos, R. H. (1996). Reduced substance-abuse-related health care costs among voluntary participants in Alcoholics Anonymous. *Psychiatric Services, 47*, 709–713.

Humphreys, K., & Moos, R. H. (2001). Can encouraging substance abuse patients to participate in self-help groups reduce demand for health care?: A quasi-experimental study. *Alcoholism: Clinical and Experimental Research, 25*, 711–716.

Hunt, G. M., & Azrin, N. H. (1973). A community-reinforcement approach to alcoholism. *Behaviour Research and Therapy, 11*, 91–104.

Hunt, W. A., Barnett, L. W., & Branch, L. G. (1971). Relapse rates in addiction programs. *Journal of Clinical Psychology, 27,* 455–456.

Iguchi, M. Y., Belding, M. A., Morral, A. R., Lamb, R. J., & Husband, S. D. (1997). Reinforcing operants other than abstinence in drug abuse treatment: An effective alternative for reducing drug use. *Journal of Consulting and Clinical Psychology, 65,* 421–428.

Ingersoll, K. S., Wagner, C. C., & Gharib, S. (2002). *Motivational groups for community substance abuse programs.* Richmond, VA: Mid-Atlantic Addiction Technology Transfer Center, Center for Substance Abuse Treatment (Mid-ATTC/CSAT).

Institute of Medicine. (1990). *Broadening the base of treatment for alcohol problems.* Washington, DC: National Academy Press.

Irwin, T. W., Morgenstern, J., Parsons, J. T., Wainberg, M., & Labouvie, E. (2006). Alcohol and sexual HIV risk behavior among problem drinking men who have sex with men: An event level analysis of Timeline Followback data. *AIDS and Behavior, 10,* 299–307.

Isenhart, C. E. (1991). Factor structure of the Inventory of Drinking Situations. *Journal of Substance Abuse, 3,* 59–71.

Isenhart, C. E. (1993). Psychometric evaluation of a short form of the Inventory of Drinking Situations. *Journal of Studies on Alcohol, 54,* 345–349.

Isenhart, C. (1994). Motivational subtypes in an inpatient sample of substance abusers. *Addictive Behaviors, 19,* 463–475.

Ito, J. R., Donovan, D. M., & Hall, J. J. (1988). Relapse prevention in alcohol after-care: Effects on drinking outcome, change process, and after-care attendance. *British Journal of Addiction, 83,* 171–181.

Jacobson, G. R. (1989). A comprehensive approach to pretreatment evaluation: I. Detection, assessment, and diagnosis of alcoholism. In R. K. Hester & W. R. Miller (Eds.), *Handbook of alcoholism treatment approaches* (pp. 17–53). New York: Pergamon Press.

Jahn, D. L., & Lichstein, K. L. (1980). The resistive client: A neglected phenomenon in behavior therapy. *Behavior Modification, 4,* 303–320.

Janis, I. L., & Mann, L. (1977). *Decision-making: A psychological analysis of conflict, choice, and commitment.* New York: Free Press.

Joanning, H., Thomas, F., Quinn, W., & Mullen, R. (1992). Treating adolescent drug abuse: A comparison of family systems therapy, group therapy, and family education. *Journal of Marital and Family Therapy, 18,* 345–356.

Johnson, J. L., & Leff, M. (1999). Children of substance abusers: Overview of research findings. *Pediatrics, 103,* 1085–1099.

Johnson, P. B., Richter, L., Kleber, H. D., McLellan, A. T., & Carise, D. (2005). Telescoping of drinking-related behaviors: Gender, racial/ethnic, and age comparisons. *Substance Use and Misuse, 40,* 1139–1151.

Johnson, V. E. (1986). *Intervention: How to help someone who doesn't want help.* Minneapolis: Johnson Institute Books.

Joint Commission on Accreditation of Healthcare Organizations. (1994). *Accreditation manual for mental health, chemical dependency, and mental retardation/developmental disabilities services.* Oakbrook Terrace, IL: Author.

Jordan, C. M., & Oei, T. P. S. (1989). Help-seeking behaviour in problem drinkers: A review. *British Journal of Addiction, 84,* 979–988.

Joseph, J., Breslin, C., & Skinner, H. (1999). Critical perspectives on the transtheoretical model and stages of change. In J. A. Tucker, D. M. Donovan, & G. A. Marlatt (Eds.), *Changing addictive behavior: Bridging clinical and public health strategies* (pp. 160–190). New York: Guilford Press.

Kadden, R., Carroll, K., Donovan, D., Cooney, N., Monti, P., Abrams, D., et al. (1992). *Cognitive-behavioral coping skills therapy manual: A clinical research guide for therapists treating individuals with alcohol abuse and dependence* (National Institute on Alcohol Abuse and Alcoholism, Project MATCH Monograph Series, Vol. 3). Rockville, MD: National Institute on Alcohol Abuse and Alcoholism.

Kadden, R. M., & Skerker, P. M. (1999). Treatment decision making and goal setting. In B. S. McCrady & E. E. Epstein (Eds.), *Addiction: A comprehensive guidebook* (2nd ed., pp. 216–231). New York: Oxford University Press.

Kaner, E. F. S., Dickinson, H. O., Beyer, F., Pienaar, E., Schlesinger, C., Campbell, F., et al. (2009). The effectiveness of brief alcohol interventions in primary care settings: A systemic review. *Drug and Alcohol Review, 28*, 301–323.

Kanfer, F. H. (1986). Implications of a self-regulation model of therapy for treatment of addictive behaviors. In W. R. Miller & N. Heather (Eds.), *Treating addictive behaviors: Processes of change* (pp. 29–47). New York: Plenum Press.

Kaskutas, L. A. (1996a). Road less traveled: Choosing the "Women for Sobriety" program. *Journal of Drug Issues, 26*, 77–94.

Kaskutas, L. A. (1996b). Pathways to self-help among Women for Sobriety. *American Journal of Drug and Alcohol Abuse, 22*, 259–280.

Kaskutas, L. A., Zhang, L., French, M. T., & Witbrodt, J. (2005). Women's programs versus mixed-gender day treatment: Results from a randomized study. *Addiction, 100*, 60–69.

Kauffman, E., Dore, M. M., & Nelson-Zlupko, L. (1995). The role of women's therapy groups in the treatment of chemical dependence. *American Journal of Orthopsychiatry, 65*, 355–363.

Kay, A., Taylor, T. E., Barthwell, A. G., Wichelecki, J., & Leopold, V. (2010). Substance use and women's health. *Journal of Addictive Diseases, 29*, 139–163.

Kendler, K. S., Gardner, C. O., & Prescott, C. A. (2011). Toward a comprehensive developmental model for alcohol use disorders in men. *Twin Research and Human Genetics, 14*, 1–15.

Kendler, K. S., Schmitt, E., Aggen, S. H., & Prescott, C. A. (2008). Genetic and environmental influences on alcohol, caffeine, cannabis, and nicotine use from early adolescence to middle adulthood. *Archives of General Psychiatry, 65*, 674–682.

Kessler, R. C. (2004). The epidemiology of dual diagnosis. *Biological Psychiatry, 56*, 730–737.

Keyes, K. M., Hatzenbuehler, M. L., McLaughlin, K. A., Link, B., Olfson, M., Grant, B. F., et al. (2010a). Stigma and treatment for alcohol disorders in the United States. *American Journal of Epidemiology, 172*, 1364–1372.

Keyes, K. M., Martins, S. S., Blanco, C., & Hasin, D. S. (2010b). Telescoping and gender differences in alcohol dependence: New evidence from two national surveys. *American Journal of Psychiatry, 167*, 969–976.

King, A. C., Bernardy, N. C., & Hauner, K. (2003). Stressful events, personality, and mood disturbance: Gender differences in alcoholics and problem drinkers. *Addictive Behaviors, 28*, 171–187.

Kirby, K. C., Marlowe, D. B., Festinger, D. S., Garvey, K. A., & LaMonaca, V. (1999). Community reinforcement training for family and significant others of drug abusers: A unilateral intervention to increase treatment entry of drug abusers. *Drug and Alcohol Dependence, 56*, 85–96.

Kirshenbaum, A. P., Olsen, D. M., & Bickel, W. K. (2009). A quantitative review of the ubiquitous relapse curve. *Journal of Substance Abuse Treatment, 36*, 8–17.

Klingemann, H. (1991). The motivation for change from problem alcohol and heroin use. *British Journal of Addiction, 86*, 727–744.

Knight, K., Hiller, M. L., Broome, K. M., & Simpson, D. D. (2000). Legal pressure, treatment readiness, and engagement in long-term residential programs. *Journal of Offender Rehabilitation, 31*, 101–115.

Krampe, H., & Ehrenreich, H. (2010). Supervised disulfiram as adjunct to psychotherapy in alcoholism treatment. *Current Pharmaceutical Design, 16,* 2076–2090.

Krampen, G. (1989). Motivation in the treatment of alcoholism. *Addictive Behaviors, 14,* 197–200.

LaBrie, J. W., Hutching, K., Tawalbeh, S., Pederson, E. R., Thompson, A. D., Shelesky, K., et al. (2008). A randomized motivational enhancement prevention group reduces drinking and alcohol consequences in first-year college women. *Psychology of Addictive Behaviors, 22,* 149–155.

Landau, J., Garrett, J., Shea, R. R., Stanton, M. D., Brinkman-Sull, D., & Baciewicz, G. (2000). Strength in numbers: The ARISE method for mobilizing family and network to engage substance abusers in treatment. *American Journal of Drug and Alcohol Abuse, 26,* 379–398.

Landau, J., Stanton, M. D., Brinkman-Sull, D., Ikle, D., McCormick, D., Garrett, J., et al. (2004). Outcomes with the ARISE approach to engaging reluctant drug- and alcohol-dependent individuals in treatment. *American Journal of Drug and Alcohol Abuse, 30,* 711–748.

Langeland, W., Draijer, N., & van den Brink, W. (2004). Psychiatric comorbidity in treatment-seeking alcoholics: The role of childhood trauma and perceived parental dysfunction. *Alcoholism: Clinical and Experimental Research, 28,* 441–447.

Lapham, S. C. (2004–2005). Screening and brief intervention in the criminal justice system. *Alcohol Research and Health, 28,* 85–93.

Lapham, S. C., C'de Baca, J., McMillan, G., & Hunt, W. C. (2004). Accuracy of alcohol diagnosis among DWI offenders referred for screening. *Drug and Alcohol Dependence, 76,* 135–141.

Lapham, S. C., C'de Baca, J., McMillan, G. P., & Lapidus, J. (2006). Psychiatric disorders in a sample of repeat impaired-driving offenders. *Journal of Studies on Alcohol, 67,* 707–713.

Lapham, S. C., & England-Kennedy, E. (2012). Convicted driving-while-impaired offenders' views on effectiveness of sanctions and treatment. *Qualitative Health Research, 22,* 17–30.

Lapham, S. C., & McMillan, G. P. (2011). Open-label pilot study of extended-release naltrexone to reduce drinking and driving among repeat offenders. *Journal of Addiction Medicine, 5,* 163–169.

Larson, C. C., & Talley, L. K. (1977). Family resistance to therapy: A model for services and therapists' roles. *Child Welfare, 56,* 121–126.

Lash, S. J., Burden, J. L., Monteleone, B. R., & Lehmann, L. P. (2004). Social reinforcement of substance abuse treatment aftercare participation: Impact on outcome. *Addictive Behaviors, 29,* 337–342.

Lash, S. J., Gilmore, J. D., Burden, J. L., Weaver, K. R., Blosser, S. L., & Finney, M. L. (2005). The impact of contracting and prompting substance abuse treatment entry: A pilot trial. *Addictive Behaviors, 30,* 415–422.

Lash, S. J., Petersen, G. E., O'Connor, E. A., & Lehmann, L. P. (2001). Social reinforcement of substance abuse aftercare group therapy attendance. *Journal of Substance Abuse Treatment, 20,* 3–8.

Lash, S. J., Stephens, R. S., Burden, J. L., Grambow, S. C., DeMarce, J. M., Jones, M. E., et al. (2007). Contracting, prompting, and reinforcing substance use disorder continuing care: A randomized clinical trial. *Psychology of Addictive Behaviors, 21,* 387–397.

Lazarus, A. A., & Fay, A. (1982). Resistance or rationalization?: A cognitive-behavioral perspective. In P. L. Wachtel (Ed.), *Resistance: Psychodynamic and behavioral approaches* (pp. 115–132). New York: Plenum Press.

Lebow, J., Kelly, J., Knobloch-Fedders, L. M., & Moos, R. (2006). Relationship factors in treating substance use disorder. In L. G. Castonguay & L. E. Beutler (Eds.), *Principles of therapeutic change that work* (pp. 293–317). New York: Oxford University Press.

Leeies, M., Pagura, J., Sareen, J., & Bolton, J. M. (2010). The use of alcohol and drugs to self-medicate symptoms of posttraumatic stress disorder. *Depression and Anxiety, 27,* 731–736.

Leigh, G., & Skinner, H. A. (1988). Physiological assessment. In D. M. Donovan & G. A. Marlatt (Eds.), *Assessment of addictive behaviors* (pp. 112–136). New York: Guilford Press.

Lemmens, P., Tan, E. S., & Knibbe, R. A. (1992). Measuring quantity and frequency of drinking in a general population survey: A comparison of five indices. *Journal of Studies on Alcohol, 53,* 476–486.

Lennox, R. D., Scott-Lennox, J. A., & Bohlig, E. M. (1993). The cost of depression-complicated alcoholism: Health-care utilization and treatment effectiveness. *Journal of Mental Health Administration, 20,* 138–152.

Lennox, R. D., Scott-Lennox, J. A., & Holder, H. D. (1992). Substance abuse and family illness: Evidence from health care utilization and cost-offset research. *Journal of Mental Health Administration, 19,* 83–95.

Levy, M. (1997). Group therapy in addictive and psychiatric disorders. In N. S. Miller (Ed.), *The principles and practice of addictions in psychiatry* (pp. 384–391). Philadelphia: Saunders.

Lewis, J. A., Dana, R. Q., & Blevins, G. A. (1988). *Substance abuse counseling: An individualized approach.* Pacific Grove, CA: Brooks/Cole.

Lewis, M. W., & Petry, N. M. (2005). Contingency management treatments that reinforce completion of goal-related activities: Participation in family activities and its association with outcomes. *Drug and Alcohol Dependence, 79,* 267–271.

Lichtenstein, E. (1971). Modification of smoking behavior: Good designs—ineffective treatment. *Journal of Consulting and Clinical Psychology, 36,* 163–166.

Lichtenstein, E., Zhu, S. H., & Tedeschi, G. J. (2010). Smoking cessation quitlines: An underrecognized intervention success story. *American Psychologist, 65,* 252–261.

Liepman, M. R. (1993). Using family influence to motivate alcoholics to enter treatment: The Johnson Institute Intervention approach. In T. J. O'Farrell (Ed.), *Treating alcohol problems: Marital and family interventions* (pp. 54–77). New York: Guilford Press.

Lincourt, P., Kuettel, T. J., & Bombardier, C. H. (2002). Motivational interviewing in a group setting with mandated clients: A pilot study. *Addictive Behaviors, 27,* 381–391.

Liotti, G. (1987). The resistance to change of cognitive structures: A counterproposal to psychoanalytic metapsychology. *Journal of Cognitive Psychotherapy, 1,* 87–104.

Litman, G. K. (1986). Alcoholism survival: The prevention of relapse. In W. R. Miller & N. Heather (Eds.), *Treating addictive behaviors* (pp. 391–405). New York: Plenum Press.

Litman, G. K., Eiser, J. R., Rawson, N. S. B., & Oppenheim, A. N. (1979). Towards a typology of relapse: Differences in relapse and coping behaviours between alcoholic relapsers and survivors. *Behaviour Research and Therapy, 17,* 89–94.

Livingston, M., Wilkinson, C., & Laslett, A.-M. (2010). Impact of heavy drinkers on others' health and well-being. *Journal of Alcohol and Drugs, 71,* 778–785.

Loneck, B., Garrett, J. A., & Banks, S. M. (1996a). A comparison of the Johnson Intervention with four other methods of referral to outpatient treatment. *American Journal of Drug and Alcohol Abuse, 22,* 233–246.

Loneck, B., Garrett, J. A., & Banks, S. M. (1996b). The Johnson Intervention and relapse during outpatient treatment. *American Journal of Drug and Alcohol Abuse, 22,* 363–375.

Loneck, B., Garrett, J., & Banks, S. M. (1997). Engaging and retaining women in outpatient alcohol and other drug treatment: The effect of referral intensity. *Health and Social Work, 22,* 38–46.

Longabaugh, R., Wirtz, P. W., Beattie, M. C., Noel, N., & Stout, R. (1995). Matching treatment focus to patient social investment and support: 18 month follow-up results. *Journal of Consulting and Clinical Psychology, 63,* 296–307.

Longabaugh, R., Woolard, R. F., Nirenberg, T. D., Minugh, A. P., Becker, B., Clifford, P. R., et al. (2001). Evaluating the effects of a brief motivational intervention for injured drinkers in the emergency department. *Journal of Studies on Alcohol, 62,* 806–816.

Lovejoy, M., Rosenblum, A., Magura, S., Foote, J., Handelsman, L., & Stimmel, B. (1995). Patients' perspective on the process of change in substance abuse treatment. *Journal of Substance Abuse Treatment, 12,* 269–282.

Lovett, L., & Lovett, J. (1991). Group therapeutic factors on an alcohol in-patient unit. *British Journal of Psychiatry, 159,* 365–370.

Lowman, C., Allen, J., Stout, R. L., & the Relapse Research Group. (1996). Replication and extension of Marlatt's taxonomy of relapse precipitants: Overview of procedures and results. *Addiction, 91*(Suppl.), 51–71.

Lowman, C., & Le Fauve, C. E. (2003). Health disparities and the relationship between race, ethnicity, and substance abuse treatment outcomes. *Alcoholism: Clinical and Experimental Research, 27,* 1324–1326.

Luborsky, L., Singer, B., & Luborsky, L. (1975). Comparative studies of psychotherapy: Is it true that "Everyone has won and all must get prizes"? *Archives of General Psychiatry, 32,* 995–1008.

Lucas, G. M., Gebo, K. A., Chaisson, R. E., & Moore, R. D. (2002). Longitudinal assessment of the effects of drug and alcohol abuse on HIV-1 treatment outcomes in an urban clinic. *AIDS, 16,* 767–774.

Ludwig, A. M., & Wikler, A. (1974). "Craving" and relapse to drink. *Quarterly Journal of Studies on Alcohol, 35,* 108–130.

Luoma, J. B., Twohig, M. P., Waltz, T., Hayes, S. C., Roget, N., Padilla, M., et al. (2007). An investigation of stigma in individuals receiving treatment for substance abuse. *Addictive Behaviors, 32,* 1331–1346.

Lutz, M. E. (1991). Sobering decisions: Are there gender differences? *Alcoholism Treatment Quarterly, 8,* 51–64.

MacAndrew, C. (1965). The differentiation of male alcoholic outpatients from nonalcoholic psychiatric outpatients by means of the MMPI. *Quarterly Journal of Studies on Alcohol, 26,* 238–246.

MacDonald, J. M., Morral, A. R., Raymond, B., & Eibner, C. (2007). The efficacy of the Rio Hondo DUI court: A 2-year field experiment. *Evaluation Review, 31,* 4–23.

Macgowan, M. J. (2008). *A guide to evidence-based group work.* New York: Oxford University Press.

Madras, B. K., Compton, W. M., Avula, D., Stegbauer, T., Stein, J. B., & Clark, H. W. (2009). Screening, brief interventions, referral to treatment (SBIRT) for illicit drug and alcohol use at multiple healthcare sites: Comparison at intake and 6 months later. *Drug and Alcohol Dependence, 99,* 280–295.

Magura, S., & Laudet, A. B. (1996). Parental substance abuse and child maltreatment: Review and implications for intervention. *Children and Youth Services Review, 18,* 193–220

Maisto, S. A., Connors, G. J., & Zywiak, W. H. (2000). Alcohol treatment, changes in coping skills, self-efficacy, and levels of alcohol use and related problems 1 year following treatment initiation. *Psychology of Addictive Behaviors, 14,* 257–266.

Maisto, S. A., Krenek, M., Chung, T., Martin, C. S., Clark, D., & Cornelius, J. (2011). A comparison of the concurrent and predictive validity of three measures of readiness to change alcohol use in a clinical sample of adolescents. *Psychological Assessment, 23,* 983–994.

Maisto, S. A., McKay, J. R., & Connors, G. J. (1990). Self-report issues in substance abuse: State of the art and future directions. *Behavioral Assessment, 12,* 117–134.

Maisto, S. A., McKay, J. R., & Tiffany, S. T. (2003). Diagnosis. In J. P. Allen & V. Wilson (Eds.), *Assessing alcohol problems: A guide for clinicians and researchers* (2nd ed., pp. 55–73). Bethesda, MD: National Institute on Alcohol Abuse and Alcoholism.

Maisto, S. A., O'Farrell, T. J., Worthen, M., & Walitzer, K. S. (1993). Alcohol abuse and dependence. In A. S. Bellack & M. Hersen (Eds.), *Handbook of behavior therapy in the psychiatric setting* (pp. 293–319). New York: Plenum Press.

Mallams, J. H., Godley, M. D., Hall, G. M., & Meyers, R. J. (1982). A social-systems approach to resocializing alcoholics in the community. *Journal of Studies on Alcohol, 43,* 1115–1123.

Marcus, B. H., Rossi, J. S., Selby, V. C., Niaura, R. S., & Abrams, D. B. (1992). The stages and processes of exercise adoption and maintenance in a worksite sample. *Health Psychology, 11,* 386–395.

Mark, F. O. (1988). Does coercion work?: The role of referral source in motivating alcoholics in treatment. *Alcoholism Treatment Quarterly, 5,* 5–22.

Marlatt, G. A. (1985a). Lifestyle modification. In G. A. Marlatt & J. R. Gordon (Eds.), *Relapse prevention* (pp. 280–348). New York: Guilford Press.

Marlatt, G. A. (1985b). Relapse prevention: Theoretical rationale and overview of the model. In G. A. Marlatt & J. R. Gordon (Eds.), *Relapse prevention* (pp. 3–70). New York: Guilford Press.

Marlatt, G. A. (1996). Taxonomy of high-risk situations for alcohol relapse: Evolution and development of a cognitive-behavioral model. *Addiction, 91*(Suppl.), 37–49.

Marlatt, G. A., & Donovan, D. M. (Eds.). (2005). *Relapse prevention: Maintenance strategies in the treatment of addictive behaviors* (2nd ed.). New York: Guilford Press.

Marlatt, G. A., & Gordon, J. R. (1980). Determinants of relapse: Implications for the maintenance of behavior change. In P. O. Davidson & S. M. Davidson (Eds.), *Behavioral medicine: Changing health lifestyles* (pp. 410–452). New York: Brunner/Mazel.

Marlatt, G. A., & Gordon, J. R. (Eds.). (1985). *Relapse prevention.* New York: Guilford Press.

Marlatt, G. A., Tucker, J. A., Donovan, D. M., & Vuchinich, R. E. (1997). Help-seeking by substance abusers: The role of harm reduction and behavioral-economic approaches to facilitate treatment entry and retention. In L. S. Onken, J. D. Blaine, & J. J. Boren (Eds.), *Beyond the therapeutic alliance: Keeping the drug-dependent individual in treatment* (pp. 44–84). Rockville, MD: National Institute on Drug Abuse.

Marlowe, D. B., Merikle, E. P., Kirby, K. C., Festinger, D. S., & McLellan, A. T. (2001). Multidimensional assessment of perceived treatment-entry pressures among substance abusers. *Psychology of Addictive Behaviors, 15,* 97–108.

Martin, G. W., & Wilkinson, D. A. (1989). Methodological issues in the evaluation of treatment of drug dependence. *Behaviour Research and Therapy, 11,* 133–150.

Martino, S., Carroll, K. M., Nich, C., & Rounsaville, B. J. (2006). A randomized controlled pilot study of motivational interviewing for patients with psychotic and drug use disorders. *Addiction, 101,* 1479–1492.

Mayer, J. E., & Koeningsmark, C. S. (1991). Self-efficacy, relapse and the possibility of post-treatment denial as a stage in alcoholism. *Alcoholism Treatment Quarterly, 8,* 1–16.

Mayfield, D., McLeod, G., & Hall, P. (1974). The CAGE questionnaire: Validation of a new alcoholism instrument. *American Journal of Psychiatry, 131,* 1121–1123.

McCambridge, J., & Strang, J. (2004). The efficacy of single-session motivational interviewing in reducing drug consumption and perceptions of drug-related risk and harm among young people: Results from a multi-site cluster randomized trial. *Addiction*, *99*, 39–52.

McCarty, D., Argeriou, M., Huebner, R. B., & Lubran, B. (1991). Alcoholism, drug abuse, and the homeless. *American Psychologist*, *46*, 1139–1148.

McConnaughy, E. A., DiClemente, C. C., Prochaska, J. O., & Velicer, W. F. (1989). Stages of change in psychotherapy: A follow-up report. *Psychotherapy*, *26*, 494–503.

McConnaughy, E. A., Prochaska, J. O., & Velicer, W. F. (1983). Stages of change in psychotherapy: Measurement and sample profiles. *Psychotherapy: Theory, Research and Practice*, *20*, 368–375.

McCrady, B. S. (1989). Extending relapse prevention models to couples. *Addictive Behaviors*, *14*, 69–74.

McCrady, B. S. (1991). Promising but underutilized treatment approaches. *Alcohol Health and Research World*, *15*, 215–218.

McCrady, B. S. (1993). Relapse prevention: A couples-therapy perspective. In T. J. O'Farrell (Ed.), *Treating alcohol problems: Marital and family interventions* (pp. 327–350). New York: Guilford Press.

McCrady, B. S., Epstein, E. E., & Hirsch, L. S. (1999). Maintaining change after conjoint behavioral alcohol treatment for men: Outcomes at 6 months. *Addiction*, *94*, 1381–1396.

McCrady, B. S., Epstein, E. E., & Kahler, C. W. (2004). Alcoholics Anonymous and relapse prevention as maintenance strategies after conjoint behavioral alcohol treatment for men: 18-month outcomes. *Journal of Consulting and Clinical Psychology*, *72*, 870–878.

McCrady, B. S., Noel, N. E., Abrams, D. B., Stout, R. L., Nelson, H. F., & Hay, W. M. (1986). Comparative effectiveness of three types of spouse involvement in outpatient behavioral alcoholism treatment. *Journal of Studies on Alcohol*, *47*, 459–467.

McCrady, B. S., Stout, R., Noel, N., Abrams, D., & Nelson, H. F. (1991). Effectiveness of three types of spouse-involved behavioral alcoholism treatment. *British Journal of Addiction*, *86*, 1415–1424.

McGue, M. (1997). A behavioral-genetic perspective on children of alcoholics. *Alcohol Health and Research World*, *21*, 210–217.

McKay, J. R. (2001). The role of continuing care in outpatient alcohol treatment programs. *Recent Developments in Alcoholism*, *15*, 357–372.

McKay, J. R. (2005). Is there a case for extended interventions for alcohol and drug use disorders? *Addiction*, *100*, 1594–1610.

McKay, J. R. (2006). Continuing care in the treatment of addictive disorders. *Current Psychiatry Reports*, *8*, 355–362.

McKay, J. R. (2009). Continuing care research: What we have learned and where we are going. *Journal of Substance Abuse Treatment*, *36*, 131–145.

McKay, J. R., Maisto, S. A., & O'Farrell, T. J. (1996). Alcoholics' perceptions of factors in the onset and termination of relapses and the maintenance of abstinence: Results from a 30-month follow-up. *Psychology of Addictive Behaviors*, *10*, 167–180.

McLellan, A. T., Alterman, A. I., Metzger, D. S., Grissom, G. R., Woody, G. E., Luborsky, L., et al. (1994) Similarity of outcome predictors across opiate, cocaine and alcohol treatments: Role of treatment services. *Journal of Consulting and Clinical Psychology*, *62*, 1141–1158.

McLellan, A. T., Arndt, I. O., Metzger, D. S., Woody, G. E., & O'Brien, C. P. (1993). The effects of psychosocial services in substance abuse treatment. *Journal of the American Medical Association*, *269*, 1953–1959.

McLellan, A. T., Kushner, H., Metzger, D., Peters, R., Smith, I., Grissom, G., et al. (1992). The fifth edition of the Addiction Severity Index. *Journal of Substance Abuse Treatment*, *9*, 199–213.

McLellan, A. T., Luborsky, L., Woody, G. E., & O'Brien, C. P. (1980). An improved diagnostic evaluation instrument for substance abuse patients: The Addiction Severity Index. *Journal of Nervous and Mental Disease, 168*, 26–33.

Meichenbaum, D. H. (1995). Cognitive-behavioral therapy in historical perspective. In B. Bongar & L. E. Beutler (Eds.), *Comprehensive textbook of psychotherapy* (pp. 140–158). New York: Oxford University Press.

Mello, M. J., Nirenberg, T. D., Longabaugh, R., Woolard, R., Minugh, A., Becker, B., et al. (2005). Emergency department brief motivational interventions for alcohol with motor vehicle crash patients. *Annals of Emergency Medicine, 45*, 620–625.

Merikangas, K. R., Li, J. J., Stipelman, B., Yu, K., Fucito, L., Swendsen, J., & Zhang, H. (2009). The familial aggregation of cannabis use disorders. *Addiction, 104*, 622–629.

Merikangas, K. R., Stolar, M., Stevens, D. E., Goulet, J., Preisig, M. A., Fenton, B., et al. (1998). Familial transmission of substance use disorders. *Archives of General Psychiatry, 55*, 973–979.

Metzger, L. (1988). *From denial to recovery.* San Francisco: Jossey-Bass.

Metzger, D. S., Woody, G. E., & O'Brien, C. P. (2010). Drug treatment as HIV prevention: A research update. *Journal of Acquired Immune Deficiency Syndromes, 55*(Suppl. 1), S32–S36.

Meyerhoff, D. J. (2001). Effects of alcohol and HIV infection on the central nervous system. *Alcohol Research and Health, 25*, 288–298.

Meyers, R. J., Dominguez, T. P., & Smith, J. E. (1996). Community reinforcement training with concerned others. In V. B. Van Hassell & M. Hersen (Eds.), *Sourcebook of psychological treatment manuals for adult disorders* (pp. 257–294). New York: Plenum Press.

Meyers, R. J., Miller, W. R., Hill, D. E., & Tonigan, J. S. (1998). Community reinforcement and family training (CRAFT): Engaging unmotivated drug users in treatment. *Journal of Substance Abuse, 10*, 291–308.

Meyers, R. J., Miller, W. R., Smith, J. E., & Tonigan, J. S. (2002). A randomized trial of two methods for engaging treatment-refusing drug users through concerned significant others. *Journal of Consulting and Clinical Psychology, 70*, 1182–1185.

Meyers, R. J., & Smith, J. E. (1995). *Clinical guide to alcohol treatment: The community reinforcement approach.* New York: Guilford Press.

Meyers, R. J., & Smith, J. E. (1997). Getting off the fence: Procedures to engage treatment-resistant drinkers. *Journal of Substance Abuse Treatment, 14*, 467–472.

Meyers, R. J., Smith, J. E., & Lash, D. N. (2003). The Community Reinforcement Approach. *Recent Developments in Alcoholism, 16*, 183–195.

Meyers, R. J., Smith, J. E., & Miller, E. J. (1998). Working through the concerned significant other. In W. R. Miller & N. Heather (Eds.), *Treating addictive behaviors* (2nd ed., pp. 149–161). New York: Plenum Press.

Milby, J. B., Schumacher, J. E., McNamara, C., Wallace, D., Usdan, S., & Michael, M. (1998). Abstinent contingent housing greatly improves outcomes for homeless cocaine abusers in behavioral day treatment. *Pharmacology Biochemistry and Behavior, 61*, 154.

Milby, J. B., Schumacher, J. E., Raczynski, J. M., Caldwell, E., Engle, M., Michael, M., et al. (1996). Sufficient conditions for effective treatment of substance abusing homeless persons. *Drug and Alcohol Dependence, 43*, 39–47.

Milby, J. B., Schumacher, J. E., Wallace, D., Freedman, M. J., & Vuchinich, R. E. (2005). To house or not to house: The effects of providing housing to homeless substance abusers in treatment. *American Journal of Public Health, 95*, 1259–1265.

Milby, J. B., Schumacher, J. E., Wallace, D., Vuchinich, R., Mennemeyer, S. T., & Kertesz, S. G. (2010). Effects of sustained abstinence among treated substance-abusing homeless persons on housing and employment. *American Journal of Public Health, 100*, 913–918.

Miller, K. J., McCrady, B. S., Abrams, D. B., & Labouvie, E. W. (1994). Taking an individualized approach to the assessment of self-efficacy and the prediction of alcoholic relapse. *Journal of Psychopathology and Behavioral Assessment, 16*, 111–120.

Miller, N. S. (1995). Group therapy. In N. S. Miller (Ed.), *Addiction psychiatry: Current diagnoses and treatment* (pp. 256–270). New York: Wiley.

Miller, P. J., Ross, S. M., Emmerson, R. Y., & Todt, E. H. (1989). Self-efficacy in alcoholics: Clinical validation of the Situational Confidence Questionnaire. *Addictive Behaviors, 14*, 217–224.

Miller, P. M., & Mastria, M. A. (1977). *Alternatives to alcohol abuse: A social learning model.* Champaign, IL: Research Press.

Miller, W. R. (1985). Motivation for treatment: A review with special emphasis on alcoholism. *Psychological Bulletin, 98*, 84–107.

Miller, W. R. (1995). Increasing motivation for change. In R. K. Hester & W. R. Miller (Eds.), *Handbook of alcoholism treatment approaches: Effective alternatives* (2nd ed., pp. 89–104). Boston: Allyn & Bacon.

Miller, W. R. (1996). *Manual for Form 90: A structured assessment interview for drinking and related behaviors* (National Institute on Alcohol Abuse and Alcoholism, Project MATCH Monograph Series, Vol. 5). Rockville, MD: National Institute on Alcohol Abuse and Alcoholism.

Miller, W. R. (Consensus Panel Chair). (1999). *Enhancing motivation for change in substance abuse treatment* (DHHS Publication No. [SMA] 99-3354; CSAT Treatment Improvement Protocol No. 35). Washington, DC: U.S. Government Printing Office.

Miller, W. R. (2001). Foreword. In M. M. Velasquez, G. G. Maurer, C. Crouch, & C. C. DiClemente (Eds.), *Group treatment for substance abuse: A stages-of-change therapy manual* (pp. ix–xi). New York: Guilford Press.

Miller, W. R. (2006). Motivational factors in addictive behaviors. In W. R. Miller & K. M. Carroll (Eds.), *Rethinking substance abuse: What science shows and what we should do about it* (pp. 134–150). New York: Guilford Press.

Miller, W. R., Benefield, R. G., & Tonigan, J. S. (1993). Enhancing motivation for change in problem drinking: A controlled comparison of two therapist styles. *Journal of Consulting and Clinical Psychology, 61*, 455–461.

Miller, W. R., Brown, J. M., Simpson, T. L., Handmaker, N. S., Bien, T. H., Luckie, L. F., et al. (1995). What works?: A methodological analysis of the alcohol treatment outcome literature. In R. K. Hester & W. R. Miller (Eds.), *Handbook of alcoholism treatment approaches: Effective alternatives* (2nd ed., pp. 12–44). Boston: Allyn & Bacon.

Miller, W. R., & C'de Baca, J. (2001). *Quantum change.* New York: Guilford Press.

Miller, W. R., & DelBoca, F. K. (1994). Measurement of drinking behavior using the Form 90 family of instruments. *Journal of Studies on Alcohol,* (Suppl. 12), 112–118.

Miller, W. R., Forcehimes, A. A., & Zweben, A. (2011). *Treatment addiction: A guide for professionals.* New York: Guilford Press.

Miller, W. R., & Hester, R. K. (1980). Treating the problem drinker: Modern approaches. In W. R. Miller (Ed.), *The addictive behaviors: Treatment of alcoholism, drug abuse, smoking, and obesity* (pp. 11–141). New York: Pergamon Press.

Miller, W. R., Leckman, A. L., Delaney, H. D., & Tinkcom, M. (1992a). Long-term follow-up of behavioral self-control training. *Journal of Studies on Alcohol, 53*, 249–261.

Miller, W. R., & Marlatt, G. A. (1984). *Manual for the Comprehensive Drinker Profile.* Odessa, FL: Psychological Assessment Resources.

Miller, W. R., Meyers, R. J., & Tonigan, J. S. (1999). Engaging the unmotivated in treatment for alcohol problems: A comparison of three strategies for intervention through family members. *Journal of Consulting and Clinical Psychology, 67,* 688–697.

Miller, W. R., & Rollnick, S. (1991). *Motivational interviewing: Preparing people to change addictive behavior.* New York: Guilford Press.

Miller, W. R., & Rollnick, S. (2002). *Motivational interviewing: Preparing people for change* (2nd ed.). New York: Guilford Press.

Miller, W. R., & Rollnick, S. (2013). *Motivational interviewing: Third edition.* New York: Guilford Press.

Miller, W. R., & Rose, G. S. (2009). Toward a theory of motivational interviewing. *American Psychologist, 64,* 527–537.

Miller, W. R., & Tonigan, J. S. (1996). Assessing drinkers' motivations for change: The Stages of Change Readiness and Eagerness Scale (SOCRATES). *Psychology of Addictive Behaviors, 10,* 81–89.

Miller, W. R., Westerberg, V. S., Harris, R. J., & Tonigan, J. S. (1996). What predicts relapse?: Prospective testing of antecedent models. *Addiction, 91*(Suppl.), 155–171.

Miller, W. R., Zweben, A., DiClemente, C. C., & Rychtarik, R. G. (1992). *Motivational enhancement therapy manual: A clinical research guide for therapists treating individuals with alcohol abuse and dependence* (National Institute on Alcohol Abuse and Alcoholism, Project MATCH Monograph Series, Vol. 2). Rockville, MD: National Institute on Alcohol Abuse and Alcoholism.

Monti, P. M., Abrams, D. B., Kadden, R. M., & Cooney, N. L. (1989). *Treating alcohol dependence.* New York: Guilford Press.

Moos, R. H., Finney, J. W., & Cronkite, R. C. (1990). *Alcoholism treatment: Context, process, and outcome.* New York: Oxford University Press.

Moos, R. H., Moos, B. S., & Timko, C. (2006). Gender, treatment and self-help in remission from alcohol use disorders. *Clinical Medicine and Research, 4,* 163–174.

Morgenstern, J., Blanchard, K. A., McCrady, B. S., McVeigh, K. H., Morgan, T. J., & Pandina, R. J. (2006). Effectiveness of intensive case management for substance-dependent women receiving temporary assistance for needy families. *American Journal of Public Health, 96,* 2016–2023.

Morgenstern, J., Neighbors, C. J., Kuerbis, A., Riordan, A., Blanchard, K. A., McVeigh, K. H., et al. (2009). Improving 24-month abstinence and employment outcomes for substance-dependent women receiving temporary assistance for needy families with intensive case management. *American Journal of Public Health, 99,* 328–333.

Morse, R. M., & Flavin, D. K. (1992). The definition of alcoholism. *Journal of the American Medical Association, 268,* 1012–1014.

Moss, H. B., Chen, C. M., & Yi, H. Y. (2010). Prospective follow-up of empirically derived alcohol dependence subtypes in Wave 2 of the National Epidemiologic Survey on Alcohol and Related Conditions (NESARC): Recovery status, alcohol use disorders and diagnostic criteria, alcohol consumption behavior, health status, and treatment seeking. *Alcoholism: Clinical and Experimental Research, 34,* 1073–1083.

Moyer, A., Finney, J. W., Swearingen, C. E., & Vergun, P. (2002). Brief interventions for alcohol problems: A meta-analytic review of controlled investigations in treatment-seeking and non-treatment-seeking populations. *Addiction, 97,* 279.

Mueser, K. T., Noordsy, D. L., Drake, R. E., & Fox, L. (2003). *Integrated treatment for dual disorders: A guide to effective practice.* New York: Guilford Press.

Muetzell, S. (1995). Are boys more vulnerable than girls in alcoholic families? *Early Child Development and Care, 105,* 43–58.

Muhleman, D. (1987). 12-step study groups in drug abuse treatment programs. *Journal of Psychoactive Drugs, 19,* 291–298.

Mullen, P. D., Velasquez, M. M., von Sternberg, K., Cummins, A. G., & Green, C. (2005,

April). *Efficacy of a dual behavior focus, transtheoretical model-based motivational intervention with transition assistance to prevent an alcohol-exposed pregnancy (AEP) after a jail term.* Paper presented at the annual meeting of the Society of Behavioral Medicine, Boston.

Muraven, M., & Baumeister, R. F. (2000). Self-regulation and depletion of limited resources: Does self-control resemble a muscle? *Psychological Bulletin, 126,* 247–259.

Murphy, C. M., & O'Farrell, T. J. (1997). Couple communication patterns of maritally aggressive and nonaggressive male alcoholics. *Journal of Studies on Alcohol, 58,* 83–90.

Myers, B., Fakier, N., & Louw, J. (2009). Stigma, treatment beliefs, and substance abuse treatment use in historically disadvantaged communities. *African Journal of Psychiatry, 12,* 218–222.

Myrick, H., & Wright, T. (2008). Clinical management of alcohol abuse and dependence. In M. Galanter & H. D. Kleber (Eds.), *Textbook of substance abuse treatment* (4th ed., pp. 129–142). Washington, DC: American Psychiatric Publishing.

Napper, L. E., Wood, M. M., Jaffe, A., Fisher, D. G., Reynolds, G. L., & Klahn, J. A. (2008). Convergent and discriminant validity of three measures of stage of change. *Psychology of Addictive Behaviors, 27,* 362–371.

Nath, A., Hauser, K. F., Wojna, V., Booze, R. M., Maragos, W., Prendergast, M., et al. (2002). Molecular basis for interactions of HIV and drugs of abuse. *Journal of Acquired Immune Deficiency Syndromes, 31,* S62–S69.

National Highway Traffic Safety Administration. (2010a). *National survey of drinking and driving attitudes and behaviors: 2008. Volume 1: Summary report* (DOT HS 311 842). Washington, DC: U.S. Department of Transportation.

National Highway Traffic Safety Administration. (2010b). *Traffic safety facts 2009 data: Alcohol-impaired driving* (DOT HS 811 385). Washington, DC: U.S. Department of Transportation.

Nelson-Zlupko, L., Dore, M. M., Kauffman, E., & Kaltenbach, K. (1996). Women in recovery: Their perceptions of treatment effectiveness. *Journal of Substance Abuse Treatment, 13,* 51–59.

Nidecker, M., DiClemente, C. C., Bennett, M. E., & Bellack, A. S. (2008). Application of the transtheoretical model of change: Psychometric properties of leading measures in patients with co-occurring drug abuse and severe mental illness. *Addictive Behaviors, 33,* 1021–1030.

Niles, B. L., & McCrady, B. S. (1991). Detection of alcohol problems in a hospital setting. *Addictive Behaviors, 16,* 223–233.

Niv, N., & Hser, Y. I. (2007). Women-only and mixed-gender drug abuse treatment programs: Service needs, utilization and outcomes. *Drug and Alcohol Dependence, 87,* 194–201.

Nochajski, T. H., & Stasiewicz, P. R. (2005). Assessing stages of change in DUI offenders: A comparison of two measures. *Journal of Addictions Nursing, 16,* 57–67.

Norcross, J. C. (Ed.). (2002). *Psychotherapy relationships that work: Therapist contributions and responsiveness to patient needs.* New York: Oxford University Press.

Norcross, J. C., & Goldfried, M. R. (Eds.). (1992). *Handbook of psychotherapy integration.* New York: Basic Books.

Norcross, J. C., & Wampold, B. E. (2011). Evidence-based therapy relationships: Research conclusions and clinical practices. *Psychotherapy, 48,* 98–102.

Nordstrom, G., & Berglund, M. (1987). A prospective study of successful long-term adjustment in alcohol dependence: Social drinking versus abstinence. *Journal of Studies on Alcohol, 48,* 95–103.

Nowinski, J. (1999). Self-help groups for addictions. In B. S. McCrady & E. E. Epstein (Eds.), *Addiction: A comprehensive guidebook* (pp. 328–346). New York: Oxford University Press.

O'Brien, C. P. (1996). Recent developments in the pharmacotherapy of substance abuse. *Journal of Consulting and Clinical Psychology, 64,* 677–686.

O'Brien, C., & Kampman, K. M. (2008). Antagonists of opioids. In M. Galanter & H. D. Kleber (Eds.), *Textbook of substance abuse treatment* (4th ed., pp. 325–329). Washington, DC: American Psychiatric Publishing.

O'Farrell, T. J. (1989). Marital and family therapy in alcoholism treatment. *Journal of Substance Abuse Treatment, 6,* 23–29.

O'Farrell, T. J. (Ed.). (1993). *Treating alcohol problems: Marital and family interventions.* New York: Guilford Press.

O'Farrell, T. J. (1994). Marital therapy and spouse-involved treatment with alcoholic patients. *Behavior Therapy, 25,* 391–406.

O'Farrell, T. J., & Bayog, R. D. (1986). Antabuse contracts for married alcoholics and their spouses: A method to maintain Antabuse ingestion and decrease conflict about drinking. *Journal of Substance Abuse Treatment, 3,* 1–8.

O'Farrell, T. J., Choquette, K. A., & Cutter, H. S. (1998). Couples relapse prevention sessions after behavioral marital therapy for male alcoholics: Outcomes during the three years after starting treatment. *Journal of Studies on Alcohol, 59,* 357–370.

O'Farrell, T. J., Choquette, K. A., Cutter, H. S., Brown, E. D., & McCourt, W. F. (1993). Behavioral marital therapy with and without additional couples relapse prevention sessions for alcoholics and their wives. *Journal of Studies on Alcohol, 54,* 652–666.

O'Farrell, T. J., & Cutter, H. S. (1984). Behavioral marital family couples groups for male alcoholics and their wives. *Journal of Substance Abuse Treatment, 1,* 191–204.

O'Farrell, T. J., Cutter, H. S., Choquette, K. A., Floyd, F. J., & Bayog, R. D. (1992). Behavioral marital therapy for male alcoholics: Marital and drinking adjustment during the two years after treatment. *Behavior Therapy, 23,* 529–549.

O'Farrell, T. J., & Fals-Stewart, W. (2001). Family-involved alcoholism treatment: An update. *Recent Developments in Alcoholism, 15,* 329–356.

O'Farrell, T. J., & Fals-Stewart, W. (2002). Behavioral couples and family therapy for substance abusers. *Current Psychiatry Reports, 4,* 371–376.

O'Farrell, T. J., & Feehan, M. (1999). Alcoholism treatment and the family: Do family and individual treatments for alcoholic adults have preventive effects for children? *Journal of Studies on Alcohol,* Suppl. 13, 125–129.

O'Farrell, T. J., Murphy, M., Alter, J., & Fals-Stewart, W. (2008). Brief family treatment intervention to promote continuing care among alcohol-dependent patients in inpatient detoxification: A randomized pilot study. *Journal of Substance Abuse Treatment, 34,* 363–369.

Office of the United Nations High Commission on Human Rights. (2005). *Report of the sixty-first session of the Commission on Human Rights.* Geneva: United Nations.

Orford, J., & Edwards, G. (1977). *Alcoholism: A comparison of treatment and advice, with a study of influence of marriage* (Maudsley Monographs No. 26). New York: Oxford University Press.

Orford, J., & Keddie, A. (1986). Abstinence or controlled drinking in clinical practice: Indications at initial assessment. *Addictive Behaviors, 11,* 71–86.

Orford, J., Natera, G., Davies, J., Nava, A., Mora, J., Rigby, K., et al. (1998). Tolerate, engage or withdraw: A study of the structure of families coping with alcohol and drug problems in south west England and Mexico City. *Addiction, 93,* 1799–1813.

Orford, J., Templeton, L., Velleman, R., & Copello, A. (2005). Family members of relatives with alcohol, drug and gambling problems: A set of standardized questionnaires for assessing stress, coping and strain. *Addiction, 100,* 1611–1624.

Ossip-Klein, D. J., & Rychtarik, R. G. (1993). Behavioral contracts between alcoholics and family members: Improving aftercare participation and maintaining sobriety after inpatient alcoholism treatment. In T. J. O'Farrell (Ed.), *Treating alcohol problems: Marital and family interventions* (pp. 281–304). New York: Guilford Press.

Ossip-Klein, D. J., Vanlandingham, W., Prue, D. M., & Rychtarik, R. G. (1984). Increasing attendance at alcohol aftercare using calendar prompts and home based contracting. *Addictive Behaviors, 9,* 85–89.

Palepu, A., Horton, N. J., Tibbetts, N., Meli, S., & Samet, J. H. (2004). Uptake and adherence to highly active antiretroviral therapy among HIV-infected people with alcohol and other substance use problems: The impact of substance abuse treatment. *Addiction, 99,* 361–368.

Palmer, R. S., Ball, S. A., Rounsaville, B. J., & O'Malley, S. S. (2007). Concurrent and predictive validity of drug use and psychiatric diagnosis among first-time DWI offenders. *Alcoholism: Clinical and Experimental Research, 31,* 619–624.

Panas, L., Caspi, Y., Fournier, E., & McCarty, D. (2003). Performance measures for outpatient substance abuse services: Group versus individual counseling. *Journal of Substance Abuse Treatment, 25,* 271–278.

Pantalon, M. V., Nich, C., Franckforter, T., & Carroll, K. M. (2002). The URICA as a measure of motivation to change among treatment-seeking individuals with concurrent alcohol and cocaine problems. *Psychology of Addictive Behaviors, 16,* 299–307.

Paolino, T. J., & McCrady, B. S. (1977). *The alcoholic marriage: Alternative perspectives.* New York: Grune & Stratton.

Penberthy, J. K., Ait-Daoud, N., Breton, M., Kovatchev, B., DiClemente, C. C., & Johnson, B. A. (2007). Evaluating readiness and treatment seeking effects in a pharmacotherapy trial for alcohol dependence. *Alcoholism: Clinical and Experimental Research, 31,* 1538–1544.

Perron, B. E., & Bright, C. L. (2008). The influence of legal coercion on dropout from substance abuse treatment: Results from a national survey. *Drug and Alcohol Dependence, 92,* 123–131.

Persons, J. B. (2008). *The case formulation approach to cognitive-behavior therapy.* New York: Guilford Press.

Perz, C. A., DiClemente, C. C., & Carbonari, J. P. (1996). Doing the right thing at the right time?: Interaction of stages and processes of change in successful smoking cessation. *Health Psychology, 15,* 462–468.

Peteet, J. R., Brenner, S., Curtiss, D., Ferrigno, M., & Kauffman, J. (1998). A stage of change approach to addiction in the medical setting. *General Hospital Psychiatry, 20,* 267–373.

Peterson, K. A., Swindle, R. W., Phibbs, C. S., Recine, B., & Moos, R. H. (1994). Determinants of readmission following inpatient substance abuse treatment: A national study of VA programs. *Medical Care, 32,* 535–550.

Petry, N. M. (2000). A comprehensive guide to the application of contingency management procedures in clinical settings. *Drug and Alcohol Dependence, 58,* 9–25.

Piazza, N. J., Vrbka, J. L., & Yeager, R. D. (1989). Telescoping of alcoholism in women alcoholics. *International Journal of the Addictions, 24,* 19–28.

Pierce, J. P., Farkas, A., Zhu, S.-H., Berry, C., & Kaplan, R. M. (1996). Should the stage of change model be challenged? *Addiction, 91,* 1290–1293.

Pirard, S., Estee, S., Kang, S. K., Angarita, G. A., & Gastfriend, D. R. (2005). Prevalence of physical and sexual abuse among substance abuse patients and impact on treatment outcomes. *Drug and Alcohol Dependence, 78,* 57–64.

Pokorny, A. D., Miller, B. A., & Kaplan, H. B. (1972). The brief MAST: A shortened version of the Michigan Alcoholism Screening Test. *American Journal of Psychiatry, 129,* 342–345.

Polcin, D. L., & Beattie, M. (2007). Relationship and institutional pressure to enter treatment: Differences by demographics, problem severity, and motivation. *Journal of Studies on Alcohol and Drugs, 68*, 428–436.

Polich, J. M., Armor, D. J., & Braiker, H. B. (1981). *The course of alcoholism: Four years after treatment.* New York: Wiley.

Powers, M. B., Vedel, E., & Emmelkamp, P. M. (2008). Behavioral couples therapy (BCT) for alcohol and drug use disorders: A meta-analysis. *Clinical Psychology Review, 28*, 952–962.

Prendergast, M. L., Messina, N. P., Hall, E. A., & Warda, U. S. (2011). The relative effectiveness of women-only and mixed-gender treatment for substance-abusing women. *Journal of Substance Abuse Treatment, 40*, 336–348.

Prendergast, M. L., Podus, D., Finney, J., Greenwell, L., & Roll, J. (2006). Contingency management for treatment of substance use disorders: A meta-analysis. *Addiction, 101*, 1546–1560.

Prevention Research Institute. (2009). *PRIME for life.* Lexington, KY: Author.

Price, R. K., Cottler, L. B., & Robins, L. N. (1991). Patterns of drug abuse treatment utilization in a general population. In L. Harris (Ed.), *Problems of drug dependence, 1990* (pp. 466–467). Washington, DC: U.S. Government Printing Office.

Prochaska, J. O. (1979). *Systems of psychotherapy: A transtheoretical analysis.* Homewood, IL: Dorsey Press.

Prochaska, J. O. (1984). *Systems of psychotherapy: A transtheoretical analysis* (2nd ed.). Homewood, IL: Dorsey Press.

Prochaska, J. O., & DiClemente, C. C. (1982). Transtheoretical therapy: Toward a more integrative model of change. *Psychotherapy: Theory, Research and Practice, 19*, 276–288.

Prochaska, J. O., & DiClemente, C. C. (1983). Stages and processes of self-change of smoking: Toward an integrative model of change. *Journal of Consulting and Clinical Psychology, 51*, 390–395.

Prochaska, J. O., & DiClemente, C. C. (1984). *The transtheoretical approach: Crossing the traditional boundaries of therapy.* Malabar, FL: Krieger.

Prochaska, J. O., & DiClemente, C. C. (1986). Toward a comprehensive model of change. In W. R. Miller & N. Heather (Eds.), *Treating addictive behaviors: Processes of change* (pp. 3–27). New York: Plenum Press.

Prochaska, J. O., & DiClemente, C. C. (1992). Stages of change in the modification of problem behaviors. In M. Hersen, R. M. Eisler, & P. M. Miller (Eds.), *Progress in behavior modification* (Vol. 28, pp. 183–218). Sycamore, IL: Sycamore.

Prochaska, J. O., & DiClemente, C. C. (1998). Comments, criteria and creating better models. In W. R. Miller & N. Heather (Eds.), *Treating addictive behaviors* (2nd ed., pp. 39–45). New York: Plenum Press.

Prochaska, J. O., DiClemente, C. C., & Norcross, J. C. (1992). In search of how people change: Applications to addictive behaviors. *American Psychologist, 47*, 1102–1114.

Prochaska, J. O., DiClemente, C. C., Velicer, W. F., Ginpil, S. E., & Norcross, J. C. (1985). Predicting change in smoking status for self-changers. *Addictive Behaviors, 10*, 395–406.

Prochaska, J. O., DiClemente, C. C., Velicer, W. F., & Rossi, J. S. (1993). Standardized, individualized, interactive and personalized self-help programs for smoking cessation. *Health Psychology, 12*, 399–405.

Prochaska, J. O., & Norcross, J. C. (1999). *Systems of psychotherapy: A transtheoretical analysis* (4th ed.). Pacific Grove, CA: Brooks/Cole.

Prochaska, J. O., & Norcross, J. (2007). *Systems of psychotherapy: A transtheoretical analysis* (7th ed.). New York: Brooks/Cole.

Prochaska, J. O., Norcross, J. C., & DiClemente, C. C. (1994). *Changing for good.* New York: Morrow.

Prochaska, J. O., Velicer, W. F., DiClemente, C. C., & Fava, J. (1988). Measuring processes of change: Applications to the cessation of smoking. *Journal of Consulting and Clinical Psychology, 56,* 520–528.

Prochaska, J. O., Velicer, W. F., Guadagnoli, E., Rossi, J. S., & DiClemente, C. C. (1991). Patterns of change: Dynamic typology applied to smoking cessation. *Multivariate Behavioral Research, 26,* 83–107.

Prochaska, J. O., Velicer, W. F., Rossi, J. S., Goldstein, M. G., Marcus, B. H., Rakowski, W., et al. (1994). Stages of change and decisional balance for twelve problem behaviors. *Health Psychology, 13,* 39–46.

Project CHOICES Intervention Research Group. (2003). Reducing the risk of alcohol-exposed pregnancies: A study of a motivational intervention in community settings. *Pediatrics, 111,* 1131–1135.

Project CHOICES Research Group. (2002). Alcohol-exposed pregnancy: Characteristics associated with risk. *American Journal of Preventive Medicine, 23,* 166–173.

Project MATCH Research Group. (1997a). Matching alcoholism treatments to client heterogeneity: Project MATCH posttreatment drinking outcomes. *Journal of Studies on Alcohol, 58,* 7–29.

Project MATCH Research Group. (1997b). Project MATCH secondary a priori hypotheses. *Addiction, 92,* 1671–1698.

Project MATCH Research Group. (1998a). Matching alcoholism treatments to client heterogeneity: Project MATCH three year drinking outcomes. *Alcoholism: Clinical and Experimental Research, 22,* 1300–1311.

Project MATCH Research Group. (1998b). Therapist effects in three treatments for alcohol problems. *Psychotherapy Research, 8,* 455–474.

Ramlow, B. E., White, A. L., Watson, D. D., & Leukefeld, C. G. (1997). The needs of women with substance use problems: An expanded vision for treatment. *Substance Use and Misuse, 32,* 1395–1404.

Randall, C. L., Roberts, J. S., Del Boca, F. K., Carroll, K. M., Connors, G. J., & Mattson, M. E. (1999). Telescoping of landmark events associated with drinking: A gender comparison. *Journal of Studies on Alcohol, 60,* 252–260.

Rapp, R. C., Otto, A. L., Lane, D. T., Redko, C., McGatha, S., & Carlson, R. G. (2008a). Improving linkage with substance abuse treatment using brief case management and motivational interviewing. *Drug and Alcohol Dependence, 94,* 172–182.

Rapp, R. C., Xu, J., Carr, C. A., Lane, D. T., Redko, C., & Carlson, R. G. (2008b). Development of the Pretreatment Readiness Scale for Substance Abusers: Modification of an existing motivation assessment. *Substance Abuse, 29,* 39–50.

Rapp, R. C., Xu, J., Carr, C. A., Lane, T., Wang, J., & Carlson, R. (2006). Treatment barriers identified by substance abusers assessed at a centralized intake unit. *Journal of Substance Abuse Treatment, 30,* 227–235.

Ray, G. T., Mertens, J. R., & Weisner, C. (2007). The excess medical cost and health problems of family members of persons diagnosed with alcohol or drug problems. *Medical Care, 45,* 116–122.

Ray, G. T., Mertens, J. R., & Weissner, C. (2009). Family members of people with alcohol or drug dependence: Health problems and medical cost compared to family members of people with diabetes and asthma. *Addiction, 104,* 203–214.

Regier, D. A., Farmer, M. E., Rae, O. S., Locke, B. Z., Keith, S. J., Judd, L. L., et al. (1990). Comorbidity of mental disorders with alcohol and other drug abuse. *Journal of the American Medical Association, 264,* 2511–2518.

Rehm, J., Taylor, B., & Room, R. (2006). Global burden of disease from alcohol, illicit drugs, and tobacco. *Drug and Alcohol Review, 25,* 503–513.

Rider, R., Kelley-Baker, T., Voas, R. B., Murphy, B., McKnight, A. J., & Levings, C. (2006).

The impact of a novel educational curriculum for first-time DUI offenders on intermediate outcomes relevant to DUI recidivism. *Accident Analysis and Prevention, 38,* 482–489.

Rider, R., Voas, R. B., Kelley-Baker, T., Grosz, M., & Murphy, B. (2007). Preventing alcohol-related convictions: The effect of a novel curriculum for first-time offenders on DUI recidivism. *Traffic Injury Prevention, 8,* 147–152.

Rinaldi, R. C., Steindler, E. M., Wilford, B. B., & Goodwin, D. (1988). Clarification and standardization of substance abuse terminology. *Journal of the American Medical Association, 259,* 555–557.

Ritter, J., Stewart, M., Bernet, C., Coe, M., & Brown, S. A. (2002). Effects of childhood exposure to familial alcoholism and family violence on adolescent substance use, conduct problems, and self-esteem. *Journal of Traumatic Stress, 15,* 113–122.

Roberts, K. S., & Brent, E. E. (1982). Physician utilization and illness patterns in families of alcoholics. *Journal of Studies on Alcohol, 43,* 119–128.

Robertson, A. A., Gardner, S., Xu, X., & Costello, H. (2009). The impact of remedial intervention on 3–year recidivism among first-time DUI offenders in Mississippi. *Accident Analysis and Prevention, 41,* 1080–1086.

Robertson, A. A., Liew, H., & Gardner, S. (2011). An evaluation of the narrowing gender gap in DUI arrests. *Accident Analysis and Prevention, 43,* 1414–1420.

Robinson, J., Sareen, J., Cox, B. J., & Bolton, J. (2009). Self-medication of anxiety disorders with alcohol and drugs: Results from a nationally representative sample. *Journal of Anxiety Disorders, 23,* 38–45.

Roe, B., Beynon, C., Pickering, L., & Duffy, P. (2010). Experiences of drug use and ageing: Health, quality of life, relationship and service implications. *Journal of Advanced Nursing, 66,* 1968–1979.

Rohsenow, D. J., Monti, P. M., Martin, R. A., Colby, S. M., Myers, M. G., Gulliver, S. B., et al. (2004). Motivational enhancement and coping skills training for cocaine abusers: Effects on substance use outcomes. *Addiction, 99,* 862–874.

Rollnick, S., & Heather, N. (1982). The application of Bandura's self-efficacy theory to abstinence-oriented alcoholism treatment. *Addictive Behaviors, 7,* 243–250.

Rollnick, S., Heather, N., Gold, R., & Hall, W. (1992). Development of a short "readiness to change" questionnaire for use in brief, opportunistic interventions among excessive drinkers. *British Journal on Addictions, 87,* 743–754.

Rollnick, S., Mason, P., & Butler, C. (1999). *Health behavior change.* London: Churchill Livingstone.

Rollnick, S., Miller, W. R., & Butler, C. (2008). *Motivational interviewing in health care: Helping patients change behavior.* New York: Guilford Press.

Room, R. (1989). The U.S. general population's experiences of responding to alcohol problems. *British Journal of Addiction, 84,* 1291–1304.

Roozen, H. G., de Waart, R., & van der Kroft, P. (2010). Community reinforcement and family training: An effective option to engage treatment-resistant substance-abusing individuals in treatment. *Addiction, 105,* 1729–1738.

Rosen, T. J., & Shipley, R. H. (1983). A stage analysis of self-initiated smoking reductions. *Addictive Behaviors, 8,* 263–272.

Rosen, D., Tolman, R. M., & Warner, L. A. (2004). Low-income women's use of substance abuse and mental health services. *Journal of Health Care for the Poor and Underserved, 15,* 206–219.

Ross, S. (2008). The mentally ill substance abuser. In M. Galanter & H. D. Kleber (Eds.), *Textbook of substance abuse treatment* (4th ed., pp. 537–554). Washington, DC: American Psychiatric Publishing.

Rotgers, F., Keller, D. S., & Morgenstern, J. (1996). *Treating substance abuse: Theory and technique.* New York: Guilford Press.

Rotgers, F., Morgenstern, J., & Walters, S. T. (Eds.). (2003). *Treating substance abuse: Theory and technique* (2nd ed.). New York: Guilford Press.

Roth, A., & Fonagy, P. (1996). Alcohol dependency and abuse. In A. Roth & P. Fonagy (Eds.), *What works for whom?: A critical review of psychotherapy research* (pp. 216–233). New York: Guilford Press.

Roth, R., Marques, P. R., & Voas, R. B. (2009). A note on the effectiveness of the house-arrest alternative for motivating DWI offenders to install ignition interlocks. *Journal of Safety Research, 40,* 437–441.

Rothfleisch, J. (1997). *Assessing different measures of stages of change with cocaine dependent clients.* Unpublished doctoral dissertation, University of Houston.

Rotunda, R. J., West, L., & O'Farrell, T. J. (2004). Enabling behavior in a clinical sample of alcohol-dependent clients and their partners. *Journal of Substance Abuse Treatment, 26,* 269–276.

Rounsaville, B. J. (1986). Clinical implications of relapse research. In F. M. Tims & C. G. Leukefeld (Eds.), *Relapse and recovery in drug abuse* (pp. 172–184). Rockville, MD: National Institute on Drug Abuse.

Rounsaville, B. J., & Carroll, K. M. (1997). Individual psychotherapy. In J. H. Lowinson, P. Ruiz, R. B. Millman, & J. G. Langrod (Eds.), *Substance abuse: A comprehensive textbook* (3rd ed., pp. 430–439). Baltimore: Williams & Wilkins.

Rubin, A., Stout, R. L., & Longabaugh, R. (1996). Gender differences in relapse situations. *Addiction, 91*(Suppl.), S111–S120.

Rush, M. M. (2002). Perceived social support: Dimensions of social interaction among sober female participants in Alcoholics Anonymous. *Journal of the American Psychiatric Nurses Association, 8,* 114–119.

Ryan, R. M., Plant, R. W., & O'Malley, S. (1995). Initial motivations for alcohol treatment: Relations with patient characteristics, treatment involvement, and dropout. *Addictive Behaviors, 20,* 279–297.

Rychtarik, R. G. (1990). Alcohol-related coping skills in spouses of alcoholics: Assessment and implications for treatment. In R. L. Collins, K. E. Leonard, & J. S. Searles (Eds.), *Alcohol and the family: Research and clinical perspectives* (pp. 356–379). New York: Guilford Press.

Rychtarik, R. G., Koutsky, J. R., & Miller, W. R. (1998). Profiles of the Alcohol Use Inventory: A large sample cluster analysis conducted with split-sample replication rules. *Psychological Assessment, 10,* 107–119.

Rychtarik, R. G., Koutsky, J. R., & Miller, W. R. (1999). Profiles of the Alcohol Use Inventory: Correction to Rychtarik, Koutsky, and Miller (1998). *Psychological Assessment, 11,* 396–402.

Rychtarik, R. G., Prue, D. M., Rapp, S. R., & King, A. C. (1992). Self-efficacy, aftercare and relapse in a treatment program for alcoholics. *Journal of Studies on Alcohol, 53,* 435–440.

Saatcioglu, O., Erim, R., & Cakmak, D. (2006). Role of family in alcohol and substance abuse. *Psychiatry and Clinical Neurosciences, 60,* 125–132.

Sacks, J. A. Y., Drake, R. E., Williams, V. F., Banks, S. M., & Herrell, J. M. (2003). Utility of the time-line follow-back to assess substance use among homeless adults. *Journal of Nervous and Mental Disease, 191,* 145–153.

Samet, J. H., & O'Connor, P. G. (1998). Alcohol abusers in primary care: Readiness to change behavior. *American Journal of Medicine, 105,* 302–306.

Sanchez-Craig, M., Annis, H. M., Bornet, A. R., & MacDonald, K. R. (1984). Random assignment to abstinence and controlled drinking: Evaluation of a cognitive behavioral program for problem drinkers. *Journal of Consulting and Clinical Psychology, 52,* 390–403.

Sandler, J., Holder, A., & Dare, C. (1970). Basic psychoanalytic concepts: V. Resistance. *British Journal of Psychiatry, 117*, 215–221.

Saunders, B., Baily, S., Phillips, M., & Allsop, S. (1993). Women with alcohol problems: Do they relapse for reasons different to their male counterparts? *Addiction, 88*, 1423–1422.

Saunders, J. B., Aasland, O. G., Babor, T. F., de la Fuente, J. R., & Grant, M. (1993). Development of the Alcohol Use Disorders Identification Test (AUDIT): WHO collaborative project on early detection of persons with harmful alcohol consumption—II. *Addiction, 88*, 791–804.

Scharff, J. L., Broida, J. P., Conway, K., & Yue, A. (2004). The interaction of parental alcoholism, adaptation role, and familial dysfunction. *Addictive Behaviors, 29*, 575–581.

Schaub, M., Stevens, A., Berto, D., Hunt, N., Kerschl, V., McSweeney, T., et al. (2010). Comparing outcomes of "voluntary" and "quasi-compulsory" treatment of substance dependence in Europe. *European Addiction Research, 16*, 53–60.

Scheidlinger, S. (2000). The group psychotherapy movement at the millennium: Some historical perspectives. *International Journal of Group Psychotherapy, 50*, 315–339.

Schermer, C. R., Moyers, T. B., Miller, W. R., & Bloomfield, L. A. (2006). Trauma center brief interventions for alcohol disorders decrease subsequent driving under the influence arrests. *Journal of Trauma: Injury, Infection, and Critical Care, 60*, 29–34.

Schober, R., & Annis, H. M. (1996). Barriers to help-seeking for change in drinking: A gender-focused review of the literature. *Addictive Behaviors, 21*, 81–92.

Schrimsher, G. W., & Filtz, K. (2011). Assessment reactivity: Can assessment of alcohol use during research be an active treatment? *Alcoholism Treatment Quarterly, 29*, 108–115.

Schuckit, M. A., Anthenelli, R. M., Bucholz, K. K., Hesselbrock, V. M., & Tipp, J. (1995). The time course of development of alcohol-related problems in men and women. *Journal of Studies on Alcohol, 56*, 218–225.

Schuckit, M. A., Daeppen, J. B., Tipp, J. E., Hesselbrock, M., & Bucholz, K. K. (1998). The clinical course of alcohol-related problems in alcohol dependent and nonalcohol dependent drinking women and men. *Journal of Studies on Alcohol, 59*, 581–590.

Schulz, J. E., & Chappel, J. N. (1998). Twelve step programs. In A. W. Graham, T. K. Schultz, & B. B. Wilford (Eds.), *Principles of addiction medicine* (pp. 693–705). Chevy Chase, MD: American Society of Addiction Medicine.

Schutt, R. K., & Garrett, G. R. (1992). *Responding to the homeless: Policy and practice.* New York: Plenum Press.

Schwartz, J. (2008). Gender differences in drunk driving prevalence rates and trends: A 20-year assessment using multiple sources of evidence. *Addictive Behaviors, 33*, 1217–1222.

Scott, J. (1993). Homelessness and mental illness. *British Journal of Psychiatry, 162*, 314–324.

Seale, P., Boltri, J. M., Shellenberger, S., Velasquez, M. M., Cornelius, M., Guyinn, M., et al. (2006). Primary care validation of a single screening question for drinkers. *Journal of Studies on Alcohol, 67*, 778–784.

Selzer, M. L. (1971). The Michigan Alcoholism Screening Test: The quest for a new diagnostic instrument. *American Journal of Psychiatry, 127*, 1653–1658.

Selzer, M. L., Vinokur, A., & van Rooijen, L. (1975). A self-administered short Michigan Alcoholism Screening Test (SMAST). *Journal of Studies on Alcohol, 36*, 117–126.

Shaffer, H. J. (1992). The psychology of stage change: The transition from addiction to recovery. In J. H. Lowison, P. Ruiz, R. B. Millman, & J. G. Langrod (Eds.), *Substance abuse: A comprehensive textbook* (2nd ed., pp. 100–105). Baltimore: Williams & Wilkins.

Sher, K. J., Gershuny, B. S., Peterson, L., & Raskin, G. (1997). The role of childhood stressors in the intergenerational transmission of alcohol use disorders. *Journal of Studies on Alcohol, 58*, 414–427.

Sheridan, M. J. (1995). A proposed intergenerational model of substance abuse, family functioning, and abuse/neglect. *Child Abuse and Neglect, 19*, 519–530.

Shiffman, S. (1989). Conceptual issues in the study of relapse. In M. Gossop (Ed.), *Relapse and addictive behavior* (pp. 149–179). London: Tavistock/Routledge.

Silverman, K., & Schonberg, S. K. (2001). Adolescent children of drug-abusing parents. *Adolescent Medicine, 12*, 485–491.

Simpson, D. D., & Joe, G. W. (1993). Motivation as a predictor of early drop out from drug abuse treatment. *Psychotherapy, 30*, 357–368.

Simpson, D. D., Joe, G. W., Rowan-Szal, G., & Greener, J. (1995). Client engagement and change during drug abuse treatment. *Journal of Substance Abuse, 7*, 117–134.

Sisson, R. W., & Azrin, N. H. (1993). Community reinforcement training for families: A method to get alcoholics into treatment. In T. J. O'Farrell (Ed.), *Treating alcohol problems: Marital and family interventions* (pp. 34–53). New York: Guilford Press.

Sitharthan, T., & Kavanagh, D. J. (1991). Role of self-efficacy in predicting outcomes from a programme for controlled drinking. *Drug and Alcohol Dependence, 27*, 87–94.

Skinner, H. A. (1982). The Drug Abuse Screening Test. *Addictive Behaviors, 7*, 363–371.

Smith, C. A., Elwyn, L. J., Ireland, T. O., & Thornberry, T. P. (2010). Impact of adolescent exposure to intimate partner violence on substance use in early adulthood. *Journal of Studies on Alcohol and Drugs, 71*, 219–230.

Smith, J. E., Meyers, R. J., & Miller, W. R. (2001). The community reinforcement approach to the treatment of substance use disorders. *American Journal of Addiction, 10*(Suppl.), 51–59.

Smith, J. E., Meyers, R. J., & Waldorf, V. A. (1999). Covering all bases: Engaging and treating individuals with alcohol problems. In J. H. Hannigan, L. P. Spear, N. E. Spear, & C. R. Goodlett (Eds.), *Alcohol and alcoholism: Effects on brain and development* (pp. 202–218). Mahwah, NJ: Erlbaum.

Smith, K. J., Subich, L. M., & Kalodner, C. (1995). The transtheoretical model's stages and processes of change and their relation to premature termination. *Journal of Counseling Psychology, 42*, 34–39.

Smith, P. C., Schmidt, S. M., Allensworth-Davies, D., & Saitz, R. (2009). Primary care validation of a single-question alcohol screening test. *Journal of General Internal Medicine, 24*, 783–788.

Snow, D., & Anderson, C. (2000). Exploring the factors influencing relapse and recovery among drug and alcohol addicted women. *Journal of Psychosocial Nursing and Mental Health Services, 38*, 8–19.

Snow, M., Prochaska, J., & Rossi, J. (1994). Processes of change in Alcoholics Anonymous: Maintenance factors in long-term sobriety. *Journal of Studies on Alcohol, 55*, 362–371.

Sobell, L. C., Cunningham, J. A., Sobell, M. B., & Toneatto, T. (1993). A life-span perspective on natural recovery (self-change) from alcohol problems. In J. S. Baer, G. A. Marlatt, & R. J. McMahon (Eds.), *Addictive behaviors across the life span* (pp. 34–66). Newbury Park, CA: Sage.

Sobell, L. C., Maisto, S. A., Sobell, M. B., & Cooper, A. M. (1979). Reliability of alcohol abusers' self-reports of drinking behavior. *Behaviour Research and Therapy, 17*, 157–160.

Sobell, L. C., & Sobell, M. B. (1992). Timeline follow-back: A technique for assessing self-reported alcohol consumption. In R. Litten & J. Allen (Eds.), *Measuring alcohol consumption* (pp. 41–72). Totowa, NJ: Humana Press.

Sobell, L. C., & Sobell, M. B. (1996). *Alcohol Timeline Followback (TLFB) users' manual.* Toronto: Addiction Research Foundation.

Sobell, L. C., & Sobell, M. B. (2008). Alcohol Timeline Followback (TLFB). In American Psychiatric Association (Ed.), *Textbook of psychiatric measures* (pp. 477–479). Washington, DC: American Psychiatric Association.

Sobell, L. C., & Sobell, M. B. (2011). *Group therapy for substance use disorders: A motivational cognitive-behavioral approach.* New York: Guilford Press.

Sobell, L. C., Sobell, M. B., & Agrawal, C. (2009). Randomized controlled trial of a cognitive-behavioral motivational intervention in a group versus individual format for substance use disorders. *Psychology of Addictive Behaviors, 23,* 672–683.

Sobell, L. C., Sobell, M. B., & Nirenberg, T. D. (1982). Differential treatment planning for alcohol abusers. In E. M. Pattison & E. Kaufman (Eds.), *Encyclopedic handbook of alcoholism* (pp. 1140–1151). New York: Gardner Press.

Sobell, L. C., Sobell, M. B., & Nirenberg, T. D. (1988). Behavioral assessment and treatment planning with alcohol and drug abusers: A review with an emphasis on clinical application. *Clinical Psychology Review, 8,* 19–54.

Sobell, L. C., Sobell, M. B., Toneatto, T., & Leo, G. I. (1993). What triggers the resolution of alcohol problems without treatment? *Alcoholism: Clinical and Experimental Research, 17,* 217–224.

Sobell, L. C., Toneatto, T., & Sobell, M. B. (1994). Behavioral assessment and treatment planning for alcohol, tobacco, and other drug problems: Current status with an emphasis on clinical applications. *Behavior Therapy, 25,* 533–580.

Sobell, M. B., Bogardis, J., Schuller, R., Leo, G. I., & Sobell, L. C. (1989). Is self-monitoring of alcohol consumption reactive? *Behavioral Assessment, 11,* 447–458.

Sobell, M. B., & Sobell, L. C. (1981). Functional analysis of alcohol problems. In C. K. Prokop & L. A. Bradley (Eds.), *Medical psychology: Contributions to behavioral medicine* (pp. 81–90). New York: Academic Press.

Sobell, M. B., & Sobell, L. C. (1993). *Problem drinkers: Guided self-change treatment.* New York: Guilford Press.

Soderstrom, C. A., DiClemente, C. C., Dischinger, P. C., Hebel, J. R., McDuff, D. R., Auman, K. M., et al. (2007). A controlled brief intervention versus brief advice for at-risk drinking trauma center patients. *Journal of Trauma: Injury, Infection and Critical Care, 62,* 1102–1112.

Solomon, K. E., & Annis, H. M. (1990). Outcome and efficacy expectancy in the prediction of posttreatment drinking behaviour. *British Journal of Addiction, 85,* 659–665.

Solomon, R. L. (1980). The opponent–process theory of acquired motivation: The costs of pleasure and the benefits of pain. *American Psychologist, 35,* 691–712.

Spinks, S. H., & Birchler, G. R. (1982). Behavioral-systems marital therapy: Dealing with resistance. *Family Process, 21,* 169–185.

Stanger, C., & Budney, A. J. (2010). Contingency management approaches for adolescent substance use disorders. *Child and Adolescent Psychiatric Clinics of North America, 19,* 547–562.

Stanton, M. D. (1997). The role of family and significant others in the engagement and retention of drug-dependent individuals. In L. S. Onken, J. D. Blaine, & F. J. Boren (Eds.), *Beyond the therapeutic alliance: Keeping the drug dependent individual in treatment* (pp. 157–180). Rockville, MD: National Institute on Drug Abuse.

Stanton, M. D. (2004). Getting reluctant substance abusers to engage in treatment/self-help: A review of outcomes and clinical options. *Journal of Marital and Family Therapy, 30,* 165–182.

Stasiewicz, P. R., & Smith, K. E. (2002). Addictions in special populations: Treatment. In M. Hersen & W. Sledge (Eds.), *Encyclopedia of psychotherapy* (pp. 9–14). New York: Academic Press.

Stein, L. A. R., Minugh, P. A., Longabaugh, R., Wirtz, P., Baird, J., Nirenberg, T. D., et al.

(2009). Readiness to change as a mediator of a brief motivational intervention on post-treatment alcohol-related consequences of injured emergency department hazardous drinkers. *Psychology of Addictive Behaviors, 23*, 185–195.

Stevens, A., Berto, D., Frick, U., Hunt, N., Kerschl, V., McSweeney, T., et al. (2006). The relationship between legal status, perceived pressure and motivation in treatment for drug dependence: Results from a European study of quasi-compulsory treatment. *European Addiction Research, 12*, 197–209.

Stewart, D., Gossop, M., & Trakada, K. (2007). Drug dependent parents: Childcare responsibilities, involvement with treatment services, and treatment outcomes. *Addictive Behaviors, 32*, 1657–1668.

Stinchfield, R., Owen, P. L., & Winters, K. C. (1994). Group therapy for substance abuse: A review of the empirical evidence. In A. Fuhriman & G. M. Burlingame (Eds.), *Handbook of group psychotherapy: An empirical and clinical synthesis* (pp. 458–488). New York: Wiley.

Stitzer, M., & Petry, N. (2006). Contingency management for treatment of substance abuse. *Annual Review of Clinical Psychology, 2*, 411–434.

Stitzer, M. L., & Vandrey, R. (2008). Contingency management: Utility in the treatment of drug abuse disorders. *Clinical Pharmacology and Therapeutics, 83*, 644–647.

Stotts, A., DiClemente, C. C., Carbonari, J. P., & Mullen, P. (1996). Pregnancy smoking cessation: A case of mistaken identity. *Addictive Behaviors, 21*, 459–471.

Stotts, A. L., DiClemente, C. C., Carbonari, J. P., & Mullen, P. D. (2000). Postpartum return to smoking: Staging a suspended behavior. *Health Psychology, 19*, 324–332.

Stotts, A. L., Schmitz, J. M., Rhoades, H. M., & Grabowski, J. (2001). Motivational interviewing with cocaine-dependent patients: A pilot study. *Journal of Consulting and Clinical Psychology, 69*, 858–862.

Substance Abuse and Mental Health Services Administration (2008). *Results from the 2007 National Survey on Drug Use and Health: National findings*. Rockville, MD: Author.

Substance Abuse and Mental Health Services Administration. (2011). *Results from the 2010 National Survey on Drug Use and Health: Summary of national findings*. Rockville, MD: U.S. Department of Health and Human Services.

Sullivan, M. A., Birkmayer, F., Boyarsky, B. K., Frances, R. J., Fromson, J. A., Galanter, M., et al. (2008). Uses of coercion in addiction treatment: Clinical aspects. *American Journal of Addiction, 17*, 36–47.

Sullivan, W. P. (1994). Case management and community-based treatment of women with substance abuse problems. *Journal of Case Management, 3*, 158–161.

Sutton, S. (1996). Can "stages of change" provide guidance in treatment of addiction?: A critical examination of Prochaska & DiClemente's model. In G. Edwards & C. Dare (Eds.), *Psychotherapy, psychological treatments and the addictions* (pp. 189–205). New York: Cambridge University Press.

Swenson, W. M., & Morse, R. M. (1975). The use of a self-administered alcoholism screening test (SAAST) in a medical center. *Mayo Clinic Proceedings, 50*, 204–208.

Szuster, R. R., Rich, L. L., Chung, A., & Bisconer, S. W. (1996). Treatment retention in women's residential chemical dependency treatment: The effect of admission with children. *Substance Use and Misuse, 31*, 1001–1013.

Tang, Z., Claus, R. E., Orwin, R. G., Kissin, W. B., & Arieira, C. (2012). Measurement of gender-sensitive treatment for women in mixed-gender substance abuse treatment programs. *Drug and Alcohol Dependence, 123*, 160–166.

Tempier, R., Boyer, R., Lambert, J., Mosier, K., & Duncan, C. R. (2006). Psychological distress among female spouses of male at-risk drinkers. *Alcohol, 40*, 41–49.

Templeton, L. J., Zohhadi, S. E., & Velleman, R. D. (2007). Working with family members in specialist drug and alcohol services: Findings from a feasibility study. *Drugs: Education, Prevention and Policy, 14,* 137–150.

Thavorncharoensap, M., Teerawattananon, Y., Yothasamut, J., Lertpitakpong, C., & Chaikledkaew, U. (2009). The economic impact of alcohol consumption: A systematic review. *Substance Abuse Treatment, Prevention, and Policy, 4,* 20–30.

Thom, B. (1987). Sex differences in help-seeking for alcohol problems: Entry into treatment. *British Journal of Addiction, 82,* 989–997.

Thomas, E. J. (1994). The spouse as a positive rehabilitative influence in reaching the uncooperative alcohol abuser. In D. K. Granvold (Ed.), *Cognitive and behavioral treatment: Methods and applications* (pp. 159–173). Pacific Grove, CA: Brooks/Cole.

Thomas, E. J., & Ager, R. D. (1993). Unilateral family therapy with spouses of uncooperative alcohol abusers. In T. J. O'Farrell (Ed.), *Treating alcohol problems: Marital and family interventions* (pp. 3–33). New York: Guilford Press.

Thomas, E. J., & Santa, C. A. (1982). Unilateral family therapy for alcohol abuse: A working conception. *American Journal of Family Therapy, 10,* 49–58.

Thomas, E. J., Santa, C., Bronson, D., & Oyserman, D. (1987). Unilateral family therapy with the spouses of alcoholics. *Journal of Social Service Research, 10,* 145–162.

Thomas, E. J., Yoshioka, M., & Ager, R. D. (1996). Spouse enabling of alcohol abuse: Conception, assessment, and modification. *Journal of Substance Abuse, 8,* 61–80.

Tiffany, S. T. (1990). A cognitive model of drug urges and drug-use behavior: Role of automatic and nonautomatic processes. *Psychological Review, 97,* 147–168.

Tiffany, S. T. (1992). A critique of contemporary urge and craving research: Methodological, psychometric, and theoretical issues. *Advances in Behaviour Research and Therapy, 14,* 123–139.

Tonigan, J. S., & Hiller-Sturmhofel, S. (1994). Alcoholics Anonymous: Who benefits? *Alcohol Health and Research World, 18,* 308–310.

Tonigan, J. S., Miller, W. R., & Brown, J. M. (1997). The reliability of Form 90: An instrument for assessing alcohol treatment outcome. *Journal of Studies on Alcohol, 58,* 358–364.

Tsoh, J. (1995). *Stages of change, drop-outs and outcome in substance abuse treatment.* Unpublished doctoral dissertation, University of Rhode Island, Kingston.

Tuchman, E. (2010). Women and addiction: The importance of gender issues in substance abuse research. *Journal of Addictive Diseases, 29,* 127–138.

Tucker, J. A. (2001). Resolving problems associated with alcohol and drug misuse: Understanding relations between addictive behavior change and the use of services. *Substance Use and Misuse, 36,* 1501–1518.

Tucker, J. A., Vuchinich, R. E., & Pukish, M. M. (1995). Molar environmental contexts surrounding recovery from alcohol problems by treated and untreated problem drinkers. *Experimental and Clinical Psychopharmacology, 3,* 195–204.

Turkat, I. D., & Meyer, V. (1982). The behavior-analytic approach. In P. L. Wachtel (Ed.), *Resistance: Psychodynamic and behavioral approaches* (pp. 157–184). New York: Plenum Press.

Urbanoski, K. A. (2010). Coerced addiction treatment: Client perspectives and the implications of their neglect. *Harm Reduction Journal, 7,* 13.

U. S. Department of Justice. (2011). *The economic impact of illicit drug use on American society.* Washington, DC: National Drug Intelligence Center.

Vaillant, G. E. (1977). *Adaptation to life.* Boston: Little, Brown.

Vaillant, G. E. (1995). *The natural history of alcoholism revisited.* Cambridge, MA: Harvard University Press.

Vanable, P. A., McKirnan, D. J., Buchbinder, S. P., Bartholomew, B. N., Douglas, J. M., Judson, F. N., et al. (2004). Alcohol use and high-risk sexual behavior among men who have sex with men: The effects of consumption level and partner type. *Health Psychology, 23,* 525–532.

Van Horn, D. H. A., & Bux, D. A. (2001). A pilot test of motivational interviewing groups for dually diagnosed inpatients. *Journal of Substance Abuse Treatment, 20,* 191–195.

Vannicelli, M. (1992). *Removing the roadblocks: Group psychotherapy with substance abusers and family members.* New York: Guilford Press.

Velasquez, M. M. (2006, June). *Incorporating the processes of change into treatment using therapist and client perspectives: Making process activity central to treatment for substance abuse.* Paper presented at the MPACT Conference, University of Maryland, Baltimore County.

Velasquez, M. M., Carbonari, J. P., & DiClemente, C. C. (1999). Psychiatric severity and behavior change in alcoholism: The relation of the transtheoretical model variables to psychiatric distress in dually diagnosed patients. *Addictive Behaviors, 24,* 481–496.

Velasquez, M. M., Crouch, C., von Sternberg, K., & Grosdanis, I. (2000). Motivation for change and psychological distress in homeless substance abusers. *Journal of Substance Abuse Treatment, 19,* 395–401.

Velasquez, M. M., Ingersoll, K. S., Sobell, M. B., Floyd, R. L., Sobell, L. C., & von Sternberg, K. (2010). A dual-focus motivational intervention to reduce the risk of alcohol-exposed pregnancy. *Cognitive and Behavioral Practice, 17,* 203–212.

Velasquez, M. M., Maurer, G., Crouch, C., & DiClemente, C. C. (2001). *Group treatment for substance abuse: A stages-of-change therapy manual.* New York: Guilford Press.

Velasquez, M. M., Stephens, N., & Drenner, K. (2013). The transtheoretical model and motivational interviewing: Experiences with a cocaine treatment group. In C. C. Wagner & K. S. Ingersoll (Eds.), *Motivational interviewing in groups.* New York: Guilford Press.

Velasquez, M. M., Stephens, N., & Ingersoll, K. (2006). Motivational interviewing in groups. *Journal of Groups in Addiction and Recovery, 1,* 27–50.

Velasquez, M. M., von Sternberg, K., Johnson, D. H., Green, C., Carbonari, J. P., & Parsons, J. T. (2009). Reducing sexual risk behaviors and alcohol use among HIV-positive men who have sex with men: A randomized clinical trial. *Journal of Consulting and Clinical Psychology, 77,* 657–667.

Velasquez, M. M., von Sternberg, K., & Stephens, N. (2011, June). *Motivational interviewing in groups: Alcohol use and reduction in a group treatment for cocaine.* Paper presented at the symposium Group Motivational Interviewing Interventions with High Risk Adolescents and Adult Populations at the annual meeting of the Research Society on Alcoholism, San Antonio, TX.

Velicer, W. F., DiClemente, C. C., Rossi, J., & Prochaska, J. O. (1990). Relapse situations and self-efficacy: An integrative model. *Addictive Behaviors, 15,* 271–283.

Velicer, W. F., Prochaska, J. O., Bellis, J. M., DiClemente, C. C., Rossi, J. S., Fava, J. L., et al. (1993). An expert system intervention for smoking cessation. *Addictive Behaviors, 18,* 269–290.

Velleman, R., Bennett, G., Miller, T., Orford, J., Rigby, K., & Tod, A. (1993). The families of problem drug users: A study of 50 close relatives. *Addiction, 88,* 1281–1289.

Voas, R. B., Blackman, K. O., Tippetts, A. S., & Marques, P. R. (2002). Evaluation of a program to motivate impaired driving offenders to install ignition interlocks. *Accident Analysis and Prevention, 34,* 449–455.

Voas, R. B., DuPont, R. L., Talpins, S. K., & Shea, C. L. (2011). Towards a national model for managing impaired driving offenders. *Addiction, 106,* 1221–1227.

Voas, R. B., & Fisher, D. A. (2001). Court procedures for handling intoxicated drivers. *Alcohol Research and Health, 25,* 32–42.

Voas, R. B., & Marques, P. R. (2004). Emerging technological approaches for controlling the hard core DUI offender in the U.S. *Traffic Injury Prevention, 5,* 309–316.

Wagner, C. C., & Ingersoll, K. S. (Eds.). (2013). *Motivational interviewing in groups.* New York: Guilford Press.

Waldron, H. B., Kern-Jones, S., Turner, C. W., Peterson, T. R., & Ozechowski, T. J. (2007). Engaging resistant adolescents in drug abuse treatment. *Journal of Substance Abuse Treatment, 32,* 133–142.

Walitzer, K. S., & Dearing, R. L. (2006). Gender differences in alcohol and substance use relapse. *Clinical Psychology Review, 26,* 128–148.

Wallace, B. B. (1989). Psychological and environmental determinants of relapse in crack cocaine smokers. *Journal of Substance Abuse Treatment, 6,* 95–106.

Wanberg, K. W., Horn, J. L., & Foster, F. M. (1977). A differential assessment model of alcoholism: The scales of the Alcohol Use Inventory. *Journal of Studies on Alcohol, 38,* 512–543.

Washton, A. M. (1987). Outpatient treatment techniques. In A. M. Washton & M. S. Gold (Eds.), *Cocaine: A clinician's handbook* (pp. 106–117). New York: Guilford Press.

Washton, A. M. (1988). Preventing relapse to cocaine. *Journal of Clinical Psychiatry, 49*(Suppl.), 34–38.

Washton, A. M. (1992). Structured outpatient group therapy with alcohol and substance abusers. In J. H. Lowinson, P. Ruiz, R. B. Millman, & J. G. Langrod (Eds.), *Substance abuse: A comprehensive textbook* (pp. 508–519). Baltimore: Williams & Wilkins.

Weisner, C., Parthasarathy, S., Moore, C., & Mertens, J.R. (2010). Individuals receiving addiction treatment: Are medical costs of their family members reduced? *Addiction, 105,* 1226–1234.

Weiss, R. D., Jaffee, W. B., de Menil, V. P., & Cogley, C. B. (2004). Group therapy for substance use disorders: What do we know? *Harvard Review of Psychiatry, 12,* 339–350.

Weissberg, J. H., & Levay, A. N. (1981). The role of resistance in sex therapy. *Journal of Sex and Marital Therapy, 7,* 125–130.

Wells, K. (2009). Substance abuse and child maltreatment. *Pediatric Clinics of North America, 56,* 345–362.

Wells-Parker, E. (1995). Mandated treatment: Lessons from research with drinking and driving offenders. *Alcohol Health and Research World, 18,* 302–306.

Wells-Parker, E., Dill, M. P., Williams, M., & Stoduto, G. (2006). Are depressed drinking/driving offenders more receptive to brief intervention? *Addictive Behaviors, 31,* 339–350.

Wells-Parker, E., Kenne, D. R., Spratke, K. L., & Williams, M. T. (2000). Self-efficacy and motivation for controlling drinking and drinking/driving: An investigation of changes across a driving under the influence (DUI) intervention program and of recidivism prediction. *Addictive Behaviors, 25,* 229–238.

Wells-Parker, E., Mann, R. E., Dill, P. L., Stoduto, G., Shuggi, R., & Cross, G. W. (2009). Negative affect and drinking drivers: A review and conceptual model linking dissonance, efficacy and negative affect to risk and motivation for change. *Current Drug Abuse Reviews, 2,* 115–126.

Wells-Parker, E., & Williams, M. (2002). Enhancing the effectiveness of traditional interventions with drinking drivers by adding brief individual intervention components. *Journal of Studies on Alcohol, 63,* 655–664.

Wells-Parker, E., Williams, M., Dill, P., & Kenne, D. (1998). Stages of change and self-efficacy for controlling drinking and driving: A psychometric analysis. *Addictive Behaviors, 23,* 351–363.

Werch, C. E., & DiClemente, C. C. (1994). A multi-component stage model for matching drug prevention strategies and messages to youth stage of use. *Health Education Research: Theory and Practice, 9,* 37–46.

West, R. (2005). Time for a change: Putting the transtheoretical (stages of change) model to rest. *Addiction, 100,* 1036–1039.

West, R. (2008). Whether and how to develop a comprehensive theory: The example of the PRIME theory of motivation. *Psychological Health, 23,* 27–28.

Whitelaw, S., Baldwin, S., Buton, R., & Flynn, D. (2000). The status of evidence and outcomes in stages of change research. *Health Education Research, 15.* 707–718.

Whitlock, E., Polen, M., Green, C. A., Orleans, T., & Klein, J. (2004). Behavioral counseling interventions in primary care to reduce risky/harmful alcohol use by adults: A summary of the evidence for the U.S. Preventive Services Task Force. *Annals of Internal Medicine, 140,* 557–568.

Wholey, D. (1984). *The courage to change.* New York: Warner Books.

Wickizer, T., Maynard, C., Artherly, A., Frederick, M., Koepsell, T., Krupski, A., et al. (1994). Completion rates of clients discharged from drug and alcohol treatment programs in Washington state. *American Journal of Public Health, 84,* 215–221.

Wieczorek, W. F., Callahan, C. P., & Morales, M. A. (1997). Motivation for change among DWI offenders. In C. Mercier-Guyon (Ed.), *Alcohol, drugs, and traffic safety—T97* (pp. 1069–1075). Annecy, France: CERMT.

Wild, T. C., Cunningham, J. A., & Ryan, R. M. (2006). Social pressure, coercion, and client engagement at treatment entry: A self-determination theory perspective. *Addictive Behaviors, 31,* 1858–1872.

Wild, T. C., Newton-Taylor, B., & Alletto, R. (1998). Perceived coercion among clients entering substance abuse treatment: Structural and psychological determinants. *Addictive Behaviors, 23,* 81–95.

Wilke, D. (1994). Women and alcoholism: How a male-as-norm bias affects research, assessment, and treatment. *Health and Social Work, 191,* 29–35.

Wilke, D. J., Kamata, A., & Cash, S. J. (2005). Modeling treatment motivation in substance-abusing women with children. *Child Abuse and Neglect, 29,* 1313–1323.

Will, D. (1983). Some techniques for working with resistant families of adolescents. *Journal of Adolescence, 6,* 13–26.

Williams, R., & Vinson, D. C. (2001). Validation of a single screening question for problem drinking. *Journal of Family Practice, 50,* 307–312.

Williams, E. C., Kivlahan, D. R., Saitz, R., Merrill, J. O., Achtmeyer, C. E., Kinsey, A. M., et al. (2006). Readiness to change in primary care patients who screened positive for alcohol misuse. *Annals of Family Medicine, 4,* 213–220.

Willoughby, F. W., & Edens, J. F. (1996). Construct validity and predictive utility of the Stages of Change Scale for Alcoholics. *Journal of Substance Abuse, 8,* 275–291.

Wilsnack, S. C. (1991). Barriers to treatment for alcoholic women. *Addiction and Recovery, 11,* 10–12.

Wilson, H. W., & Widom, C. S. (2009). A prospective examination of the path from child abuse and neglect to illicit drug use in middle adulthood: The potential mediating role of four risk factors. *Journal of Youth and Adolescence, 38,* 340–354.

Wise, R. A. (1988). The neurobiology of craving: Implications for the understanding and treatment of addiction. *Journal of Abnormal Psychology, 97,* 118–132.

Witkiewitz, K., Hartzler, B., & Donovan, D. (2010). Matching motivation enhancement treatment to client motivation: Re-examining the Project MATCH motivation matching hypothesis. *Addiction, 105,* 1403–1413.

Witkiewitz, K., & Marlatt, G. A. (2004). Relapse prevention for alcohol and drug problems: That was zen, this is tao. *American Psychologist, 59,* 224–235.

Witkiewitz, K., & Marlatt, G. A. (2007). Overview of relapse prevention. In K. Witkiewitz & G. A. Marlatt (Eds.), *Therapist's guide to evidence-based relapse prevention* (pp. 3–17). New York: Academic Press.

Woodall, W. G., Delaney, H. D., Kunitz, S. J., Westerberg, V. S., & Zhao, H. (2007). A randomized trial of a DWI intervention program for first offenders: Intervention outcomes and interactions with antisocial personality disorder among a primarily American-Indian sample. *Alcoholism: Clinical and Experimental Research, 31,* 974–987.

World Health Organization. (2010). *The Alcohol, Smoking and Substance Involvement Screening Test (ASSIST).* Geneva: Author.

World Health Organization. (2011). *Global status report on noncommunicable diseases: 2010.* Geneva: Author.

World Health Organization ASSIST Working Group. (2002). The Alcohol, Smoking and Substance Involvement Screening Test (ASSIST): Development, reliability and feasibility. *Addiction, 97,* 1183–1194.

Xu, J., Rapp, R. C., Wang, J., & Carlson, R. G. (2008). The multidimensional structure of external barriers to substance abuse treatment and its invariance across gender, ethnicity, and age. *Substance Abuse, 29,* 43–54.

Xu, J., Wang, J., Rapp, R. C., & Carlson, R. G. (2007). The multidimensional structure of internal barriers to substance abuse treatment and its invariance across gender, ethnicity, and age. *Journal of Drug Issues, 37,* 321–340.

Yalom, I. (1995). *The theory and practice of group psychotherapy* (4th ed.). New York: Basic Books.

Yonas, M., Baker, D., Cornwell, E. E., Chang, D., Phillips, J., Paradise, J., et al. (2005). Readiness to change and the role of inpatient counseling for alcohol/substance abusing youth with major trauma. *Journal of Trauma Injury, Infection, and Critical Care, 59,* 464–467.

Yoshioka, M. R., Thomas, E. J., & Ager, R. D. (1992). Nagging and other drinking control efforts of spouses and uncooperative alcohol abusers: Assessment and modification. *Journal of Substance Abuse, 4,* 309–318.

Yu, M. M., & Watkins, T. (1996). Group counseling with DUI offenders: A model using client anger to enhance group cohesion and movement. *Alcoholism Treatment Quarterly, 14,* 47–57.

Yuma-Guerrero, P. J., Lawson, K. A., Velasquez, M. M., von Sternberg, K., Maxson, T., & Garcia, N. (2012). Screening, brief intervention, and referral for alcohol use in adolescents: A systematic review. *Pediatrics, 130,* 115–122.

Zilberman, M. L., Tavares, H., Andrade, A. G., & El-Guebaly, N. (2003). The impact of an outpatient program for women with substance use-related disorders on retention. *Substance Use and Misuse, 38,* 2109–2124.

Zilberman, M., Tavares, H., & El-Guebaly, N. (2003). Gender similarities and differences: The prevalence and course of alcohol- and other substance-related disorders. *Journal of Addictive Diseases, 22,* 61–74.

Zimmerman, G. L., Olsen, C. G., & Bosworth, M. F. (2000). A "stages of change" approach to helping patients change behavior. *American Family Physician, 61,* 1409–1416.

Zywiak, W. H., Connors, G. J., Maisto, S. A., & Westerberg, V. S. (1996). Relapse research and the Reasons for Drinking Questionnaire: A factor analysis of Marlatt's taxonomy. *Addiction, 91*(Suppl.), 121–130.

Zywiak, W. H., Kenna, G. A., & Westerberg, V. S. (2011). Beyond the ubiquitous relapse curve: A data-informed approach. *Frontiers in Psychiatry, 2,* 1–6.

Index